Autistic Intelligence

Autistic Intelligence

Interaction, Individuality, and the Challenges of Diagnosis

DOUGLAS W. MAYNARD AND JASON TUROWETZ

The University of Chicago Press

Chicago and London

The University of Chicago Press, Chicago 60637
The University of Chicago Press, Ltd., London
© 2022 by The University of Chicago
Published 2022
Printed in the United States of America

31 30 29 28 27 26 25 24 23 22   1 2 3 4 5

ISBN-13: 978-0-226-81598-5 (cloth)
ISBN-13: 978-0-226-81600-5 (paper)
ISBN-13: 978-0-226-81599-2 (e-book)
DOI: https://doi.org/10.7208/chicago/9780226815992.001.0001

Library of Congress Cataloging-in-Publication Data

Names: Maynard, Douglas W., 1946– author. | Turowetz, Jason, author.
Title: Autistic intelligence : interaction, individuality, and the challenges of diagnosis /
    Douglas W. Maynard and Jason Turowetz.
Description: Chicago : University of Chicago Press, 2022. | Includes bibliographical
    references and index.
Identifiers: LCCN 2021037124 | ISBN 9780226815985 (cloth) | ISBN 9780226816005
    (paperback) | ISBN 9780226815992 (ebook)
Subjects: LCSH: Autism spectrum disorders in children—Diagnosis. | Autism
    spectrum disorders in children—Diagnosis—Case studies. | Communication in
    medicine. | Ethnomethodology.
Classification: LCC RC553.A88 M37 2022 | DDC 618.92/85882—dc23
LC record available at https://lccn.loc.gov/2021037124

Contents

Common Sense and the
Interaction Order of the Clinic

This is a book about autism spectrum disorder (ASD). More specifically, it is a book about the interactions in clinics where children go to be evaluated for a possible autism diagnosis. The clinic is the site where a history of odd or troublesome behavior may be assigned a name, one that will follow the bearer through the school system, through the offices of therapists and physicians, through friendships and relationships, and sometimes into the courtroom and welfare system. Yet for all its importance, and despite the dramatically rising prevalence of autism diagnoses around the world, there has been little research about the clinic and its human operations per se—how testing gets done and how diagnosis is actually accomplished on the ground, by actual participants dealing with one another in real time. Our research has involved spending time with clinicians, children, and families in the clinic, observing how children are evaluated for autism and how clinicians decide whether or not to give a life-changing label to what, up to that point, had been an amorphous cluster of missed milestones, behavioral problems, and seemingly inexplicable or even mysterious conduct.

Though our focus on interaction and the phenomenon of commonsense knowledge is quite specific, we expect that our audiences will be diverse. Sociologists with an interest in medicine and diagnosis; scholars of science, technology, and disability; linguists and psycholinguists; and anthropologists may all find something of interest in this book's pages. Not least, we hope that people with autism and their families will find parts of the text that resonate with them. In particular, we describe how autism as a form of sensemaking has its own logic, coherence, and intelligibility. Understanding this will not only enhance appreciation for the many strengths children on the autism spectrum exhibit but also prompt further examination—and perhaps expansion—of common sense itself.

Finally, clinicians and mental health practitioners may find something of value in the book. Although it is primarily a work of academic sociology rather than a set of practical suggestions for reforming diagnosis or improving the lives of those on the spectrum, we attempt to identify crucial but tacit features of interaction that end up mattering for the outcomes of autism cases. Whether an understanding of these features can enhance diagnosis is not for us to decide, although we offer suggestions along those lines. At the same time, we attempt to convey something of the very real demands that clinicians face as they go about the work of understanding children and helping families, educators, and others handle the challenges that bring children to the clinic in the first place.

The Search for Answers

When Dan Chapman[1] was nine years old, he was arrested at school. Though it was not the first time the school had called the police on Dan, the incident nonetheless stood out from the others, as it ended with five officers pinning him to the ground, handcuffing him, and tying his feet together. This was the last straw for Dan's parents, who for some time had been unhappy with the school's punitive responses to their son's behavior and administrators' refusal to listen to advice about how to deescalate tense situations before they became explosive. The Chapman family had recently moved their son to a new school, where he was doing better overall. Still, he had already been suspended several times and was only attending classes on a half-day schedule.

Dan's family was seeking answers, searching for a diagnosis that would explain their son's behavior and help him access the support services he so desperately needed. This search brought them to Central Developmental Disabilities Clinic (CDDC),[2] the site where we conducted field research for four years. In some ways, Dan stood out from other children we observed. For example, while meltdowns and tantrums were commonplace, these children rarely if ever became violent, much less had encounters with police. Nonetheless, all the children, including Dan, engaged in disruptive behavior that seemed to defy common sense; all had problems that could not be settled or explained by laypeople alone, leading their families to seek out the advice of professionals. In these respects, their journeys to and experiences at the clinic share important similarities.

These similarities constitute our focus in this book, which examines the trajectory that culminates in an autism diagnosis for Dan and children like him. More precisely, within that trajectory, we focus on the methods clinicians use to decide whether to give the diagnosis. Unpacking that trajectory allows us, as sociologists, to deal with a host of issues that the now vast literature on autism has not fully explored. For any child, what does an experience at the clinic entail? Mostly, of course, it means being subjected to a variety of assessments: medical, cognitive, speech and language, behavioral, and so forth. But how do clinicians from various disciplines conduct these assessments? How do they generate and use the results to determine—fatefully—whether a child does or does not qualify for the autism diagnosis? And how do children and families respond to that decision?

Such questions signify that, although we know a good deal about what happens after a child is diagnosed with autism, the diagnostic process itself remains something of a black box. Our aim in this study is to open that box and inspect its workings. Doing so will establish a basis for addressing a broader set of questions that get at the heart of current discussions about autism: When all is said and done, what *is* autism? Is it "real"? And if so, to what degree are its roots to be found in biology (genetics and genomics) and neurology (structures of cognition)? Can we even say whether autism is intrinsic to someone like Dan as an individual? To what degree are the *social environments*—family, school, clinical, and other institutions—in which Dan (or any other child with autism) exists implicated in autistic behavior? What are the social dynamics within the professional decision-making context where the diagnostic decision is made and then conveyed? What analytic tools do we have to address these matters, and how do we use them? Finally, given the documented high prevalence of autism, what can be done to ameliorate the challenges it presents for diagnosed children and their social environments?

This chapter begins to answer such questions by following Dan's path to and experience in the clinic. As we do this, we explain our sociological understanding of autism in terms of conduct that violates or disrupts *common sense*—the tacit assumptions by which we continually measure social competence in the everyday world. We suggest that, in challenging commonsense assumptions, autistic behavior can make those assumptions *strange*, bringing to the surface deep sensemaking practices that are invisible when interactions go smoothly. Drawing on an example from Prizant (2015:114), when a teacher asks a question of her class, then must instruct an autistic student that he should not just blurt out an answer but should raise his hand so that she can call on him, and then must further explain that she cannot call on him every time because she sometimes needs to let another student talk, she in effect exposes the taken-for-granted rules of the classroom, articulating them in ways that are usually unnecessary.

Common sense is the pervasive but largely invisible foundation for everyday thought and action, although participants must demonstrate their commitment to its assumptions whenever they sanction others for violating them or defend an action of their own. Even so, common sense is far from static. As we explain below, commonsense actors are capable of widening their repertoires of understanding to accommodate a child's seeming strangeness. This involves grasping the logic behind otherwise odd or challenging behavior and incorporating that logic into one's repertoire of ordinary comportment—as when another teacher (Prizant 2015:143), aware that an autistic student frequently visits the zoo and talks to the animals, makes approving animal sounds (meowing like a cat) whenever the student goes beyond their rigid habit of drawing cartoon characters to engage in other forms of drawing. In other words, rather than judging the child as incompetent for failing to properly participate in the neurotypical world, a teacher may *make the strange familiar* (Grinker 2007) by entering the child's world, becoming competent in their methods of sensemaking, and using those methods to create an intersubjective space where child and adult can *make sense together*.

The themes of common sense and possibilities for its expansion are explored throughout the book in the context of evaluating and diagnosing autism, both being core activities in what we call the *interaction order of the clinic*. In this chapter, we explain what we mean by the concept of an interaction order and how it structures the experiences children like Dan have in the clinic. We then describe our data and data collection and set the stage for subsequent chapters, all of which stress the centrality of *social interaction* for understanding autism and the diagnostic process. Finally, we conclude with a brief summary of each of the book's chapters. Overall, we suggest that taking an interactional approach to evaluation and diagnosis creates possibilities for enhancing appreciation of autistic children's *competence* and *intelligence*— rather than their deficits and challenges—in both the clinic and the broader society.

Arriving at a Diagnostic Clinic for Autism

Dan Chapman was first seen at a county mental health center when he was five. At that time, he was diagnosed with a "disruptive behavior disorder" and other conditions. The problems continued, and by the time he was nine and in the third grade, Dan had been suspended from school sixteen times in a single semester. According to Dan's mother, the incidents that led to his suspensions escalated after the principal "got in Dan's face" and demanded that he leave the premises. School personnel frequently called for police intervention, which led to incidents like the one that resulted in his arrest. According to his medical records, during that incident Dan had "pulled two fire alarms, threatened someone with a 2 by 4 [piece of lumber], and flipped over a table. There was police involvement." The report immediately continues: "It is noted that the precipitating factor that was identified in this recent incident was a change in schedule." Events like this seemed to happen without warning, frequently leaving bystanders upset, confused, and at a loss for explanations.

We first met Dan in the winter of 2014. A stocky boy with dark hair and eyebrows, he was one of forty-nine children we followed over four years of fieldwork at CDDC, a large diagnostic center in a medium-sized US city.[3] Dan had been referred to the clinic by his pediatrician, who recommended an assessment for "cognitive disability as a possible factor for behavioral outbursts." By that time, Dan had already seen numerous mental health professionals who, per his medical record, commented on his poor social skills. Dan was prescribed various courses of treatment: most recently, psychiatrists at the county mental health center had put him on a combination of the powerful antipsychotic drug Seroquel and the mood stabilizer lithium, medications whose side effects are known to include slurred speech, sluggishness, and weight gain.

These disparate labels and interventions attest to how challenging it can be for professionals to explain the troubles experienced by children such as Dan. By the time they are evaluated at a clinic like CDDC, children often have had contact with a variety of institutions and agents, including teachers, therapists, physicians, and sometimes, as in Dan's case, the police. To adapt Goffman's (1959a) study of mental hospitalization, these experiences can be considered aspects of the children's preclinical, incipient career as a person with autism. As used by sociologists, the term *career* describes a common sequence of stages that people experience as they acquire identities associated with established institutions in the society, whether for typical or problematic behavior.

Because he was concerned with mental hospitals in particular, the career stages Goffman (1959a) identified were "pre-patient," "in-patient," and "ex-patient." These statuses, he argued, are acquired by mental patients regardless of differences in their backgrounds. Similarly, in our study, we find that despite differences (described in chap. 3) in age, race, ethnicity, and social class, the children we observed had all begun to accrue the preclinical status of person with autism. For these children, what we call the "in-clinic" (rather than "in-patient") phase involved an evaluation to determine whether or not they qualified for the diagnosis.

Like Goffman (1959a), who focused primarily on the middle stage, we concentrate on the in-clinic experience of diagnosis—the stage that has thus

far been explored in least detail. And like Goffman (1959a), whose study did
not extend to ex-patient processes, we do not follow the postclinic part of a
child's career after autism diagnosis. That career unfolds in family, school,
and employment contexts and may involve further clinic visits, hospitals, insurance determinations, welfare bureaucracies, and criminal justice agencies
(cf. Maynard 2019; Maynard and Turowetz 2020)—all of which merit research
in their own right but are beyond the scope of our present investigation.[4]

Nevertheless, we can say a little more about the preclinic career of an autistic child. Most of the children we observed came to a point where behaviors or developmental delays became concerning enough that their parents
decided to seek professional help. In some cases, the parents themselves suspected something was not quite right. For example, some noticed that their
child was behind other children in motor or speech development or that the
child was stuck in what the parents had initially dismissed as a developmental "phase" that would eventually pass. In other cases, it was a friend, family
member, or teacher who first raised concerns about the child's development.
In still other cases, it was the child's pediatrician who suspected something
was amiss. Sometimes these early red flags prompted a quick referral to
CDDC for an autism evaluation. Other children followed a more circuitous
path to the clinic, one that might have run through the offices of occupational
therapists, neurologists, and psychologists before someone recommended or
made a referral to CDDC. During this time, parents might have begun to
reinterpret the child's early troubles as signs of a possible psychological disorder, even if they did not yet have a name for it. In doing so, they started the
process of reorganizing the child's biography around turning points that led
to professional intervention.

By the time they arrived at CDDC, many parents had stories about differences they had noticed in their child early on, such as repetitive behavior, tantrums, and failure to meet developmental milestones like walking and talking. In Dan's case, his mother reported that he was a fussy baby who by age
one was constantly inserting objects into outlets, throwing things, and having
meltdowns. Although granting that such challenges "are typical toddler behaviors," Betsy Chapman, Dan's mother, also stated (as paraphrased in Dan's
medical report), "The frequency and severity was greater than would be expected for a child at this age." She explained that Dan required everything—
such as his collection of Hot Wheels cars—to be put in order and became
upset otherwise. Betsy also shared concerns about his limited social interactions: the playdates she arranged between Dan and other children were unsuccessful, and he usually preferred to play by himself, leaving him without
any friends apart from his sister, with whom he often quarreled.

A Day at the Clinic

We met Dan and his mother in the early morning hours, shortly before his evaluation was to begin. As they sat in the clinic's waiting room, the professionals with whom they would be working handled administrative matters and prepared examination materials. At CDDC, things tend to move at a fast pace. Schedules are tight and often need to be rearranged at a moment's notice to accommodate families arriving late to their appointments or cases that take longer than expected. Working in teams, clinicians usually juggle two or three cases a day, frequently leaving an exam or interview with a child they had met just an hour earlier to attend to a different case. They worked diligently, under considerable time and resource constraints, to make a dent in the six-month-long list of families waiting for an appointment while at the same time trying to balance considerations of efficiency against the careful attention each child required. Then there was the daily emotional labor involved in working with children, arriving at a diagnosis, and breaking potentially life-changing news to families—who entered the clinic with expectations, fears, and hopes of their own. Having long endured the frustrations that come with raising an unusually challenging child, these families were understandably eager for diagnostic information. They wanted answers. Unfortunately, the answers clinicians provided were not always the ones families wanted to hear.

As we spoke to Dan and his mother, we explained that we were researchers interested in better understanding how clinicians make diagnostic decisions, and we requested permission to record their visit. Betsy listened and occasionally asked questions before signing the consent form we had reviewed with her. Dan also assented to participate, though he did not ask any questions and seemed bored. We chatted a bit more with Betsy, making small talk until Sheila, the clinic coordinator, entered the room. As one of two coordinators at CDDC, Sheila guided families through their appointments. She told Betsy and Dan that their first meeting of the day would be with Dr. Leah Grant,[5] a developmental pediatrician, and explained that Dr. Grant would be working with her colleague Jennifer Erickson, a child psychologist, to evaluate Dan. The team would be completed by Norah Gonzalez, a social worker whose role was to advise families about insurance, community services, and educational and therapeutic resources.

In the Examination Rooms

As Sheila guided Dan and his mother to their meeting with Dr. Grant, we followed them down a fluorescent-lit corridor with white floors, yellow walls, and rows of wooden doors that led to examination rooms, observation rooms, and offices. When Dan and his mother entered one of the rooms with Dr. Grant, we assumed a position in an adjoining room, where we could observe and videotape the session from behind a one-way mirror.

While Dan sat on the floor and worked on a puzzle that Sheila brought him, Dr. Grant asked Betsy questions about her son's developmental history and the family's present concerns. Her questions were from a structured interview called the *Autism Diagnostic Interview–Revised* (ADI-R; cf. Rutter, LeCouteur, and Lord 2003), a standardized instrument designed to solicit symptoms of autism as defined by the *Diagnostic and Statistical Manual of Mental Disorders* (DSM-5; APA 2013).[6] The official compendium of psychiatric diagnosis, the DSM is in its fifth edition as of 2013.

In response to a question about when she began to have concerns about Dan's development, Betsy recalled, "It was early, I mean even when he was baby, all he did was cry, and cry, and cry. . . . I noticed a lot of these behaviors even at age one, sticking things in outlets, throwing objects, and of course as a toddler you're gonna do that, but I mean it's more than usual. . . . At age four it got even worse, where I did have to hold him and get him to stop." She then raised the issue of Dan's problems at school, saying, "The reason we had moved is the school, I don't think they were able or capable of handling the situations that would occur. There's always police, always, nonstop." She reported that following one incident, personnel at Dan's previous school had wanted him committed to an inpatient psychiatric facility, but she was able to stop this by getting disability rights advocates from a local clinic involved.

As the interview continued, Betsy discussed Dan's lack of social relationships and regular fights with his older sister and elaborated further on his difficulties at school. For nearly an hour, Dr. Grant listened attentively, took notes, and asked follow-up questions. Next, she guided Dan into a nearby room, where she performed a physical exam and asked him questions, particularly about his imaginative play and friendships, before returning mother and son to the waiting room. After a few minutes passed, Sheila came to retrieve them, leading them down the hallway to a different room, where Dr. Erickson would do a psychological assessment for autism. Dan's pediatrician, who made the referral, had asked for this kind of assessment.

The centerpiece of Dr. Erickson's evaluation was an instrument called the *Autism Diagnostic Observation Schedule—Second Edition* (ADOS-2; cf. Lord et al. 2012). Frequently used in conjunction with the ADI-R, cognitive testing, and school and medical reports, the ADOS is widely considered the gold standard for autism diagnosis. The ADOS is a *play*-based (rather than cognitive) exam, during which the clinician creates a "simulated social world" and observes the child's participation along a number of dimensions. As explained to us when we underwent ADOS training, the instrument "creates a 'social world' in which behaviors related to the autism spectrum can be observed."[7] There are four core modules, graded according to age and verbal ability, and a fifth module for use with toddlers as young as eighteen months. Dan was administered Module 3, which is for children capable of speaking in flexible, full sentences.

As clinicians lead children through a series of tasks, including imaginary play, back-and-forth conversation, storytelling, and questions about emotions and relationships, they monitor for indications of trouble with social interaction, communication, and behavior—the major diagnostic criteria for autism listed in the DSM. For each task, the clinician uses a coding scheme to score behaviors such as joint attention, eye contact, enthusiasm, and asking/answering questions. She later sums these scores and uses an algorithm to convert them into an overall age-normed score. If that overall score exceeds the threshold for autism—the exact cutoff depends on the child's age group—it supports an autism diagnosis. That is, higher numbers on the exam may qualify a child for the label.

Autism and Commonsense Reasoning

At various times during his interviews and examinations, Dan appeared to depart from ordinary, or commonsense ways of acting and reasoning. For example, as Dr. Grant talked to Dan and his mother about whether Dan engaged in "imagination play like pretending," his mother explained, "He has ghost friends," at which point Dan chimed in: "They're real . . . one of them burned down the house where we used to live, except that one wasn't my friend." Then he offered, "My ghost friends always moved wherever I go, they listen to me." Dr. Grant asked, "So are they nice friends?" After Dan answered, "They don't hurt anyone," she queried about whether he had "friends at school." Dan answered, "The whole entire class." Yet when she followed up by asking, "Do you know anybody's name that is a friend of yours at school?" Dan replied, "Not really. But everyone knows my name." Common sense would lead us to expect that most nine-year-old children will have at least a few real, as opposed to imaginary, friends (particularly ghosts) and not equate the fact that classmates know their name with friendship as such.[8]

Later, Dr. Erickson would report on Dan's "unchanged" facial expressions, "limited gestures," and "flat intonation" during her time with him. She also described an incident in which Dan seemed to interrupt an exam in progress by standing up, walking to a corner, and crouching behind a chair (see chap. 5).

Although he eventually returned to finish the exam, he never did complete the task that triggered his withdrawal. Again, we might ordinarily expect that by age nine children will be able to articulate feelings in at least a rudimentary way, participate in an exam without incident, and animate talk with facial expressions, hand gestures, and prosodic inflections.

Pervasive though these expectations may be, they remain tacit and implicit in everyday life. As such, they are not easily articulated. Indeed, they usually come to the surface only when violated, particularly through the sanctions they incur.[9] In the clinic, as opposed to everyday life, the ADOS is specifically designed to bring commonsense expectations to the surface and make violations explicit for diagnostic purposes. Of course, this description is a sociological and not a clinical one. (More about the ADOS and its design as a clinical instrument can be found in later chapters.) Our point here is that clinicians and laypeople share a tendency to explain disruptive behavior in terms of the child's psychological state or disposition while at same time *disattending* circumstances that occasioned it and their own reactions to the behavior. Mental health practitioners, in particular, are trained to look for psychological explanations for odd-seeming behavior, making the child's putative deficits and psychopathology the basis for clinical understanding.

Our position in this book is different. Rather than looking at the child's actions from the inside out (in a psychological sense), our approach is to examine them *from the outside in*: to explore the interactions through which professionals may prompt a child's behavior, act in response to it, and fit assessments to strict diagnostic definitions. Accordingly, our interest is not only in what these interactions say about the child but also in what they can tell us about social organization and the properties of commonsense reasoning that pervade that organization.[10]

Disrupting Common Sense

The relation between autism and common sense is already well recognized in the literature. Temple Grandin (1995:37–38), the professor of animal science who writes about her own autism and others with the condition, gives us this report: "Ted Hart, a man with severe autism, has almost no ability to generalize and no flexibility in his behavior. His father, Charles, described how on one occasion Ted put wet clothes in the dresser after the dryer broke. He just went on to the next step in a clothes-washing sequence that he had learned by rote. He has no common sense." And Uta Frith (2003:47), a psychologist who has published extensively about autism, writes, "Even in very able people with autism, whose high verbal ability and abstruse knowledge may be impressive, the lack of common sense can be striking."

In 1943, Leo Kanner, a physician émigré from Germany who came to Johns Hopkins University, first gave the diagnosis of autism to children who had come to his attention and seemed to suffer from a lack of common sense—although he did not use that phrase per se. In his groundbreaking paper, "Autistic Disturbances of Affective Contact," Kanner (1943) described in great detail eleven children who were referred to him because of his growing reputation in the field of child psychiatry. One of those children was a boy named Donald Triplett (identified only as "Donald T" in Kanner's paper), who was born in September 1933. In 2010, when Donald was seventy-seven, two journalists (Donvan and Zucker 2010) tracked him down and wrote about his life subsequent to the encounters he had with Kanner. Although still showing oddities of various kinds—distinctive gait and posture, ritualistic behaviors, repetitive phrases, halting conversational interactions—he was leading a quiet and meaningful life on his own, traveling internationally, driving a car, playing golf, and meeting community friends for breakfast. As Donvan and Zucker (2010) observe, "This is the same man whose favorite pastimes, as a boy, were spinning objects, spinning himself, and rolling nonsense words around in his mouth." These behaviors, by taken-for-granted (commonsense) standards, are out of bounds. In fact, the commonsense perspective is deeply entrenched in Kanner's (1943:219–20) report on Donald:

(a) Words to him had a specifically literal, inflexible meaning. He seemed unable to generalize, to transfer an expression to another similar object or situation.

(b) He paid no attention to persons around him. When taken into a room, he completely disregarded the people and instantly went for objects, preferably those that could be spun.

(c) Most of his actions were repetitions carried out in exactly the same way in which they had been performed originally. . . . And his mother had to conform or else he squealed, cried, and strained every muscle in his neck in tension. This happened all day long about one thing or another.

Kanner is assuming that we should be able to (a) use words and expressions across circumstances—for example, use the word *glass* to refer to any beverage container, rather than having a *water glass* and a *milk glass* (Kanner 1943:220); (b) orient to others in social situations; and (c) show flexibility in everyday actions. In Fitzgerald's (2017:136, original emphasis) terms, "It often seems impossible to talk about autism, as either a diagnosis or an experience, without *also* talking about the specific understandings, meanings, and sensations that mediate some person's social environment." Although they are often vague rather than "specific," such understandings are what we mean by common sense.

Because autism can throw common sense into relief, it raises questions about our usual ways of doing things. How are we able to generalize, show co-orientation, and act flexibly? What everyday, concrete practices in talk and embodied conduct implement such features? We pursue answers to these questions from an ethnomethodological perspective, which means investigating commonsense knowledge itself and the use of what Garfinkel (1967:37) called the "seen but unnoticed" assumptions about how the world should work with its "life as usual character." Life as usual is undergirded by a sense of trust and reciprocity, or what the social phenomenologist Alfred Schutz (1962) called the "attitude of daily life," his gloss for the unquestioned and unchallenged presumptions about the objective reality of the commonsense social world.

Although based in sociology, our approach is consistent with what the arts, whether they involve music, paintings, sculpture, drama, or other forms, accomplish by "making strange," or providing experiences of "defamiliarization," so that devotees can become more aware of self, others, and the world (Kumagai and Wear 2014). Nearly a century ago, the Russian literary critic Viktor Shklovsky (1990[1929]) proposed that perceptual experience, as it becomes habitual in everyday experience, also becomes automatic. A role for art is to bring us back to knowledge of the familiar by rejuvenating the work of perception—arresting our attention, as it were—to encompass the special and detailed nature of our usual ways of talking and doing things. Similarly, Pinchevski (2005) highlights the work of the philosopher Emmanuel Levinas to suggest the importance of "interruption" in providing a basis for an ethics of communication. Indeed, Pinchevski (2005:164) cites autism as a perspicuous example for the way it exposes the "epistemological boundary" between effective communication and its breakdown. Crucially, such interruption also means opportunities for exploring the *other side* of ordinary communication—the exact manner in which it is conducted. Ethnomethodology, even as it is a rigorous social science, aims to rejuvenate perception, interrupt automaticity in social practices, and reveal how those practices, in the collaborative actions of participants, organize the world of everyday life and experience.

Autism enables us to explore what common sense presumes, what it imposes, and how malleable or not it may be as a real feature of ordinary experience. Equally, our inquiries into testing and diagnosis can be informative about how to work with and enhance the learning and understanding of those with autism so that they may be better woven into the social fabrics in home, school, and many such settings—or so that these settings can be rewoven to fit different individuals and their particularities. In short, we suggest how there can be *mutual adjustments* between autistic individuals[11] and the clinical and ordinary settings they occupy.

Making Everyday Life Strange

Our approach to the relationship between common sense and autism has its roots in Garfinkel's sociologically famous ethnomethodological breaching demonstrations, which show what happens when people break with the unspoken assumptions of everyday life. In fact, Garfinkel (1967:9, 36) described his goal with ethnomethodological studies as making the structures of commonsense knowledge "anthropologically strange." Because of their taken-for-granted or tacit nature, and because of our "sluggish imaginations"—a term that Garfinkel (1967:38) borrowed from Herbert Spiegelberg—the practices of everyday life that constitute taken-for-granted ways of comporting ourselves during interactions often seem impermeable. We are typically on what seems like automatic pilot, enabling us "to solicit enthusiasm and friendliness" from others and "avoid anxiety, guilt, shame, or boredom" (Garfinkel 1967:49) that may result when we stray from usual ways of saying and doing things.

So how is it possible to break into the autopilot mode and gain access to the structures of commonsense knowledge? Garfinkel (1967:42) devised some innocuous-seeming but highly disruptive tactics. For example, he directed his students (as with E below) to question what their friends, acquaintances, or partners (S below) "meant" by their most commonplace remarks:

> The subject was telling the experimenter, a member of the subject's car pool, about having had a flat tire while going to work the previous day.
>
> S: I had a flat tire.
> E: What do you mean, you had a flat tire?
>
> She appeared momentarily stunned. Then she answered in a hostile way: "What do you mean, 'What do you mean?' A flat tire is a flat tire. That is what I meant. Nothing special. What a crazy question!"

Such purposeful disruptions show the properties of ordinary discourse, such as the context-embeddedness of everyday references and their "specific vagueness," on which actors rely for making sense together. In this case, the mention of "flat tire" between friends and acquaintances should stand as a perfectly intelligible announcement about trouble with a familiar object and not require further explanation.

When one party seems differently oriented to commonsense properties or structures, other participants can quickly turn hostile and begin constructing the talk as "crazy," even questioning the health of the participant (Garfinkel 1967:42–44):

> S: Hi, Ray. How is your girlfriend feeling?
> E: What do you mean, "How is she feeling?" Do you mean physical or mental?
> S: I mean how is she feeling? What's the matter with you?
>   (He looked peeved.)
> E: Nothing. Just explain a little clearer what do you mean?
> S: Skip it. How are your Med School applications coming?
> E: What do you mean, "How are they?"
> S: You know what I mean.
> E: I really don't.
> S: What's the matter with you? Are you sick?

Whereas the health status of someone who departs from taken-for-granted expectations is quickly called into question, common sense itself is seldom, if ever, investigated or probed for its assumptions and perversities.

This matter—the unquestioned status of commonsense knowledge—is not one of normative orientation, as if the student-experimenters in the preceding examples were breaking a rule and being "deviant." The matter is more fundamental. Taken-for-granted knowledge has the features that (a) participants assume its pervasive relevance for themselves and (b) for others, *and* (c) they expect that others reciprocally assume likewise. If parties to interaction assume that reference to "a flat tire" should be plain enough, or that a routine inquiry of the form "How is X feeling?" needs no explication, it is because they presuppose that the recipients of such utterances know the same routine things that they themselves know. When their recipient challenges such a presupposition, it is not just adherence to some cultural rule about how to talk that is at stake but also the very basis for mutual intelligibility, cooperative understanding, and overall socially organized trust.

Trust is about reciprocation in what we take for granted. For example, when a life partner has an affair, it can throw our assumptions about fidelity in the relationship to the wind. But that is only one example of how the violation of commonsense knowledge, rather than being superficially deviant (e.g., sneezing without covering one's mouth, cutting into a queue, or being late for a meeting or appointment), goes very deep into social being. This is because the very foundations for "life as usual" are disrupted. Going against what everyone—and therefore what *anyone*, even if it is only in a two-way partnership—is presumed to know and take for granted undermines community intimacy and evokes strongly felt emotions—bewilderment, consternation, confusion, anger, indignation—on the part of recipients (Garfinkel 1967:36–38). Hence the references to a recipient appearing "stunned" and "hostile" in the first example above and the recipient's utter indignation in the second example.

Autistic Breaching of Common Sense

As is well documented in autism biography and autobiography, or what Hacking calls "autism narrative" (Hacking 2009), behaviors associated with ASD have effects like those in Garfinkel's breaching demonstrations. Consider two examples, both from John Robison's (2007) autobiographical memoir, *Look Me in the Eye: My Life with Asperger's*, about his experiences growing up with undiagnosed autism (he did not receive a diagnosis until he was in his forties).

In the first example, Robison violates a taken-for-granted rule of interaction, a rule specified by Sacks, Schegloff, and Jefferson (1974) in their foundational study of conversational turn taking. We can call this rule the *display of reciprocity*: in speaking after another participant, the current speaker is expected to display reciprocity by acknowledging and exhibiting their understanding of the prior speaker's talk, even if the current speaker goes on to develop the topic in a different direction. Robison reports that when he was young, he might try to befriend a playmate by telling her everything he knew about dinosaurs. Although he could not figure out the problem with his approach at the time, he eventually came to understand that it was because "successful conversations require a give and take between both people" (Robison 2007:10–11). This realization happened when he and his family moved to a new community and Robison (2007:20) "figured out how to talk to other children":

> I suddenly realized that when a kid said, "Look at my Tonka truck," he expected an answer that made sense in the context of what he had said. Here were some things I might have said prior to this revelation in response to "Look at my Tonka truck":
>
> a) "I have a helicopter."
> b) "I want some cookies."
> c) "My mom is mad at me today."
> d) "I rode a horse at the fair."
>
> I was so used to living inside my own world that I answered with whatever I had been thinking. If I was remembering riding a horse at the fair, it didn't

matter if a kid came up to me and said, "Look at my truck!" or "My mom is in the hospital!" I was still going to answer, "I rode a horse at the fair." The other kid's words did not change the course of my thoughts. It was almost like I didn't hear him. But on some level, I did hear, because I responded. Even though the response didn't make any sense to the person speaking to me.

Displaying one's grasp of a prior turn of talk is how participants achieve a sense of coherence and mutuality in interaction. To be a friend or make a friend, Robison had to learn how to acknowledge another's world before reporting on his own.

In our second example, Robison subverts another taken-for-granted conversational rule, this time regarding the receipt of bad news. His mother had invited her friend Betsy over to their home, and he "wandered in" on a conversation in which Betsy was reporting that a mutual friend's son had been playing on the train tracks and was hit by a train and killed (Robison 2007:30):

> I smiled at her words. She turned to me with a shocked expression on her face. "What! Do you think that's funny?"
>
> I felt embarrassed and a little humiliated. "No, I guess not," I said as I slunk away. I didn't know what to say. I knew they thought it was bad for me to be smiling, but I didn't know why I was grinning, and I couldn't help it. I didn't feel joy or happiness. . . .
>
> As I left, I could hear Betsy. "What's the matter with that boy?"

With her reaction to Robison's smile, Betsy embodies commonsense knowledge about how one should react to the interpersonal delivery of news. Recipients of an announcement are expected to respond in a way that shows verbal and affective alignment with the speaker's stance toward the news (Freese and Maynard 1998; Maynard 2003; Maynard and Freese 2012). By reacting to *bad* news with *positive* affect, the young Robison violated interactional expectations, occasioning the angry response from Betsy evident in her indignant question to Robison's mother. Although Robison (2007:30–31) says that in the situation he did not know why he was grinning, much later in life he was able to "figure out" his reaction:

> I didn't really know Eleanor [the mother of the child who was killed]. And I had never met her kid. So there was no reason for me to feel joy or sorrow on account of anything that might happen to them. Here is what went through my mind that summer day:
>
> Someone got killed.
> Wow! I'm glad I didn't get killed.
> I'm glad [my brother] or my parents didn't get killed.

I'm glad all my friends are okay.
He must have been a pretty dumb kid, playing on the train tracks.
I would never get run over by a train like that.
I'm glad I'm okay.

And at the end, I smiled with relief. Whatever killed that kid was not going to get me. I didn't even know him. It was all going to be okay, at least for me. Today my feelings would be exactly the same in that situation. The only difference is, now I have better control of my facial expressions.

Robison's retrospection is useful because it is otherwise difficult to understand the behavior of an individual who appears willfully to defy what is taken for granted and *should be* "'automatic,' 'immediate' or 'instinctive'" (Hacking 2009:1471). But it is not that autistic people do not feel so much as that they feel differently. Or, if they have feelings that fit the situation, they may not convey them. Our overall point is that exploring the matter of common sense in relation to autism tells us not only about autism but also about the very local, interpersonal organization of society in which it is manifested.

Common Sense: Threatened by Autism, but Capable of Adjustment

How can autism reveal things about the local organization of society and relationships? Consider the following example involving a mother, Sue Lehr, and her autistic son, Ben, from Solomon's (2012:247) exquisite treatise on human difference, *Far from the Tree*:

When Ben was a teenager, Bob and Sue took him to Radio Shack, his favorite store. He panicked on the escalator, and at the bottom he sat down cross-legged and began smashing himself in the head with his hands and screaming as a crowd gathered. Sue always carried a keyboard device, and when she took it out, Ben typed, hit me. "And I thought, 'Oh, yeah, in the middle of the mall with a security guard, and you're a kid and I'm a grownup,'" Sue recalled. "And then he typed out, like a record player." Sue suddenly flashed on a stuck needle; she struck him on the edge of the shoulder with the heel of her hand and said, "Tilt." Ben stood up and they walked calmly on across the mall.

One way of reacting to Ben would have been with panic and sanctioning (even asking the security guard for help). Such a reaction would be embedded in common sense: Ben's actions are ordinarily not at all acceptable in a public place, such as a mall, and *anyone* (i.e., any competent member of society) knows this. Instead of exhibiting this approach to Ben, however, Sue realized "his behaviors were a way of communicating" (Solomon 2012:247), and she was thereby able to adjust her orientation to understand the language her son was using, its analogical basis, and respond in kind. Another mother of a child with limited verbal abilities has said: "If you start from the premise that every utterance is meaningful and that Charlie, though severely limited in his speech, is bursting with communicative intent, you start to see how much he is communicating, however little he speaks in recognizable words" (Chew 2013:309). This quotation points to what has been called the *language of autism*.[12] Both Sue Lehr and Kristina Chew show an understanding of the concrete ways in which their children may communicate comprehensible social messages in the very midst of their challenging conduct. Importantly, they do not assume that the child is prima facie incompetent or doing something nonsensical. Instead, they recognize that the child is making sense in their own way and try to learn what that sense could be. They adjust their forms of knowledge to the child, rather than requiring the child to adjust to them and their taken-for-granted ways of acting and interacting. It is in this way—through adjustment on the part of the commonsense actor, that they and the child are able to make sense together.

When individuals do not seem to fit the group or the group's commonsense forms of being, we can be as reflectively interested in *those* forms as we are in the ill-fitted individual or behavior. Furthermore, *there may be just as much logic to the individual's incongruous behavior as there is to common sense*, and that logic can be brought to commonsense appreciation. In other words, just as there is a jarring strangeness to autism that can reveal our commonsense structures of everyday life—our tacit assumptions about proper behavior—there is a flip side to this that, as Grinker (2007:13) has put it, involves coming to appreciate the complexity of human behavior by rendering autism as less exotic, and thereby as "unstrange." The flip side of autism's ability to *defamiliarize* what we take for granted is the possibility of entering the world of the autistic individual in ways that render *familiar* what was formerly so distant and difficult to understand. This may mean expanding common sense and developing new parameters for what we take for granted.

Parents may come upon the language of autism in accidental ways. An impressive and famous example of this is how the Suskind family, including parents Ron and Cornelia and brother Walt, learned something unexpected about Owen, the younger child in the family. Owen was diagnosed with a regressive form of autism in which the child develops normally for his first two or three years and then seems to retreat into a remote world of his own. Owen's world came to incorporate Disney movies, which he watched obsessively. Eventually, when Owen was about four years old, the family discovered that he was so immersed in the dialogue of Disney movies that they could communicate with him and form social bonds by embracing characterological talk. First was his mother's discovery that a repetitively used mysterious word of Owen's, *juicervose*, was a phrase from the movie *The Little Mermaid*, in which the sea witch, Ursula, promises to turn Ariel (the "little mermaid") into a human, but at a price. Ursula sings,

> Go ahead—make your choice!
> I'm a very busy woman
> And I haven't got all day
> It won't cost much
> Just your voice!

As the family gathers around the TV and watches Owen replay this segment for the nth time, Cornelia Suskind realizes that Owen's *juicervose* is his version of "Just your voice." At this point, Owen's father, Ron, reports:

> I grab Owen by the shoulders. "Just your voice! Is that what you're saying!" He looks right at me—first real eye contact in a year.
> "Juicervose! Juicervose! Juicervose!"
> Walt [Owen's brother] starts to shout, "Owen's talking again!" (Suskind 2014:24)

Momentarily elated, the family felt there was a breakthrough, until a speech therapist told Ron and Cornelia that Owen's usage was an example of "echolalia" (Suskind 2014:27), a condition that involves the mechanical repetition of words and that is known to be associated with autism but that is not particularly meaningful in its own right.[13]

Talking to the Suskinds, the doctors and teachers labeled such echolalia "perserverative behavior" and "self-talk" and recommended that they limit Owen's movie watching. Fortunately, the family elected not to do so, realizing that the movies potentially represented a "way in" to Owen's world. Consequently, another dramatic thing happened one day when Ron found Owen in his room, flipping through a Disney book. Carefully, Ron grabbed a Iago puppet (a character from the movie *Aladdin*), slid under the bedspread, crawled up to Owen, and put the puppet close to his son (Suskind 2014:54):

> Then, a thought: be Iago. What would Iago say?
> I push the puppet up through the crease in the bedspread. "So, Owen, how ya' doin'?" I say, doing my best Gilbert Gottfried. "I mean, how does it feel to be you!?"
> Through the crease, I can see him turn toward Iago. It's like he was bumping into an old friend. "I'm not happy. I don't have friends. I can't understand what people say."
> I have not heard this voice, natural and easy, with the traditional rhythm of common speech, since he was two.

Staying with the Iago voice, Ron managed to elicit a *conversation* with Owen, who deployed his own as well as Disney voices in reply. To make a longer story short (for a more detailed account, see Ron Suskind's [2014] compelling book, *Life, Animated*, and the documentary movie of the same name), this breakthrough opened the door to much wider and more consistent engagement with Owen and eventually to a string of hard-won successes for his further education and engagement in the ordinary social world.

Although it could be said that early on Owen and his behavior were strange from the standpoint of common sense, his family's strategy—the use of Disney dialogue and related approaches—not only succeeded in engaging him but utterly widened the taken-for-granted world of everyday life for the Suskind family and others who surrounded Owen when he was a child and adolescent.[14] They learned to speak his language in a variety of ways and to enter his world, rather than waiting for him or otherwise insisting that he enter theirs. Importantly, they did not dismiss his sensemaking methods as mere echolalia or treat them as deficient relative to their own. Instead, they recognized that he was making sense in his own way and found methods for *making sense with him.* Just as Owen eventually became a competent participant in their world, so too did they—in the first place—become competent participants in his.

Such an accomplishment reverses the usual relationship between the stranger and the group, wherein the former "has to place in question nearly everything that seems to be unquestionable to the members of the approached group" (Schuetz 1944:502). Instead, to the degree that mutual understanding is wanted or needed, members of the commonsense group—family, educators, clinicians, and others—may have to question their own assumptions relative to the oddness of the person in their midst. They will need to learn the language of autism. They may be transformed more than the stranger, and if that happens, it makes for meaningful interaction that enriches both parties. Indeed, as Simmel (1950:402) points out in his own essay on this topic, the stranger combines elements of both nearness and remoteness, is already an "element" of the group, and "imports qualities" into the group "which do not and cannot stem from the group itself."

There is no better example of the stranger importing valued qualities to social groupings than Greta Thunberg, a Swedish girl who, when she was in fifth grade, according to her mother (Thunberg et al. 2020:15), "was slowly disappearing into some kind of darkness and little by little, bit by bit, she seemed to stop functioning." She was becoming strange. Then she was diagnosed with autism and began to improve. But, as her mother (Thunberg et al. 2020:36) reports, "What happened to our daughter can't be explained simply by a medical acronym, a diagnosis or dismissed as 'otherness'. In the end, she simply couldn't reconcile the contradictions of modern life. Things simply just didn't add up." As a result, Greta "saw what the rest of us did not want to see": "the colourless, scentless, soundless abyss that our generation has chosen to ignore" (Thunberg et al. 2020:262). Greta became an environmental activist and voice on climate change. At sixteen, in 2019, she became the youngest person to earn *Time Magazine*'s Person of the Year award, and she has effected environmental change through speaking tours and other forms of advocacy that have earned her a nomination for a Nobel Peace Prize. Not only her family but also significant figures and groups around the world have opened up to her language, her forms of alarm and advocacy. Our book draws on these more global pictures of autism language from Suskind, Thunberg, and others, but with attention to the fine details of everyday talk and social interaction.

After Testing: Determining, Conveying, and Recording Diagnosis

The stories about what we are calling the language of autism demonstrate how caretakers may learn to appreciate and use a child's competence and skill, even in the midst of disruptive behavior that is troublesome from a common-sense point of view. Taken differently, such behavior, in our view, can exhibit *first-order, fundamental competence* and *autistic intelligence*, so long as they are appreciated as such.[15] In chapter 4, we define these terms more precisely, but for now we return to Dan Chapman and his testing and diagnosis to set the stage for the analysis in subsequent chapters.

At the CDDC, once each clinician working on a case completes their evaluation, the team meets for a conference called a pre-staffing. Usually, this meeting takes place in one of the team member's offices, although multiple smaller meetings may occur if not all of the clinicians can be present. Depending on time constraints and case complexity, such meetings can vary in length from about five minutes to a half hour or more. It is in these meetings that the clinicians share their results and impressions, interpret findings, and collaboratively decide on a diagnosis (or rule one out).

In Dan's case, Dr. Erickson and Dr. Grant met together and determined that he qualified for the diagnosis. Then they saw Betsy Chapman for an informing interview (which at CDDC is called a "staffing"), and Dr. Erickson presented her results from the ADOS, noting that Dan's score of thirteen exceeded the cutoff—which is nine or higher in Dan's age group—for an autism diagnosis. As the conversation continued, the clinicians reported further test results and shared stories about Dan, building a narrative that supported their conclusions. As we discuss in chapter 6, clinicians organize diagnostic discussions among themselves, and then with family members, through forms of narrative: reporting and storytelling, weaving accounts of a child's performances into a discursive arc that speaks for or against a particular diagnosis.

Parents have varied reactions to hearing that their child has autism. In Dan's case, his mother responded by saying, "It's been since he was four that I felt he had autism. It's been really—just every year it got tougher and tougher."[16] She recalled how she contacted a doctor and said, "There's something wrong with him." When that doctor did not do anything, she sought out another doctor, who, she said, "was like try this, see if this works, and that doesn't—it was just like he was giving him [Dan] so many medications to try, and nothing really helped." She then expressed concern about what a new diagnosis would mean for the services Dan was currently receiving through the county in which the family resided: Would he still be eligible for them? Social worker Norah Gonzalez, who was sitting in on the meeting, assured Betsy that he would be, and spent much of the remainder of the discussion talking through the details, going over the family's insurance, Dan's school individualized education plan (IEP), and programs for which an autism diagnosis would qualify him. Especially when children receive a new diagnosis, these conversations are common during informing interviews and often take up a majority of the session—one of the many ways participants in the clinic show an orientation to the larger matrix of institutions that regulate and define autism for various communities (Eyal and Hart 2010).

As the informing interview drew to a close, the participants made plans for a follow-up appointment to gauge Dan's progress. Drs. Erickson and Grant also informed Dan's mother that they would be providing written evaluation reports, which she would be receiving in the mail shortly. In the meantime, they gave her a brief preliminary report that she could use immediately to procure new services for her son. These official documents had become part of Dan's permanent medical record and would now form a crucial part of his autistic career and institutional identity.

Interaction Order of the Clinic

Children like Dan are evaluated every day at clinics across the United States. When we began our fieldwork at CDDC in 2011, we wanted to investigate autism as a diagnostic phenomenon by seeing how these evaluations are organized: how clinicians establish whether a child has autism, how they produce findings that they and their colleagues consider valid and reliable, and how they deliver diagnoses to families. As one of the largest clinics specializing in autism in the state where we conducted our study, CDDC serves a great many families from both rural and urban areas, making it a rich site for observing the diagnostic process in action.

After gaining access through contacts in the clinic and its administration, we spent four years talking with clinicians and families, watching evaluations, and participating in events and (as mentioned) training seminars sponsored by CDDC. Our effort resulted in video recordings of forty-nine autism evaluations, which we tracked from intake through testing to diagnosis. Our approach permitted what is called "maximum variation sampling" (Miles and Huberman 1994:28–29). By this we mean that, although we were fundamentally obtaining an opportunity sample by taking any and all families who consented during the data collection period, the number of children supplied us with gender, age, and limited ethnic variation according to the distributions of families who availed themselves of CDDC services. Additionally, in some cases we were able to record later postdiagnosis visits, during which families updated clinicians on their children's progress and sought further advice. Because one of the authors (Maynard) had conducted a separate, but related, study of diagnostic news delivery at CDDC in 1985, we also had access to thirteen cases from that period, including two where children were diagnosed with autism, which was then considered a rare condition estimated to affect four to five in ten thousand children (Merrick, Kandel, and Morad 2004)—in stark contrast to the current rate of one in fifty-four (CDC 2020). Further data came from an unrelated study of a psychiatric clinic on the East Coast. Assembled in 1972, the collection included at least one case where a child was diagnosed with autism, at that time considered a form of "childhood psychosis."[17] These various data sources furnish us with a unique collection of audio and video recordings, case histories, and medical records spanning distinct eras in the development of the autism diagnosis (Maynard and Turowetz 2019).

We entered CDDC during a period when the category of autism was in transition. The committee working on the fifth edition of the *Diagnostic and Statistical Manual of Mental Disorders* (DSM-5) was just then debating whether to collapse the categories that made up the family of autism spectrum disorders—including Asperger's, around which a growing community of "Aspies" has forged a strong collective identity (Singh 2011)—into a single continuum, graded by symptom frequency and severity. Although we did not anticipate it, our study found us moving into highly contested and controversial territory. Even those who are relatively sympathetic to the reality of autism observe that its diagnosis, as in many psychiatric disorders, "is interpretive and sometimes unreliable" (Grinker 2007:112), while others in the

vein of critical autism studies highlight how "autism is far from settled" and
that "naming it, containing it, or diagnosing it is marked with controversy
and deep disagreement" (Orsini and Davidson 2013:7; also see chap. 7 in this
volume).

Situating autism in the interactional spheres where it is enacted, we aim to
enable a holistic understanding of the phenomenon. In other words, we are
more capable of forming a complete picture of the now well-known, exponen-
tial increase in autism diagnoses by understanding how they are assembled
at the point of ascertainment and application. If, as Silverman (2012:194) has
said, "the work that constructs autism as a stable population occurs largely at
the level of behavioral observations, diagnostic questionnaires, and checklists" (see also Brown 1990:395; Singh 2016:25), then attention needs to be paid
to the domain of everyday talk and embodied conduct by which clinicians
make sense of such materials among themselves and for others. Diagnoses
are not straightforwardly applied to children in such a way as to enable reliable large-scale counting: on the ground, in the clinic, symptoms must be
elicited, enumerated, and interpreted. This socially organized process relies
on secondhand reports from referral agents, often schools and pediatricians,
followed by extensive face-to-face interactions among clinicians, children,
family members, educators, and others.

By saying these interactions are socially organized, we mean that they are
finely patterned in what, following Goffman (1983), we call *the interaction order of the clinic*. This is a realm where participants cooperate in the practices
of talk and conduct through which clinical phenomena, such as diagnoses,
are produced. These practices have an orderliness and coherence that is independent of external social structures and identities, such as race, class, and
gender, though they interact with these externalities in various ways (Duneier and Molotch 1999, Molotch and Boden 1985, Schegloff 1987b). Stated
differently, what we mean by orderly and coherent practices is that clinicians
possess shared, professionalized forms of knowledge regarding ordinary ways
of testing and diagnosis (Peräkylä and Vehviläinen 2003), but they do not
explicitly remark on or acknowledge those practices in the course of their everyday work. Rather, clinicians simply engage in examinations, in narrating
their findings for diagnosis, in drawing conclusions, and in record keeping,
while consigning taken-for-granted practices that make these activities possible to a tacit, unnoticed background as they go about their overt business.

Because clinical work is inseparable from a background of enabling practices, however, the specification of such practices promises to illuminate not
only how the diagnoses that are represented in aggregate, statistical trends
are assembled in the first place but also "what more" (Garfinkel 2002) there

is to the official accounts of this process. In our analysis, capturing this "what more" involves explaining precisely how the "singularity" of autism is accomplished through a "praxiography" of disability (Mol 2002:119–21). *Praxiography* refers simply to the everyday, taken-for-granted methods for referring patients, intake, testing, discussing results, determining diagnosis, and consulting and contributing to records.

Moreover, insofar as this "what more" captures an individual child's ways of reasoning, sensemaking, and acting in the world, the possibility of retrieving insights from the clinic about a *particular* child, rather than a *generic* child with autism, is important to consider. Such knowledge could be used not only to help integrate the child into the wider society—at home, in school, in the workplace, and elsewhere—but also, more radically, to adapt society to the child, especially by expanding common sense to include the child's own (but different) methods of sensemaking. Could the procedures used to evaluate a child such as Dan Chapman be enhanced to incorporate aspects of his behavior that ordinary diagnosis conceals or overlooks? Would this make it possible to inform family members, educators, therapists, and others in postclinical environments about how to achieve more viability not only for the child but for those very social environments? Finally, to what degree is Dan's conduct in need of alteration, and to what degree do the commonsense environments he inhabits require adjustment?

A Map for the Rest of the Book

Our approach to autism highlights social interaction, viewing it as disrupting taken-for-granted practices and expectations. If commonsense participants allow for reflection rather than reaction, they might come to appreciate how those on the autism spectrum render ordinary ways of doing things strange. In this way, commonsense participants may gain insights into their own usual, and usually invisible, forms of producing direct, local social organization. Common sense is capable of adjustment, so that what was at first strange can become more familiar. These matters—common sense, strangeness, familiarity, and most especially the *practices* of talk and embodied action situated in the "interaction order" (Goffman 1983) of everyday and clinical settings—are what occupy us in the rest of the book.

In chapter 2, we address the history of autism and its diagnosis. We align to the view that the differences now taken to be characteristic of autism or autism spectrum disorder are not new, although they may be newly recognized. In addition, because investigations of the neurobiology of autism have exploded in response to its increased prevalence, we raise questions about what we have learned from recent studies of genetics, genomics, and the brain and suggest that a better understanding of what we define as the *interactional phenotype of autism* is sorely needed.

In chapter 3, we describe our data and lay out the specifics of our interactional approach and its grounding in the sociological subfields of ethnomethodology, conversation analysis, and the sociology of the interaction order. We suggest that, although our database is by some standards limited, the patterns of testing and diagnosis we identify and analyze reach beyond the clinics we have investigated and the data we have collected from them. We also introduce the system of transcript notation that we use for excerpts from the audio and video recordings in our data corpus.

Chapters 4 and 5 explicate what we mean by autistic intelligence, first-order (or fundamental) competence, and second-order (or structural) competence. They also document the phenomenon of autistic intelligence, which involves atypical ways of sensemaking that can interfere with the successful performance of tasks that children are asked to do. As well, we show that both the assessment instruments themselves and the actions of the clinician are important features of children's performances—though these performances are, as a matter of course, attributed to the child alone.

Chapter 6 takes us from the organization of testing to that which is dependent on the formal assessment process: the achievement of diagnostic conclusions. We analyze the narrative ways in which clinicians collectively achieve a diagnosis and subsequently deliver it to family members. But is autism itself a narrative construction? To put the question more provocatively: Is autism real? We address this and related questions in chapter 7, where we examine how clinicians themselves deal with the often ambiguous nature of their own evidence.

Finally, chapter 8 draws matters to a conclusion, returning to the problems of common sense, strangeness, the interactional phenotype, autistic intelligence, and diagnosis. Here, we expand on the significance of our argument for studies of science and technology, the sociology of diagnosis, and the sociology of autism more generally. Additionally, we contribute to the field of disability studies by further developing the notion of getting into the child's world—metaphorically entering their abode and learning about it in sufficient detail that, rather than us attempting removal, the child escorts *us* out into the world of common everyday life. Finally, we discuss how our interaction-based research can enable better specification of what has come to be called the "prosthetic environment," one that empowers the development of the child by being built to accommodate that child's unique forms of intelligence. To put our argument in different words, this endeavor requires adjustment on the part of commonsense actors as much as it means chang-ing the child's behavioral repertoire. For families and clinicians, it may mean deriving more about the particular characteristics of a specific child in a way that can be embodied in diagnostic findings and the recommendations that follow.

A Brief History and Biology of Autism Diagnosis:
Why We Need an Interactional Approach

When Dan Chapman visited the CDDC, he was evaluated by two professionals, a psychologist and a developmental pediatrician. As we know from chapter 1, the clinicians eventually diagnosed Dan with autism spectrum disorder. But how they arrived at that conclusion immediately raises questions about the history and neurobiology of the disorder. Is autism a new disorder, or has it always been with us? Would it now make sense to say that someone like Dan was autistic, even though the diagnosis did not exist in earlier decades or centuries? Would he have been noticed, possibly even stigmatized, or just regarded as awkward and shy? Would he have been consigned to an asylum or other "total institution" (Goffman 1961)? These questions are difficult to answer, not only because they ask about counterfactuals but because diagnosis in the current era is itself no simple matter. Straightforward neurological, genetic, or other markers do not define the disorder, whose diagnosis remains fraught with complications and controversy.

Historical, genetic, and neurobiological studies have deepened our understanding of autism, even in the absence of definitive conclusions. However, our purpose in this chapter is to consider the history, genetics, and neurobiology of autism in order to make an argument for why studies of interaction are important. Interactional studies probe the "more complex and richer thing[s]" (Harrington 2005) of human experience, a deep reservoir whose surface neurobiology only scrapes. Yet interaction studies are comparatively undervalued and underfunded. And it is not just in genetics, neurology, and history that interaction is neglected. Interaction-based research is also below the radar of autism studies even in the *social* sciences, which have concentrated either on the epidemiology of autism and its gigantic rise in prevalence over recent decades or on the psychology, psychiatry, and related nonbiological cognitive processes located "within the individual minds of those diagnosed" (Fein 2020:33). Taken together, neurobiology and social science largely posit what Ortega (2009) calls a "cerebral subject" whose central identity is cognitively determined. Crucially, such an orientation fails to recognize that any individual is an indelible part of a social and interactional environment. In a fundamental point that needs wider appreciation, Solomon (2010:251) puts it simply: autism "is less a property of the individual and more a property of social interaction."

In this chapter, we revisit the case of Dan Chapman to illustrate the challenges that can arise in autism diagnosis. Like those of many other children we observed, Dan's case was far from straightforward. The clinicians who diagnosed him had to reconcile sometimes conflicting pieces of information as they worked to determine whether autism was an appropriate label for his problems. From Dan's experience in the clinic, we then zoom out to provide a historical overview[1] of autism and its cultural components, followed by a detailed discussion of current trends in autism research, particularly its disproportionate emphasis on genetics and neurobiology. We argue that this research, though important, is limited in what it can tell us about autism as a social phenomenon that exists in the spaces between actors—the realm of interaction—rather than "inside" any particular individual.

If we can conceive of autism, in this spatial sense, as something existing outside the individual, then what we call an *interactional phenotype* may be worthy of analytic appreciation. In genetics, a phenotype is the set of observable traits that are characteristic of an organism. Whereas the autism phenotype is usually defined in terms of static traits, we propose the interactional phenotype as a dynamic alternative capable of capturing the constitutive role of behavior, specifically *behavior-in-interaction*,[2] in producing autism as a recognizable social and clinical phenomenon. Before getting to the interactional phenotype, however, we need to cover some background. First we consider Dan Chapman's case in more detail. Then we discuss autism's history, its recent surge in prevalence, explanations for that surge, and demographic distributions of the diagnosis, as well as current research into its biological and neurological bases. Along the way, we address what has been called the "economics of autism" before returning to the clinic to see how matters of biology and genetics were made relevant for Dan Chapman and his family.

Difficulties with Diagnosis

In all, psychologist Jennifer Erickson used four different instruments to assess Dan. First, both Dan's mother and his teacher completed a form called

TABLE 2.1. CBCL Results

Scales	Mother	Teacher
Anxious/Depressed	72	50
Withdrawn/Depressed	82	64
Somatic Complaints	67	50
Thought Problems	67	59
Attention Problems	71	64
Attention Problems	71	50
Rule-Breaking Behavior	67	59
Aggressive Behavior	76	68

the Child Behavior Checklist (CBCL), which is a way of identifying a child's potential problem areas. Table 2.1 is an exact reproduction of what was reported in Dan's medical record. Scores on the CBCL have an average of fifty, and those greater than seventy are considered to be "in the clinical range of significance." At a glance, it is apparent that the scoring discrepancies between Dan's mother and teacher are large. While the figures from Dan's mother show "significant concerns across multiple areas," as the record states it, his teacher's ratings are all below the threshold of clinical significance.

Second, Dan's mother and teacher also completed the Social Communication Questionnaire (SCQ), which specifically screens for autism. It consists of a series of yes-no questions, such as whether a child offers to share, engages in social smiling, has appropriate eye gaze and facial expressions, and participates in imaginative play with other children. Dan's medical record states (*our emphasis*), "On both forms, Dan's total score on the SCQ was *just below* the cutoff typically used to indicate that further evaluation for ASD is warranted." Thus, in contrast to their CBCL ratings, Betsy Chapman and the teacher are in agreement that Dan is not clinically impaired.

Third, however, on another rating scale filled out by parents, the Vineland II, which assesses an individual's adaptive behaviors and everyday living skills, Betsy's ratings of Dan produced scores of 74 for communication, 79 for daily living skills, 69 for socialization, and 84 for motor responses. For children Dan's age, scores between 85 and 115 are in the average range. Accordingly, Jennifer Erickson writes in her evaluation report that "Dan's adaptive skills [on the Vineland] are generally below average for his age based on the information provided." Note that these ratings are consistent with Betsy's CBCL scoring but not with her or Dan's teacher's SCQ evaluations.

Finally, Dan's score on the centrally important ADOS showed that he meets the criteria for autism. As Jennifer puts it in her evaluation report, Dan "exceeded the cutoff for a classification of autism." Yet again, the picture here is remarkably mixed. Discussing her findings with Dr. Leah Grant, the developmental pediatrician who also examined Dan, Jennifer said, "So he came up with a thirteen . . . and the cutoff was a nine. So he actually came up a little higher on the ADOS than I thought he would, just because he did so many nice things" (a higher score means more symptoms of autism). Elsewhere in the conversation, she says that she was "a little surprised" about Dan's "solid" score because he did have a number of "pretty nice" responses and moreover did not have any "inappropriate social gestures."

In later chapters, we analyze the interactions between Jennifer and Dan in more detail. For the time being, though, we can observe that Dan's mixed clinical picture may be characteristic of people on the autism spectrum generally, especially those considered "high" functioning. It is well recognized, for example, that in the area of cognitive functioning, autistic people often show widely discrepant patterns on different measures of intelligence (Dawson et al. 2007). Additionally, cognitive traits (as compared with physical ones) are highly complex, making them difficult to measure (Conley and Fletcher 2017:99). Autistic individuals characteristically score low on measures of communicative competence and high on measures of visual and spatial skills (Frith 2003:130–40). As Eyal and colleagues (2010:32) succinctly put it, "autistic children are typically described as children with uneven abilities, delayed in some areas, normal or even advanced in others." In chapters 4 and 5, we suggest that this unevenness can mask various forms of competence, which we term autistic intelligence, that children display in the clinic and elsewhere. These competences are frequently unrecognized and unrecorded and are regularly mistaken for incompetence.

In all, a warranted conclusion to our original counterfactual question about whether Dan would have received a diagnosis in another era is necessarily equivocal: *it depends*. In a different social and institutional environment, Dan might not have received any diagnosis, might have been considered as having attention deficit disorder, or oppositional defiance disorder, or at most appeared as an insignificant blip on the diagnostic radar. Even in a time and place where autism was recognized and diagnosed, Dan may not have been a candidate for it: past criteria for the diagnosis were much more restrictive than they are today, and it is unlikely that they would have been considered—much less applied—in Dan's case. However, in twenty-first-century America, where there is a broad goal of inclusiveness for persons with disability (and autism in particular) (Fein and Rios 2018), effective and accurate diagnosis is considered extremely important. Autism is more broadly defined than in the past, and children are routinely monitored for developmental differences and referred to professionals as soon as red flags are detected. It was thus that Dan found himself at a clinic for disabilities, whereas in earlier eras he might have been shunned for his anomalous behavior, consigned to an institution for the "mentally retarded," or, more optimistically, regarded as merely eccentric.[3]

A Brief History of Autism

The term *autism* was coined in 1908 by the Swiss psychiatrist Eugene Bleuler, who used it to describe symptoms of withdrawal seen in patients with schizophrenia. In the early decades of the 1900s, scholars and therapists as diverse as Sigmund Freud, Melanie Klein, and Jean Piaget drew on *autism* and related terms to describe developmental experiences in the cognitive life of children where egocentric fantasies, and even hallucinations, seemed to predominate (Evans 2013). Slightly later than Bleuler, Leo Kanner (1943), the physician at Johns Hopkins University (see chap. 1), coined the term "infantile autism" to classify a group of eleven children who exhibited several distinctive behaviors, including rigidity, insistence on sameness, and lack of interest in social interaction and engagement. As Eyal (2013:879) observes, Kanner's conception of autism complicated the distinction between mental illness, then considered to be temporary and amenable to cures, and mental retardation, thought to be permanent, intractable, and necessitating institutionalization. As a hybrid disorder combining elements of illness and retardation, infantile autism was a form of "apparent feeblemindedness" that could be ameliorated with the right interventions.

Just one year after Kanner's highly influential publication, Hans Asperger (1991[1944]), a psychiatrist who worked in Vienna, Austria, and from whom the condition with that name derives, published an account of what he called autism that also drew on Bleuler's use of the term.[4] In recent years, both Kanner and Asperger have been criticized for various failures—Kanner for apparently suppressing Asperger's nearly parallel work on the syndrome (Silberman 2015), and Asperger for his tie-ins to the Nazi regime in Vienna (Sheffer 2018). We do not address either of these controversies here. Instead, our focus is on the category of autism and its diagnostic parameters over the years.

Although the children he described had higher IQs than the ones in Kanner's sample, Asperger's account of "autistic psychopathy" was remarkably similar to Kanner's description of "infantile autism." Still, as Grinker (2007:64, original emphasis) writes, "Neither Kanner nor Asperger truly *discovered* autism. They *described* it." And Baker (2013:1090) similarly posits, "Kanner did not so much define as portray autism, in the course of a series of memorable case histories." Subsequently, debates about the relationship between the two conditions have proliferated. Although Asperger's syndrome was an official diagnosis for a time (1994–2013), in the most recent edition of the American Psychiatric Association's (APA) Diagnostic and Statistical Manual (DSM-5), it has been collapsed into a more general "autism spectrum" (Barker and Galardi 2015).[5]

Contemporary Spread of Autism Diagnosis

Given the morphing of Kanner's and Asperger's descriptions and definitions into autism spectrum disorder, a broad and persistent increase in the prevalence of ASD is well documented, at least in the United States and Great Britain (Croen et al. 2002; Fombonne 2003; Liu, King, and Bearman 2010; Yeargin-Allsopp et al. 2003). Such increase has dramatically affected public awareness of the disorder in its own right. In the early 2000s, anthropologist Roy Grinker (2007:20) wrote, "Autism is more familiar and visible than ever before." Three years later, social epidemiologists Ka-Yuet Liu, Marissa King, and Peter Bearman (2010:1390) could say, "Autism increasingly appears in the everyday life of American families." Now, after another decade, autism is so prevalent that everyday contact between those who are "neurotypical" (NT) and autistic individuals is commonplace. As mentioned in chapter 1, the prevalence of autism among children at age eight in the United States is currently one in fifty-four. People with autism are acquaintances, family members, friends (or children of friends), and coworkers. Moreover, in addition to regular newspaper stories reporting on experiences or incidents involving autistic individuals, there are countless blogs, YouTube videos, online testimonials, and other sources that provide various contemporary experiential accounts of autism.

Rather than constituting an "epidemic" in the usual sense of a contagious disease, the increase in autism has been linked to factors such as higher parental age, which increases the probability of germ cell mutations (Durkin et al. 2008), diffusion of social influence through parental networks (Liu, King, and Bearman 2010), changes in environmental toxins and stressors (Ozand et al. 2003), the possible involvement of microbiota or gastrointestinal organisms (Sharon et al. 2019), and especially (as we discuss below) the broadening of diagnostic criteria and heightened awareness of autism's heterogeneity (Gernsbacher, Dawson, and Goldsmith 2005).[6]

Diagnostic changes occurring in the United States during the 1990s and early 2000s contributed to the growth in autism. "Diagnostic substitution," write King and Bearman (2009:1224), "occurs when an individual, net of changes to diagnostic standards, practices and procedures, or individual condition, is diagnosed with one condition at one time and subsequently with another condition at some further point in time." For example, substitution is evident in a study by the California Health and Human Services Agency, which showed that the rate of autism increased from 5.78 per 10,000 in 1987 to 14.89 in 1994, while the rate of mental retardation of unknown cause decreased from 28.26 to 19.52 during the same period. The growing prevalence of autism has also been driven by accretion, which involves the addition of other diagnoses to autism: "an individual initially diagnosed with one disorder subsequently acquires a second diagnosis, but retains the first diagnosis as a co-morbidity" (King and Bearman 2009:1225). Accretion takes place when autism is co-diagnosed alongside other medical and genetic conditions—such as ADHD, Down syndrome, fragile X syndrome, Tourette's syndrome, or cerebral palsy (Gernsbacher, Dawson, and Goldsmith 2005:55–56; Grinker 2007: 161–62). And so autism now encompasses a wider range of cases (Eyal et al. 2010; King and Bearman 2009), not only in the United States but also in other countries around the world (Eyal 2013:47–48).

The huge upsurge in ASD diagnosis raises the question of whether environmental influences, such as the use of vaccinations (a discredited idea), have created an epidemic. The issues here have to do with both incidence (the rate of new cases relative to the population) and prevalence (the proportion of known cases in the population). One way of formulating the matter is to ask whether, compared to previous eras, there has been an increase in the incidence of "true" cases of autism (according to some reliable definition of the disorder) or if its incidence has been stable over time but better methods of detection have resulted in more cases being identified, so that what we are seeing is an increase in prevalence.

Given the upsurge, our position leans more toward investigators (Frith 2003:59; cf. Lord et al. 2020:2) who have argued that there has been no real increase in incidence but that there is a sharp upsurge in prevalence. To put this point differently, we can use somewhat controversial characterizations[7] from the psychological literature on autism, which posits autism as being characterized by weak central coherence (difficulties in organizing details), impulsivity (due to deficits in executive function—the "planning" part of activity), and deficits in the "theory of mind," or the ability to ascertain others' intentions. Such characteristics or ones like them may have been long recognized, but in accordance with categories indigenous to their historical and community contexts. Scholars give numerous examples of people who may have had what we now recognize as autism, including the "alien children" found in forests during the Middle Ages (Grinker 2007:52); the "blessed fools" of Russia, whose existence is documented from the sixteenth century (Frith 2003:22); Victor "the wild boy of Aveyron" circa 1800; and Hugh Blair of Borgue, Scotland, circa 1828 (Frith 2003:chap. 3). To these cases, we can add myriad other anonymous children whom Europeans and Americans indulged as "eccentric"—at least up until the twentieth century—if they could otherwise contribute socially or economically to their communities (Grinker 2007:51–53).

Even today, autism "without a name" can be found in cultures such as Senegal, with its "marvelous children" (Grinker 2007:51) or Korea, where the designation may be that of "border children" (Grinker and Cho 2013), or closer to home, among Navajo Indian youth who "are seen simply as perpetual children" (Grinker 2007:52). Historically, the attitude toward autism in the United States and other English-speaking countries (e.g., the United Kingdom and Canada) has been much less charitable: many children were not so much tolerated as labeled "mentally deficient," "mentally retarded," or "feebleminded," and shunted away to institutions (Eyal 2013:879; cf. Grinker 2007:55–56). Although this attitude has changed a great deal with time, what has not changed is a tendency to treat autism as a personal deficit and cause of dysfunction. As we will see, this deficit-centered view of autism is built into the instruments used to evaluate autism and the diagnostic criteria on which they are based.

A Network of Expertise

Related to (or even prompting) substitution and accretion are changes in US social institutions. As thousands of former inmates poured out of America's mental asylums during the deinstitutionalization initiative of the 1970s, educators, social workers, and assorted other actors created new diagnostic classifications to accommodate a growing clientele (Eyal et al. 2010). Similar processes and effects occurred in Britain during this period (Evans 2013). Coincidentally, the traditional authority of child psychiatrists over autism also began to erode, being gradually replaced by a horizontal network of parents and paraprofessionals who influenced autism's definition and diagnosis (Evans 2013; Eyal 2013). These various developments coalesced into the institutional "matrix" or expanded "network of expertise" (Eyal et al. 2010) within which autism is currently immersed.

This network of expertise began its development in the 1960s, as parents and paraprofessional groups in the United States—including occupational and speech therapists, special education teachers, nurses, and psychologists—challenged the stigmatizing notion that mothers are responsible for their children's condition (Silverman 2012). The pioneering parental advocate Bernard Rimland (1964) developed checklists that other parents could use to screen their children for autism, and parent advocacy groups, such as the National Society for Autistic Children (NSAC, circa 1965), raised awareness of autism and redefined it as a lifelong disorder distinct from other developmental disorders (Eyal 2013).

Besides raising awareness, advocacy groups adopted and popularized the innovative treatment technique known as Applied Behavior Analysis (ABA). Developed by behavioral psychologist Ivar Lovaas at UCLA, ABA targets specific autistic behaviors and replaces them with more normative or commonsense ones. Because ABA is extremely time-consuming and labor intensive, professionals could not do it alone and were prompted to enlist parents in the treatment process. This transformed parents from subordinates into collaborators (Lovaas 1987), with the result that "the new autism expert was no longer the clinician, but neither was it the behavioral psychologist, it was rather a team or an actor-network[8] composed of therapists, psychologists, psychiatrists, and parents, with the latter occupying the leading role" (Eyal 2013:886).[9]

Distribution of Autism Diagnoses

An autism matrix has not meant an even distribution of the diagnosis in the population. For example, at higher levels of socioeconomic status (SES), there is an increased likelihood of ASD diagnosis (Durkin et al. 2010). This may be due to "ascertainment" bias; in other words, high-SES parents have access to information and resources that make it easier to obtain diagnostic services, and clinicians may be more willing to give their children the diagnosis. However, Durkin and colleagues (2010) find only mixed evidence for this bias.

Race also affects who gets the diagnosis. Previous research (Mandell et al. 2009) on racial disparities reported that African American, Hispanic, and other non-White children are less likely than White children to receive an autism diagnosis. This disparity held for African American children regardless of IQ level and was concentrated among those with IQs lower than seventy in other non-White groups—Asian and Hispanic. An earlier Institute of Medicine report (2002:497), quoted in Mandell and colleagues (2009), suggests that these racial differences may be attributable to institutional factors (see also Gourdine, Baffour, and Teasley 2011), including access to health care, general prejudices held by clinicians, the way clinicians and families interpret children's symptoms, and clinicians' application of erroneous algorithms on the likelihood of a child having autism (i.e., clinicians having different expectations about the probability of autism occurring in White vs. non-White children).

According to a recent report from the Centers for Disease Control (Maenner et al. 2020), however, such diagnostic disparities are starting to even out. In particular, the report cites prevalence estimates that are approximately identical for White, Black, and Asian/Pacific Islander children but lower for Hispanic children. However, Black children with autism were less likely to have a first evaluation by age thirty-six months than were White children with autism (40% versus 45%). Previously, African American children were more likely than White children to be misdiagnosed with conduct or adjustment disorders and to receive an autism diagnosis later than their White counterparts (Mandell et al. 2007). Thus, what Grinker, Yeargin-Allsopp, and Boyle (2011:122) have asserted about diagnostic differences internationally is also true regarding disparities *within* a given society: "Autism may be universal, but the contexts in which it occurs are distinctive."

The starkest asymmetry in the distribution of autism diagnoses is by gender. Current estimates suggest that the odds of having autism are at least 3.5 times higher for boys than girls (e.g., Kogan et al. 2009; Loomes, Hull, and Mandy 2017). Reasons for this disparity are mostly speculative. One hypothesis is that at early ages, girls are less disruptive than boys, better at imitating typical behaviors, and more socially oriented (cf. Bazelon 2007). In Werling and Geschwind's (2013:151) terms, it may be that "females present the autistic phenotype differently than males." Still, this global pattern masks significant variation among girls. Girls at the low-functioning end of the spectrum are almost as likely as boys to be diagnosed with autism (the ratio may be as low as 1.95:1), while at the higher-functioning end, the disparity widens to approximately 5.5:1 (Fombonne 2003; Gillis-Buck and Richardson 2014). Also, at later ages, girls may be more susceptible to depression and anxiety than boys, encouraging diagnoses that focus on those symptoms rather than autism (Lainhart and Folstein 1994).

Another hypothesis about gender disparities, initially put forth by Baron-Cohen (2002), follows Asperger's (1991[1944]:44) argument that the "autistic personality" is an "extreme variant of male intelligence." In this view, autism reflects the male brain's hardwired tendency to systematize, and females with autism have male brains. Other research, however, reports that males and females with autism are actually more likely to have "androgynous" brains, which accords with evidence (Shumer 2016) that children and adolescents with gender dysphoria have higher than expected rates of ASD. Still other commentators caution that there are no "male" and "female" brains as such: these brains are artifacts of statistical aggregation. In reality, each individual brain is different, and comparing one to the "average" brain for a given category can be misleading (Jordan-Young 2011).

Whatever the truth of different-brain hypotheses turns out to be, Bishop (2015) and Lord and colleagues (2020) suggest the need for new scoring instruments, observations in peer-group settings that compare autistic and nonautistic girls, and a more nuanced understanding of social and communication differences by gender. Along these lines, Sturrock and colleagues (2020) suggest that females diagnosed with high-functioning autism outperform males with ASD in pragmatic (socially oriented) tasks and semantic understandings (knowledge of word meanings), including those involved with emotions. The authors suggest that understanding such differences may mean more accuracy in diagnosis and more targeted therapies. Although our study cannot specify particular changes to the diagnostic process, we do advocate for more nuance by capturing the individuality of a child coming under the diagnostic lens.

Neurology, Biology, Genomics

Gender disparities in autism diagnosis raise questions about the relationship among the brain, biology, and genomics and their complex entanglements with behavior in the laboratory, clinic, and broader society (Freese and Shostak 2009; Fujimura, Duster, and Rajagopalan 2008). Given this complexity, issues related to the biology and neurology of autism, as might be expected, are murky and controversial. In the remainder of this chapter, we first review studies that focus on the brain and then address the rapidly expanding field of autism genetics. Especially important are the matters of genomic designation, an approach to gene-behavior research that starts with genes and works backward to behavior (a reversal of the traditional approach, which starts with behavior), and temptations to climb on the bandwagon of genetic research. These topics raise an issue related to what has been called the economics of autism. Next, we return to the case of Dan Chapman to bring neurological and genetic issues into the clinic. After that, we consider the interactional phenotype of autism and its relationship to what Freese (2008) calls the "phenotypic bottleneck."

RESEARCH ON THE BRAIN AND ITS CLINICAL IMPLICATIONS

As Silverman (2012:153–54) has reported, "Studies of the brain in autism consistently failed to locate any specific impaired structures, even on a microscopic level." Things have not changed much. It has been proposed that impaired structures may include missing cerebellum cells and mirror neurons—neural substrates responsible for empathy and "theory of mind," or the purported ability to know one's own cognitive state and infer another person's point of view. These ideas are largely discredited: theory-of-mind deficits are far from universal in populations of individuals with autism; the sites of the brain regions purportedly responsible for theory of mind number in the dozens, with no definitive one having been identified; and theory-of-mind features are not innate, but rather correlated with developmental difficulties stemming from specific language impairment. In fact, training in grammatical acuity improves performance on theory-of-mind tasks (Gernsbacher and Frymiare 2005).

Investigations of neurology offer two avenues for studying autism. *Structural* approaches examine the volume or size of the brain, its gray and white matter, and anomalies in distinct neurological areas such as the cerebellum, limbic system, amygdala, and others. *Functional* investigations focus on cognitive tasks such as face perception, linguistic skill, and executive functions. Both approaches use an impressive array of neuroimaging technologies, including EEGs, PET and CAT scans, MRIs, and fMRIs (Nadesan 2005:152). However, the sheer number of correlations generated by this research has made findings hard to integrate and interpret. A PubMed review covering forty-five years of research up to 2010 suggested that structural and functional MRI studies "meaningfully informed our understanding of brain structure, composition, and function" in autism but that "existing investigations have been fraught with limitations such as small sample sizes, cross-sectional designs, heterogenous subject characteristics, and varying methodologies" (Stigler et al. 2011:14). Additional problems derive from contradictory findings related to the heterogeneity of autism, differences in diagnostic criteria and subject characteristics (e.g., age, measures of intelligence, gender), and the variety of imaging technologies (Stigler et al. 2011:3, 7).

The problem is one of reliability. Related to this is the practical work of neuroscience—literally, the hands-on, embodied ways in which neuroscientists deal with the ambiguity of digital images (Alac 2008; cf. Nelson 2018). A researcher in Fitzgerald's (2017:72) study of brain scientists decried the difficulty in finding a "point in the brain that is dysfunctional and this is causing autism," further stating, "I don't think that's ever going to happen." Therefore, it should not be surprising to find a senior investigator saying, "Quite a good pub game is [to] name a region of the brain that hasn't been associated with autism, by somebody or some paper. It's quite impossible" (Fitzgerald 2017:72). Still, despite the fact that brain research has yet to produce findings that would help in diagnosis or treatment (Lord et al. 2020:7; Silverman 2012:155–60; Singh 2016:93), the view of autism as a neurological disorder has prevailed, not only in a drive to establish the validity of the diagnosis (Schnittker 2017:243–45) but in an attempt to reduce complexity and gain control over a puzzling region of human experience (Nadesan 2005:144–45; Silverman 2012:145).

Even if, as Fitzgerald (2014:255, original emphasis) has shown, brain scientists evince enormous ambivalence and low expectations—"hope *and* deflation"—for their research, "the question has been not whether a cause for autism can be found, but how long it will take" (Silverman 2012:160).[10] We can see this decidedly optimistic (rather than ambivalent) view about the biology of autism expressed in a paper in *Science* (State and Šestan 2012:1301): "Recent advances in genetics, genomic, developmental neurobiology, systems biology, monogenic neuro-developmental syndromes, and induced pluripotent stem cells (iPSC) are now offering remarkable insights into their etiologies and converging to provide a clear and immediate path forward from the bench to the bedside." This optimistic stance concurs with what science and technology studies of neurobiological research on mental disorders document more generally. Researchers find not only a historic preoccupation with biological causes (Moncrieff and Crawford 2001) but also an increasing biologization of psychiatry by way of a "neuromolecular"—akin to Foucault's (1973) "medical"—gaze. According to Rose (2013), this "style of thought" (cf. Fleck 1979), or what Fujimura and Chou (1994) call "style of practice," has constituted a "neurochemical self" through the conceptual and material dissection of cells, genes, and other such entities while the social environment is ignored or minimized.

In fact, DSM-5 (APA 2013) came under heavy criticism in the months before its publication for not being sufficiently grounded in neurobiological research. At that time Thomas Insel, then director of the National Institute of Mental Health (NIMH), announced that NIMH would begin using something called the Research Domain Criteria Document (RDoC), either as a competitor to the DSM or as a companion (Halpin 2016:154). The aim was to incorporate neurobiological measures, neurocognitive brain imaging, and physiological findings into the diagnosis of mental disorders and disabilities.[11] However, for psychiatrists and other clinicians, RDoC usage is not the straightforward matter it was conceived to be (Halpin 2016; Pickersgill 2019). Among other things, the approach neglects how indeterminate or uncertain genetic and genomic findings may be (Fujimura 2006) and how, in the clinic, considerable interpretive work involving both geneticists and their recipients (e.g., parents) is required to make sense of this uncertainty (Stivers and Timmermans 2016). Nevertheless, researchers continue to take the brain as the centerpiece for almost any and all psychiatric conditions, correlating neurobiology with measurable outputs such as test scores and questionnaire results and asserting its primacy as a causal factor (Halpin 2020). The effect of the neurobiological preoccupation is to "disavow" and flatten sociality (Decoteau and Sweet 2016:428–29)—the role of social experience in relation to disability, disorder, and their neurobiological determinants.

In emphasizing the reductionist tendencies of current neurobiological approaches to autism, our purpose is not to "show up neuroscience in some way" (Fitzgerald 2017:9). Rather, it is to propose a way of thinking about autism that can recognize the importance of neurobiological processes while granting primacy to the more holistic social interactional environment that embeds those processes.[12] In fact, a social interactional approach does not necessarily go against the grain of how neuroscientists themselves understand their enterprise, at least to the extent that they emphasize the heterogeneity of autism and the need for interdisciplinary research into the pathways that influence its expression (Fitzgerald 2013:46–53).[13] It does, however, challenge the notion that autism can be reduced to brain and biology in any meaningful, unitary sense. The issue is not whether brain and biology play a role in autism—they surely must—but how that role depends on the collective practices and expectations through which autism is produced as a recognizable social phenomenon in the clinic and in everyday life.

If autism cannot be separated from the social milieus where it is entrenched, then surely these milieus need systematic scrutiny to understand what it is as a lived (as opposed to laboratory) phenomenon. For example, while John Robison's behavior when playing with other children or reacting to bad news (chap. 1) was anomalous, it was not so in a social vacuum. Rather, coparticipants treated it as anomalous. In his extensive ethnographic investigations of autism in the United States and Morocco, Hart (2014:298) illustrates this point by showing that any child's "personhood" is something that is "co-performed." Consider one of his examples from Morocco:

> One Sunday morning, I sat around a table in Youssra's family living room. I was sitting with Mounir, her non-verbal autistic teenage son, his sister, a behavioral therapist and a speech therapist. The speech therapist was new, and she asked why certain therapeutic programs introduced years ago had stalled out. Just then, Mounir laughed loudly. His mother laughed too and added, "he's responding to you, saying, 'oh, you guys don't know why it's not working?'" Youssra's interpretation established Mounir as an active, understanding participant in the interaction. She considered his laugh meaningful, even sardonic. Instead of considering Mounir as too disabled to benefit from therapy, Youssra's interpretation positioned him as a cunning resistor of therapeutic intervention.

Understanding events like these in terms of sequentially organized actions and responses (which we define in chap. 3) belies the notion that one person's behavior can be a decontextualized unit of analysis. Instead of behavior simplex, we need an understanding of action-in-social interaction complex. As Hart (2014:298) puts it, "It is through brokered interactions and joint movement through the world that the child's sociability or 'thickness' is established."

The Geneticization of Autism

Ever since Kanner (1943:250) noted striking similarities between autistic children and their parents—whom he described as "highly intelligent" people with "a great deal of obsessiveness in the family background" and with "very few really warmhearted fathers and mothers," people who were "strongly preoccupied with abstractions of a scientific, literary, or artistic nature"—investigators have strongly suspected that autism has a genetic basis. However it was a parent—Bernard Rimland, whose advocacy and writings as a "parent-activist-researcher" (Eyal et al. 2010:136) ramped up the preoccupation with genetic hypotheses. His laudable purpose was to defy parent blaming, especially Bruno Bettelheim's (1967) once-influential claim that "refrigerator-mothers" who could not form emotional bonds with their children were responsible for autism. Additionally, the advent of studies showing that siblings of autistic children were at higher risk for the diagnosis lent fuel to the genetic fires, despite early cautionary notes to the effect that such determination "constitutes a small subgroup of autistic disorders" (Rutter and Bartak 1971). In the 1980s, studies of monozygotic or identical twins showed concordance rates of more than 90 percent, but still there were reservations, as researchers continued to advise that even though heredity can play a role in autism, genetic heterogeneity is operative as well (Silverman 2012:149), and, indeed, strongly so (Navon 2019:chap. 4).

In the 1990s, genetics researchers paid more attention to siblings and their susceptibility to autism because they constituted genetically similar populations. The use of the Autism Diagnostic Interview (ADI) and the Autism Diagnostic Observation Schedule (ADOS), which increased the reliability of diagnosis, also helped to create standardized populations for study, in effect bringing new categories of people into being. The process here is akin to what Lippman (1991) calls "geneticization," what Hacking (2006a) calls "the genetic imperative," and what Rabinow (1992) calls "biosociality," all phrases that describe how groups with distinct identities or their advocates can form around the promotion of genetic identifiers.

To date, however, efforts toward geneticizing or biosocializing autism have met with only limited success: "By 2008, even the most successful studies using genome scans of multiplex families could use their findings to explain 1 percent of autism cases at best" (Silverman 2012:148; cf. State and Šestan 2012:1301). Indeed, despite high hopes, as the geneticist Miles (2011:281–82) has observed, "the major genome-wide and candidate gene association studies, which are used to test for common variants contributing to risk, did not identify consistent genomic areas of interest," a matter that is true not only of autism but also of many other psychiatric disorders over time (Arribas-Ayllon, Bartlett and Lewis 2019; Horwitz 2002). More recently, as Waye and Cheng (2018:238) report, "despite the progress made in the discovery of a few genes that are well established as having important associations with autism . . . it does not explain the majority of cases of autism or ASD, and many unknown genetic factors remain to be discovered, thus hampering the progress of clinical testing as a diagnostic test for autism." Similarly, Thapar and Rutter (2020:9) note that, while it is acknowledged that "much progress has been made" in autism genetics, it is also recognized that "autism shows enormous clinical as well as genetic heterogeneity," and that "there is a need to link this work with clinical research."

We wonder if the preoccupation with the genetics of autism will turn out like the enthusiasm in the 1990s for finding oncogenes thought to be causative of cancer (Fujimura 1996). Certainly research like that which identified the BRCA1 gene that is strongly associated with breast cancer is hugely valuable and may help patients in making complex therapeutic decisions, but touting human gene *therapy* as a promising cure for the variety of cancers can lead to disappointment, as was apparent by the early 2000s (Lindee 2005:199). In any case, efforts to locate the genetic causes of autism continue to proliferate (Bumiller 2008; Silverman and Herbert 2003; Singh 2016). As a result, per Navon and Eyal's (2016:1433) review, "no less than 124 gene mutations and 55 chromosomal anomalies have been associated with autism spectrum disorders."

GENOMIC DESIGNATION AND THE BANDWAGON OF GENETICS RESEARCH

The traditional approach to studying the genetics of disease begins with a phenotype/diagnosis and tries to correlate it with specific genes. For example, Down syndrome (DS) and fragile X syndrome (FXS), both of which have been linked to autism, were described clinically before their genetic cause was discovered through chromosomal analysis. The same logic holds in newborn

screening for genetic diseases. If an initial blood test detects anomalies, geneticists and lab analysts identify disorders known to be associated with
those anomalies and screen for them using exome sequencing technology
(Timmermans 2015).

By contrast, a popular approach in modern biomedicine, which Navon
(2011; 2019) describes as *genomic designation*, is first to identify abnormalities
at the level of DNA and *then* look for their phenotypic correlates. In effect,
genomic designation reverses the traditional logic of diagnosis and genetic
causation, making it an instructive example of the "molecular gaze" (Rose
2007). That gaze, made possible by technological innovations that allow for
whole-genome mapping (as opposed to single-chromosome analysis), enables the examination of numerous DNA microarrays, profiling multiple
genes and their expression at ever finer levels of detail. And yet discerning the
path from risk genes to pathophysiology is problematic. For example, there
has been debate over whether autism is caused by a common or a rare variant
on the genome (Miles 2011:290).

The result of whole-genome mapping, in any case, is big data—"unprecedented
levels of sequence data" that present "new challenges in terms of data management, query and analysis" (O'Driscoll, Daugelaite, and Sleator 2013:774), including resources for computing and data processing.[14] Investigators might
initially use these resources to generate a whole-genome map in pursuit of a
specific clinical syndrome (or one of its characteristics).[15] In doing so, however, they frequently discover mutations that have not yet been correlated
with known syndromes. While these discoveries sometimes provide for the
refinement (or complication) of the biomedical picture of the original syndrome, they can also lead to the delineation of entirely new syndromes.[16]
Thus, the retrospective diagnostic logic of genomic designation, proponents
of which include not only researchers and clinicians but also parent and other
advocacy groups (Navon and Eyal 2016), creates the possibility for "new categories of persons" on the basis of their genomic profiles (Navon 2011:206).
It also lends to an increase in the genetic heterogeneity of conditions such as
autism. Navon and Eyal (2016:1432–33), drawing on Hacking's (1995, 2006b)
notion of "looping," argue that it is as if new "kinds of people" emerge from
prior genomic identification, bringing "a raft of previously unrelated mutations into the autism population." In this way, genetic heterogeneity expands.

Such expansion also involves a "bandwagon effect" (Fujimura 1996; Fujimura 1988:261)—the way that "large numbers of people, laboratories, and
organizations commit their resources to one approach to a problem." In her
research on the ascendance of oncogene studies in cancer research, Fujimura
(1988) shows how a "package" of technologies, especially recombinant DNA,

made it possible for molecular biology to invade scientific studies of cancer causation in the 1970s and 1980s and to some degree supplant erstwhile traditions in immunology, classical genetics, biochemistry, and chemotherapy.

Although tracing the bandwagon effect in genetic autism research is beyond our present focus or expertise (but see Singh 2016:52–68), we can observe that genomic designation in autism research is analogous to the "standardized technologies" (Fujimura 1988) that operated across many social worlds of scientific research to simplify, routinize, and delete the contexts of technology development that facilitated an oncogene approach to cancer. In autism research, standardization has involved the incorporation of "devices, concepts, and institutional, discursive, and spatial arrangements" (Navon and Eyal 2016:1439) into the project of genomic designation. Spurred by diverse interest groups that include researchers, clinicians, and families whose members have identified mutations, the genomic designation movement has forged complex networks and "biosocial communities"[17] (Silverman 2012; Singh 2016) that have transformed investigations into the relationship between autism's phenotype and genotype—in other words, between a clinical autism diagnosis and its potential genetic causes.

While genome mapping and genomic designation have multiplied biosocial groups and created new links between them, they have not produced clinical applications proportionate to their expense. Or at least it can be said that the use of genome and exome sequencing is not yet cost-effective in relation to diagnosis determination (Amendah et al. 2011; Yuen et al. 2018). However, straightforward economic considerations, beyond the significant monetary outlay for genetic research and testing (Amendah et al. 2011; Yuen et al. 2018), rarely take into account the costs associated with forgoing other forms of inquiry, which can be considerable.

As Fujimura (1988:272–73) shows, when molecular genetics came into vogue at the federal level in the United States, it attracted huge investments from organizations like the National Cancer Institute. Though this incentivized research on oncogenes, it produced a corresponding *disinvestment* from more traditional scientific research on cancer causation. Comparably, in recent decades, dramatic increases in research funding for autism have primarily targeted genetics, genomics, and neurology (Singh et al. 2009:792; Singh 2016:98–99), with corresponding shifts away from the study of phenotypes per se. At best, phenotypes are of interest as manifestations of genotypes or brain processes, rather than as *socially organized phenomena in their own right*. Traditional phenotypes, in other words, are like unidimensional dependent variables: cognitively driven, isolated behaviors of the individual and not courses of action in interaction.

In the following section, we discuss the implications of this neglect and its relation to what Grinker (2018) has called "the economics of autism," which encompasses the many financial aspects of autism, including its roots; its effects on individuals and families; investments in laboratories, clinics, and schools; proliferation of new disciplines; and the development of complementary and alternative medicines.

The Economics of Autism

If some of the resources currently devoted to genomics and biomedicine were reallocated to the study of lived behavior in interaction, we can only imagine what the benefits might be. Although we know from twin studies that there is strong evidence for the role of genetic factors in autism, much less is known about which genes are implicated or how they translate into risk parameters. This is because answering such questions requires adequate DNA sample sizes and sufficient resources for "the time-consuming and labor-intensive approaches" involved in detailed phenotyping (O'Roak and State 2008:14). In addition, there is only limited evidence from health economics (Schwarze et al. 2018) to support more widespread use of whole-exome and whole-genome sequencing (WES and WGS, respectively), both of which are very expensive (Yuen et al. 2018). The usefulness of genetic testing for diagnosis is also questionable, since it is ex post facto and reveals little about cognitive function, language use, or social abilities as such (Ungar 2015). Moreover, estimated time frames from referral to completion of posttest genetic counseling can be prohibitively long (Yuen et al. 2018).

As investment in sequencing technologies advances and becomes more complex, the demand for subspecialties and subspecialists increases, resulting in longer wait times and potentially circuitous paths to treatment (Ungar 2015). And then there are opportunity costs: money spent on genetic testing or brain research—the latter surpassed the former in the first decade of the twenty-first century (Singh et al. 2009)—could instead be made available for health programs and services most relevant to families and individuals (cf. Pellicano, Ne'eman, and Stears 2011; Singh 2016:99).

Those diagnosed with autism and their family members are often well aware of these matters. For example, in a documentary about autism and autism research, John Robison, autism advocate and author of *Look Me in the Eye: My Life with Autism* (Robison 2007; see chap. 1), says, "We need to shift towards delivering benefits to us today. It's great to think that we can head off really profound disability at some far future date, but we have the ability to solve problems right now, if we deploy the resources to do it."[18] The imbalance in resources can be seen in data from 2010, which shows that only 16 percent of federal funding for autism went to services—and three-quarters of that went to practitioner training programs (Pitney 2015:431, 146n52).

We know that expenditures to support individuals with autism over the course of their lives are higher than for the general population and for people with other mental health conditions (Rogge and Janssen 2019). Current estimates put the cost at nearly one and half million dollars in the United States and close to one million pounds in the United Kingdom, with the largest expenses deriving from special education services and parental productivity loss (Buescher et al. 2014) rather than from medical or health care (cf. Amendah et al. 2011; Rogge and Janssen 2019).

Given these costs, doing what Fitzgerald (2013:119) has called "learning to trace, much more carefully, the connections between what matters in the scanner and what takes place in the world outside" could provide a low-cost alternative avenue for understanding and ultimately improving the experience of those diagnosed with autism and their families. Compared with the hundreds of millions spent on genetic and neurological research (see note 7), research on "what takes place in the world," such as the social spaces in which interaction occurs, has the potential to improve life for those on the spectrum here and now, and at a high benefit-cost ratio. Particularly in the era of the RDoC and related attempts to convert psychiatry into a neurobiological enterprise, the transfer of public resources toward neurobiological approaches (Halpin 2016) at the expense of social scientific and interactional approaches is both dramatic and narrow (Halpin 2020:11). As Solomon and Bagatell (2010:2) lament, "there is less and less attention in autism research to phenomena that cannot be studied at the neurobiological or molecular level, such as human experience, social interaction, and cross-cultural variation."

Genetic Testing in the Clinic

Although the millions of dollars spent on autism genetics research can seem removed from the everyday concerns of families with autistic children, its proximate effects are readily apparent in conversations between caregivers and clinicians about genetic testing. In the clinic, there is perhaps less preoccupation with the neurology of autism than with its genetics. From a practical standpoint, this is understandable. The cost of brain imaging is prohibitive at present. Furthermore, because of conflicting research findings, it is not clear exactly how detecting structural or functional brain anomalies would inform diagnosis, much less treatment. Genetic testing is relatively cheaper and more pervasive.

As with other disorders—especially schizophrenia (Hedgecoe 2001)—the "geneticization" (Lippman 1991) of autism is rife with complexities and mixed results. Its limited successes to date have mostly involved establishing relationships between autism and well-understood conditions like fragile X syndrome (FXS), a single-gene disorder that is often comorbid with autism, rather than identifying autism-specific genes. Indeed, the prevalence of ASD in those with FXS may be on the order of 50 percent.[19] Fragile X syndrome is diagnosed with a blood test that detects mutations in a gene responsible for brain development. In addition to testing for FXS, clinicians sometimes recommend that autistic children be given an array comparative genomic hybridization (CGH) test to screen for other genetic susceptibilities. Designed to identify de novo copy number variations (CNVs), this lab-based procedure involves looking at thousands of sections of DNA to determine whether any are either missing (deletions) or present in extra copies (duplications) and if so what the size and effects of such anomalies may be.

At our research site, the clinical stance toward genetics was consistent with the patterns we have been describing. This can be seen in the case of Dan Chapman. Leah Grant, the developmental pediatrician who evaluated Dan, interviewed his mother, Betsy, about Dan's behavior and health, including questions about headaches, sleep patterns, stomach problems, and allergies. Later, at the informing interview and in her written report, Dr. Grant not only noted Dan's ASD diagnosis (established through her own and Jennifer Erickson's evaluations) but also recommended genetic testing of the two types. Although Dan did not have the physical characteristics associated with fragile X, Dr. Grant explained that not all children who have FXS display those symptoms, so she recommended testing for it. As a "second test," Dr. Grant also recommended the array CGH to see if Dan had any chromosomal abnormalities.

TRANSCRIPT 2.1 (24.STF:16)

DR. G: And then there's a second test that's called a CGH or micro array analysis that's another genetic test that looks at sorta broad spectrum looking at the DNA. And looking for little bits where when DNA gets copied to make a new person, sometimes a little piece of the copying gets missed.

MS. C: Okay.

DR. G: And so we call that a deletion, or there's an extra copy of the little part of the DNA that's called the duplication. And those can sometimes be significant and help us understand more about what's going on.

MS. C: Okay.

DR. G: Um especially with the CGH, in the vast majority of cases there's nothing we can do to treat that. I mean we can't treat genetic conditions per se. But sometimes there are medical issues that are associated or other things that help us understand more about the child that are helpful to have.

MS. C: Right.

DR. G: Um, those tests take prior authorization. Through insurance.

Because the insurance issues were not resolved during the discussion, we do not know whether, in fact, these tests were done or what the outcomes may have been. However, the attempt to find a genetic basis for ASD is extremely common, and there is "growing acceptance of the idea that clinicians should order exploratory genomic tests in order to help diagnose an expansive range of clinical presentations, especially in children" (Navon 2011:210). This dialogue shows a pattern in which, at present, genetic testing is done *after* diagnosis, not as an aid to diagnosis, and that a positive test is not helpful for *treating* autism per se, although it may lend to understanding and dealing with other symptoms that the microarray analysis reveals.[20]

It is difficult to find cost information for the CGH test, although an earlier study (Manning and Hudgins 2007) estimated expenses in the range of $1,500–$1,800. That study also noted the difficulty of determining whether an abnormality is a pathological change, which may require parental testing or obtaining a general population screen involving microarrays, either of which could mean additional costs. Testing for fragile X is less expensive, but of course it can add to the overall expenditures for laboratory work.

The Autism Phenotype and Its "Bottleneck"

Putting aside economic issues (to which we make a partial return in chap. 8), when we study behavior, we are in the realm of what genetics calls the phenotype: the characteristic set of observable traits displayed by an organism. Diabetes, alcoholism, obesity, and other disorders have distinctive (albeit heterogeneous) phenotypes. However, when phenotypes extend to such matters as educational attainment, aggressive/antisocial conduct, or even relatively passive conditions such as loneliness, depression, or neuroticism, we not only confront the problem of connecting genetic influences to behavior (Schnittker 2017:246) but find ourselves in the realm of social-behavioral regularities, as opposed to "conditions." *Actual social behavior*, including the ways in which such behavior occurs in diverse groups, cultural settings, and interactional environments, is easily overlooked in part because the concept of the phenotype is so rarely defined at anything other than the most general level, where it is said to manifest aspects of both genotype and environment. As neurobiologist Rose (2006:526) puts it, phenotypes overwhelmingly involve a "reification of complex human interactions into presumed phenotypes with a biological locus in the individual."

Besides Grinker's (2007:121) characterization of ASD phenotypes as "the actual physical, behavioral manifestations of the disorder," one of the few more-precise definitions appears in Freese's (2008:S8) exploration of social science theory and biology, where he refers to phenotype "in the relatively restrictive sense of characteristics that are embodied—that is, materially realized as part of the organism."[21] Importantly, such characteristics have interactional dimensions. That is, if genes have causal effects, those are "in the first instance causal effects upon the material body," such as height, psychology, or skills (Freese 2008:S13). But by themselves, such effects do not explain a person's "outcomes" in the social sphere. So-called phenotypes, therefore, do not determine one's fate as a social actor. In fact, genetically caused variations in body and mind "change in response to *events*"—or the "external action of the *substrate*" in which the "unfolding" of phenotypical behavior occurs (Freese 2008:S15–S16, our emphasis).

Events can encompass such things as the social milieu of actions, and this milieu may include "stressors" (Freese 2008:S23), which in turn implicate *responses* (Freese 2008:S16). Accordingly, from a sociological point of view, if events and their substrates are not taken into account, attempts to explain individual-level outcomes encounter a problem that Freese (2008:S13) has identified as the "phenotypic bottleneck." Phenotypes do not tell us how the characteristics they embody affect what happens to us in social life. For that, we need an understanding of how a characteristic may lead participants to select themselves, or be selected, into particular social environments and how those environments can reinforce the characteristic, whether it be one considered "positive" (e.g., intellectual flexibility) or "negative" (e.g., disability or emotional instability).

As Freese (2008:S25) puts the matter when discussing behavioral genetics, "dynamics of social interaction and organization affect the influence of genes on outcomes" (and the same could be said for how neurology in general affects what happens to individuals).[22] To capture these dynamics in a phrase, we refer to the problem of discerning what we earlier called an *interactional phenotype*. As we have seen from Hart's (2014) ethnographic study, an individual's moves are always and everywhere part of a fabric of interrelated actions and interactions, rather than a solitary output of some kind.

Our research is not about "outcomes" traditionally conceived—things like attitudes, behaviors, and attainments—nor is it about modeling causal relations between the genome and human behavior. Instead, it is about the local effects of action and interaction when individuals with autism participate in social relations with more neurotypical coparticipants (in our data, mainly clinicians). The point that Freese (2008) makes regarding distal relationships between genes and behavior applies equally to the more local effects that are the focus of our inquiry. We want to know how the characteristics of children, especially those embodied characteristics (phenotypes) associated with autism, become observable in the turn structure of interactions between child and clinician and how clinicians transform them into evidence for an autism diagnosis.

At this point, we have to say that knowledge about phenotypes and their embeddedness in actual social worlds—which is where behavioral consequences occur in relationships with others—is primitive at best. It remains unclear how the autism phenotype, at present defined reductively in terms of autistic behaviors (e.g., gaze, impulsivity, repetitive movements, lack of reciprocity), is constituted as a social and interactional phenomenon. This is a problem because autism does not reside only inside autistic individuals but in the interactional space between those individuals and the relevant others who respond to their embodied actions. As Mukherjee (2016:264), drawing on the work of Victor McKusick, known as the "father of medical genetics," has put it, disorder has to do with "an incongruity between an individuals' genetic endowment and his or her current environment." This notion of incongruity implies the necessity of understanding the relationship between the individual and others, a relationship that constitutes what we are calling an interactional phenotype. If we want a more complete understanding of autism, we must move from conceptualizing it as a static entity to viewing it as a dynamic process nested in particular social environments and what actually happens within them. We also need to consider reciprocal changes among individuals and their environments over space and time and how these may introduce new incongruities or modify existing ones.[23]

Phenomenon or Epiphenomenon?

Understanding autism as an interactional phenotype can provide new insights into the question of how genes and behavior are related. The biomedical perspective treats the autism phenotype as an epiphenomenal manifestation of its corresponding genotype. On this view, the arrow of causation runs from genetic abnormalities to neurocognitive deficits and autistic behavior, in that order (Nadesan 2005:149). When the primary locus of inquiry is the genome and the secondary locus is the brain, it becomes all too easy to ignore *actual* behaviors and dismiss them as unworthy of direct analysis in their own right. Yet, because the social organization of autism is inseparable from what autism *is*, the reductionist impulse that identifies it with genes and brain structures loses precisely the phenomenon it attempts to pin down. Bearman (2013:S11) makes a similar point following his review of studies that treat "environments as settings in which genetic things can happen." He writes, "It would be great to think about ways to make them come alive; that is, to identify mechanisms by which humans in interaction with one another constitute, through their interaction, genomic influence." In our view, Bearman is putting his finger on the problem of the phenotypic bottleneck and calling for greater appreciation of social interactional phenotypes.

In a more critical vein, Rose and Abi-Rached (2013:140) recite a list of dilemmas that neurobiology has not been able to solve: how severe a disorder is, how much distress the individual or the family will experience, what the course of problems will be, what sorts of care will be needed, and others. They conclude: "It is clear that neuropsychiatry has a long way to go in developing a style of thought adequate to the complexity of its object, when that object is an ailment suffered by an individual human being living in a social world." And Schnittker (2017:288–89), invoking the distinction between *explaining* and *understanding*, reminds us that while explanation pertains to causal accounts, understanding means comprehending the "significance or meaning of behavior" for those most involved and is a valid scientific endeavor in its own right.[24]

We think that an important step in the direction of making phenotypes come alive and doing justice to autism's complexity is to investigate it as a site of social organization in its own right. This entails treating interaction as the phenomenon, as opposed to a mere epiphenomenon. To paraphrase Schegloff's (2003a:46) remarks about what he calls the "neurobiology of behavior," it is only possible to establish links between the brain and human sociality when neurobiology is combined with an accurate, valid description and analysis of lived behavior, which is predominantly "conduct in interaction." This is what we mean by the social interactional phenotype.

Our research closely aligns with the pioneering studies of Ochs and Solomon (2004) and colleagues (Ochs et al. 2004; Ochs and Solomon 2010; Solomon 2010), whose "ethnography of autism" project thoroughly highlights the role of interaction and the *social* environment in differentiating manifestations of autism. It also aligns more broadly with the work of authors who have stressed the importance of social organization, as opposed to the abstracted individual, for understanding autism. This group includes Biklen (2002:67); Decoteau and Sweet (2016); Fein (2015:18, for example); Eyal et al. (2010:262, for example); Sterponi, de Kirby, and Shankey (2015); and many others who recognize that the quality of what individuals say and do is deeply rooted in the concreteness of their social relations.

What we add to this sensibility is a focus on interactional sequences. Thus, in chapters 4 and 5, we show how practices for assessing autism simultaneously constitute autism as an interactional object, one that is diagnosable according to clinical criteria. In particular, we show how the conduct of the clinician, the design features of assessment instruments (e.g., the way tasks are phrased and organized), and other social environmental factors can deeply affect what a child says or does. Taking the social interactional phenotype seriously means analyzing such factors for how they enter into children's actions and reactions. And this is as important outside the clinic as it is inside. To return to Hart's ethnographic example from Morocco, if what seems like a haphazard laugh can be analyzed for its subterranean understanding of and comment on a visitor's question, such intelligence needs analytic appreciation. And if it does not have direct implications for diagnosis, it can nonetheless be informative for what happens to a child and to the social environments that the child occupies after diagnosis.

To be sure, in neurobiological approaches, there is an impulse toward linking biology with other facets of human life and expression. However, these other facets tend to be internal to the individual, rather than social and interactional, if only because scientists in the field often learn psychology (Fitzgerald 2013:119) but not any other social sciences. This has meant that behavior is mostly framed in psychological and cognitive terms, with a focus on the underlying neurochemistry and structures of cognition instead of the integrity of human life and experience as they take place in the social world. Per Schegloff (2003a), understanding "conduct in interaction" requires getting out of the neurobiological brain *and* out of the psychological and cognitive brain to study real activity and action in the social world. Likewise, as Goodwin (2003a:8) has stated more specifically, the "basic unit of analysis" can be "sequences of talk constructed through the collaborative actions of multiple parties." This attention to sequential organization and interactional collaboration does not have to be done in an exclusive way but can take the form of what Rose (2013:24) calls "critical friendship": a "non-reductionist biology of human beings and other organisms in their milieu." The point, as we see it, is not to dismiss neurobiology and psychology but rather to situate them in the interactional spaces between people—the only spaces where they can have any social significance.

Conclusion

At the beginning of this chapter, we raised the question of whether Dan Chapman would have been diagnosed as autistic in another historical era. Of course, such a question is impossible to answer definitively because autism is not like, say, diabetes, which was recognized as early as 3,500 years ago but not well understood until the late nineteenth and early twentieth centuries (Tattersall 2010). Autism does not have a clear physiological substrate, and the meanings given to its characteristics vary across time. They also vary across space: if Dan lived in a place like Senegal, or in a society like that of the Navajo of the American Southwest or the Somalis in Toronto, would he have been diagnosed with autism? We can only wonder.

What is clear about Dan's case—and many of the others we observed during the course of our fieldwork—is that it is not clear-cut. Those who are skeptical about autism as a diagnosis might interpret this ambiguity as grist for their skepticism. Beyond the ambiguity of diagnosis, social constructionists and disabilities studies scholars (Linton 1998; Linton 2005) have critiqued the essentializing, person-centered, and marginalizing aspects of present-day medical approaches to autism. In a similar vein, the neurodiversity movement (Bumiller 2008) promotes a positive understanding of autism through web-based discussions (most especially at www.neurodiversity.com), social events, and other avenues. Activists argue that autism is not a deficit but a valid genetic variation that can produce important contributions to society. The movement's point is not to change the diagnosis but to appreciate it as a cognitive style.

Our own orientation is neither constructionist nor critical. Our aim is not to contest the diagnosis, to question its validity (especially in our own data), or to celebrate it. Rather, we simply wish to capture the "how" of autism diagnosis, raising questions about the collaborative practices involved in testing (chap. 4 and 5) and clinicians' methods of ruling autism in or out (chap. 6) even in the face of ambiguous presentations (chap. 7). In doing so, we draw from Pollner's (1974:37) observation that those who "do" diagnosis view themselves as "confronting an order of events whose character . . . is presupposed as independent" of their own responses. Or, in Latour's (2004:246; cf. Mol 2002) idiom, we can say that our investigation is "realist" in the sense that it examines how diagnosis is a "matter of concern" for both professionals and laypersons—something they treat as real and consequential in their everyday lives. In short, we focus on the orientations of practitioners themselves to objects in their social worlds.[25] This helps us avoid the tendency in science studies of "trying to detect the real prejudices hidden behind the appearance of objective statements" (Latour 2004:227). Instead, the aim is to explain how such statements are assembled and grounded in the ethical, affective, and practical perspectives of a setting's participants.

The matter of how clinicians and children interact in the clinic, and how their interactions become the basis for ascriptions of autism, requires close attention to autism as an interactional phenotype. Analytic consideration of behavior as jointly constructed, no matter how anomalous one or the other contribution may seem, better allows us, in turn, to deal with the forms of common and uncommon sense displayed and embodied by individuals, as opposed to members of a generic diagnostic category. Among other things, it positions us to appreciate first-order, fundamental competence and autistic intelligence and thereby bring actions and reactions that initially seemed strange into the realm of the familiar. Then, determining and reporting a diagnosis, without losing sight of official categories, may be particularized to the individual child. Making the strange familiar has consequences not only for diagnostic practice but also for the integration of autistic individuals into their social environments and the construction of those environments themselves.

An Interactional Entrance to Autism Diagnosis

In chapter 1, we noted that Dan Chapman's first appointment at CDDC was with Dr. Leah Grant, a developmental pediatrician who examined Dan and interviewed his mother about his developmental history and current functioning. When that exam was complete, Dan and his mother, Betsy Chapman, were guided to another room, where his psychological evaluation was to be held.

That evaluation began as Dr. Jennifer Erickson entered the examination room and, on a clipboard, handed a Social Communication Questionnaire (SCQ) to Betsy. At CDDC, caregivers often fill out an SCQ, which is a document with yes-no questions that help screen for autism. Then, Jennifer moved to a chair that faced both Dan and his mother. Dan had also just shifted from a lounge-type chair to a table chair with wheels. Initially Dan's chair was facing away from Jennifer. But as she took her seat, he moved his chair around to face her, all the while directing his gaze toward the floor (fig. 3.1). Jennifer explained what she was "gonna be" doing (with the Autism Diagnostic Observation Schedule [ADOS]): "playing with some toys together . . . to look at social communication skill." Meanwhile, Dan was folding his hands together and swinging his feet back and forth slightly as his gaze shifted to the middle distance, to his mother, to the floor, and only fleetingly to Jennifer. Let us see what happened in the interaction and what an analysis of its social organization can tell us.

Hesitating as she changes topics, Jennifer moves from explaining the ADOS to asking Dan about having his mom "in the room for this"[1] (lines 1–2; numbers in parentheses indicate silences in tenths of a second; at line 4, the note in double parentheses is about nonvocal behavior occurring during the silence):

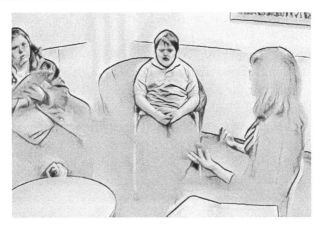

FIGURE 3.1

TRANSCRIPT 3.1: (CASE 24 PY:1)

```
 1  Jen:    Um (1.0) Dan it's up to you, do you want your mom, uh, in the room
 2          for this? Do you want her to watch behind in the observation room?
 3          It's up to you.
 4          (2.0) ((Dan looking down, hands folded))
 5  Jen:    You can think about it.
 6          (13.0)
 7  Jen:    Whadya think? Ya want Mom in here?
 8          (0.3)
 9  Betsy:  You want me in here buddy?
10          (0.4)
11  Dan:    I don't know.
12          (1.5)
13  Jen:    Well why don't we get started, and then if you want your mom not in
14          here you'll let me know, okay?
15          (3.0)
16  Jen:    That sound like a good plan to you, Betsy?
17  Betsy:  Yeah.
18  Jen:    Okay.
```

One way of characterizing this short exchange is to say that Jennifer (in lines 1–3) politely gives Dan a choice about whether to have his mother in the room, and he avoids answering until his mother intervenes (line 9), at which point he produces only a noncommittal response (line 11). Then Jennifer proposes a solution (lines 13–14), but Dan still withholds any response (line 15), prompting Jennifer to ask his mother for assent (line 16) so that things are able to proceed (lines 17–18). The administration of the ADOS begins almost immediately afterward.

In this triadic relationship, we can say that Dan is minimally involved. Indeed, there may be a *self*-involved character to his manner, of the sort that is often characterized as autistic (cf. Frith 2003:5, chap. 4). In Goffman's (1963:70) terms, it is as if he has been in an "away" state—"an inward emigration from the gathering."[2] From a commonsense standpoint, these would all be valid descriptions. However, if we look at the details of the interaction and their organization by the participants, a different picture of their interrelationships and of Dan's orientation starts to emerge.

First, there is the matter of Jennifer changing topics from explaining the ADOS to asking Dan about his mother's presence. Her hesitation at the beginning of her turn at line 1 may display an in-course recognition that the change of topic could not have been very well anticipated (Lerner 2013:103–4). Second, Dan is almost immediately nominated ("it's up to you") as the responsible party for a task that has not yet been defined. Third is the form of Jennifer's entreaty. She uses "do you want" (DYW) syntax, which in ordinary conversation is used for making an offer about something that has become relevant *during the previous interaction*. Curl (2006) gives the example of two friends, Zoe and Claire, who have been talking about an upcoming bridge party that Zoe is hosting. Near the end of the telephone call, Claire says, "Do you want me to bring the chairs?" (Curl 2006:1266). The DYW syntax suggests the possibility that Zoe needs something that has not been articulated but that can be inferred from the overall conversational topic.

However, on the face of it, there seems to be nothing in the interaction among Jennifer, Mrs. Chapman, and Dan that suggests an issue in need of resolution. Nothing, at least, that is available to all participants. Jennifer, however, does have a need to resolve something. The ADOS instructs clinicians in how to handle the presence of parents during the exam, and the instructions vary according to the age of the child (see note 1). Thus, the issue of parental presence is part of her agenda, its relevance deriving from her role as a clinician. It is her knowledge about, and responsibility for, the matter that makes it relevant for discussion with clients.

Dan does not have knowledge of the clinician's agenda, though, and so from his perspective, he is being given a matter to resolve that Jennifer, with her DYW question format, seems to be introducing from out of the blue. We can therefore understand Dan's silence at line 4, during which he holds his head and orients his gaze to the floor, as fitted to a local context of inexplicability. Still, Jennifer keeps her offer in play by proposing that Dan can "think about it" (line 5), and there follows an exceptionally long silence (line 6) as Dan continues gazing downward. After moving her file to the table at her left, Jennifer gazes back at Dan before issuing a third version of the query (line 7).

Following Dan's continued silence (line 8), his mother solicits response, using what is called a "yes-no inquiry" with positive language ("Ya want Mom in here?" and "You want me in here buddy") that tacitly pursues affirmation. But Dan does not provide an answer: his "I don't know" (line 11) is a common device for resisting the action force of a question (Stickle, Duck, and Maynard 2017). In this instance, it displays a neutral stance toward a possibly awkward feature of the interaction—having to make a choice about his mother's continued presence during the examination. During the ensuing silence (line 12), in which Dan removes his gaze from the floor, glancing up toward the ceiling and then back down again, Jennifer suggests going ahead with the examination (lines 13–14) and tells Dan to notify her if he wants his mom "not in here." Finally, when Dan remains silent (line 15), Jennifer and Mrs. Chapman resolve the matter by agreeing on how to proceed (lines 16–18).

Common Sense and Uncommon Sense, Socially Organized Actions and Responses

Although the exchange between Jennifer, Dan, and Mrs. Chapman is brief, it is dense with *socially organized actions and responses* that resonate with the themes we pursue in this book: common sense, intelligence, interaction, and the world of autism. Here is how Jennifer makes sense of the exchange as she reports on the awkward interaction to developmental pediatrician Leah Grant: "So I offered the option [about Mrs. Chapman staying in the room] and he didn't like directly respond; he sort of seemed uncomfortable at responding, um and then Mom asked if it would be okay if I was in here, and he said like, 'I don't know—I don't wanna think about it,' or some (heh) thing heh like that." Jennifer remarks on the absence of a "direct" response to her offer, Dan's apparent discomfort, and what she characterizes as his stumbling "I don't know" response to his mother. Jennifer's descriptions and subsequent laugh tokens treat Dan's behavior as strange in relation to her own common-sense understanding of the situation.

From our ethnomethodological point of view, we can observe that Dan's behavior represents a withdrawal from normative expectations about how to complete simple conversational sequences. This can occasion bewilderment, anxiety, or even chagrin on the part of others (see chap. 1), and Jennifer's humorous treatment can be understood as one of a range of common emotional responses to such experiences (Garfinkel 1967:38, 55, 112). Yet there is more to be said, specifically about the interactional context in which the offer of his mom's presence or absence is made and about how Dan responds to it.

By shutting down (via nonresponse) upon receiving Jennifer's offer, Dan may be allowing himself more time to grasp what is being asked of him. He also manages to shift responsibility for answering the question elsewhere.[3]

He may also be showing sensitivity to the fact that he is being asked about including or excluding his mother *in her very presence*. And he may be registering his awareness of the delicacy embodied in Jennifer's own utterance, particularly in her hesitations before producing the offer.

Those convinced that Dan is a troublemaker, such as the teachers and principal at his old school, may be tempted to see responses (or nonresponses) like those to Jennifer as manifestations of difficult and resistive behavior of the sort described in his medical records. Alternatively, because his responses go against what common sense would demand (a yes or no response to an explicit offer), they could be treated as a benign but awkward violation of social norms. This is Jennifer's interpretation. She treats Dan's actions as strange. However, they also present an opportunity to *make the strange familiar*, to grasp the uncommon sense embodied in Dan's actions and make it accessible to commonsense understanding. To do so, we need to examine his responses in the *sequences* where they occur. This will make it possible to see Dan's behavior as skillful, rather than deficient.

What do we mean by sequences? They are central to what we mean by the interactional phenotype (chap. 2), and we define them more systematically later in this chapter. For now, we can say that we mean that Dan's behavior does not stand on its own. At every point in our social interactional analysis of extract 3.1, we referred to what he did *in relation to* initiations on the part of the clinician or his mother. Those initiations are what conversation analysts call *actions*, as are the responses. By and large, situated conduct consists of such actions and return actions, which stand in a reflexive relationship to each other, meaning that they are co-constitutive: an offer is constituted as an offer not only by its design features but by whether and how a recipient treats it. If an intended offer is received as something else—for example, an insult—then it's not an offer, unless the participants engage in corrective or repair work, over a series of turns, to clear it up. So if Dan were to respond to Jennifer's question with something like, "I'm not a little kid. Why would I need my mom with me!?" this would indicate his reception of the utterance as an insult rather than an offer, and she would need to clarify the meaning of her original utterance, which Dan could then accept or reject, and so forth. The point is that what an action turns out to be depends, in part, on how a coparticipant treats it and on what happens over the course of a given interaction. Actions and responses, or "re-actions," form a socially organized basis for meaningful talk and embodied behavior.

In terms of socially organized actions, Jennifer abruptly changed topics, and Dan retreated from the change. She offered him the options of having his mother in the exam room or in the observation room and pursued an answer—articulation of a choice—as Dan avoided giving one. And when Mrs. Chapman presented the options to Dan through questions that inexplicitly asked for affirmation, his "I don't know" effectively demurred. Finally, Dan dealt with a last try by the clinician, who now framed the matter as contingent ("if you want . . . you'll let me know, okay?"), by demurring again.

When we consider this episode in social organizational terms, we see the series of action-response sequences in which Dan's "behaviors" are lodged and which are glossed by descriptions such as Jennifer's "he didn't like directly respond, he sort of seemed uncomfortable." From this analytic perspective, it is clear that the meanings of Dan's actions are phenomenologically tied to prior actions—his own and those of his coparticipants—and to the future courses of action that his actions make relevant (or more technically, that they *project*). In other words, as a coparticipant, Dan shows a kind of competence belied by unitary and psychological descriptions of his behavior. We will have more to say about this matter in chapter 4.

We are not suggesting that Dan is typical or that he is not "really" autistic.[4] Nor are we claiming that the way he participated in the interaction with Jennifer and his mother was commonsensical after all. Most especially, our analysis is not meant to be ironic toward Jennifer or Mrs. Chapman and their ways of talking to Dan, as if they could have done things differently or better. We have discussed this matter in chapter 2 as a "realist" (Latour 2007) approach, and take it up again in chapter 7 (see especially note 5), where we explain that clinicians, parents, and others operate in a way that necessarily consigns any explicit awareness of the reflexive relationship between actions and responses to an unseen, taken-for-granted backdrop or substrate of practical actions that make ordinary, commonsense activities possible. However, we *are* proposing that in order to fully understand the social meaning of any behavior and course of action, autistic or otherwise, it is necessary to ground them in the relational context of their production. In this way, we can get access to aspects of sensemaking—uncommon as well as common, concrete as well as abstract—that we discuss in detail in chapters 4 and 5.

Studying Language Use and Social Interaction

Our approach to the study of interaction partly stems from developments in what is called ordinary language philosophy, which conceives of language as a site of social activity, as opposed to a mere receptacle for transmitting information. It is a matter of *language in use*—talk and its interrelations with gesture and other forms of embodied conduct—in contrast to the "view that language, in its essence, is a referential system and a reflection of the individual's cognition" (Sterponi, de Kirby, and Shankey 2015:517). In the ordinary language tradition, a variety of researchers, including speech act philosophers such as John Austin (1962), Gilbert Ryle (1949), and John Searle (1969), recast the referential view, avoiding the problem of connecting abstract cognitive processes to words and objects. Instead, they examined words in concrete, *rule-governed* contexts where their meaning depends on the action or actions they perform.

With its focus on rules and rule-governed behavior, however, ordinary language philosophy neglects the constitutive conditions for rule use in actual situations. The work of Ludwig Wittgenstein (1958) represents a partial exception, particularly his argument that the "meaning" of words and utterances consists in their *use*, and his corresponding emphasis on how participants employ language in practice, as opposed to how they fit words to normative (rule-governed) environments.[5] In other words, for Wittgenstein, meaning does not precede action according to linguistic structures of one kind or another but is created through action.

Erving Goffman, whose studies of the interaction order figures prominently in this book, is a special case with regard to language use. We return to his research first, then move on to an overview of our primary orientation in ethnomethodology (EM) and conversation analysis (CA). A major provision of EM and CA approaches, partly under the influence of Wittgenstein, is to avoid rule-based approaches that attempt to *explain* human behavior. Instead, these approaches document the practices through which words and talk, as well as other embodied actions such as gestures (e.g., hand, arm, and facial manipulations), proxemics (i.e., human spatial patterning), prosody (i.e., speech stress, pacing, and intonation), and gaze contribute to meaningful forms of conduct.

In the chapters that follow, we apply ethnomethodology and conversation analysis (EMCA) to the analysis of assessment or testing situations, decision-making about diagnosis, and informing interviews (when clinicians tell parents about their findings), explicating interactional patterns of language and gesture use in these clinical contexts to specify how diagnosis is accomplished in vivo.

GOFFMAN AND THE INTERACTION ORDER

Goffman's work can be located in traditions that take normative environments of human conduct as the main target of sociological analysis. However, this is a complex matter. First of all, Goffman (1983) proposes that the corporeal and interactional "face to face" or "body to body" *situation*—whether in public or private, institutional or everyday contexts, and independent of socioeconomic class, gender, or racial and ethnic categories—should be the primary focus for understanding social interaction. That is, the rules and expectations that govern turn taking, physical distance between speakers, and other matters derive from the requirements of face-to-face conduct, regardless of its broader context. In this sense, the rules and conventions are essentially sui generis and self-organizing. For example, any "contact" ritual, such as a service encounter where customers may form a queue as they await their turn to be helped, has its own logic of conduct. Although the queue could be organized according to externally structured attributes of involved parties (e.g., age, race, gender, or class), normal queuing "blocks" or filters out the effects of such variables in favor of an egalitarian "first-come, first-served" ordering principle.

These matters are extremely important because what Goffman (1964:135) calls the "social situation"—"an environment of mutual monitoring possibilities . . . whenever two or more individuals find themselves in one another's immediate presence"—has suffered from extreme neglect in the social sciences. And while Goffman (1964:133) recommends analytic appreciation of the "human and material setting" in which talk and gesture occur, and of the need to incorporate the situation "in some systematic way," he (Goffman, 1964:135) goes on to recommend, "Cultural rules establish how individuals are to conduct themselves by virtue of being in a gathering, and these rules for commingling, when adhered to, socially organize the behavior of those in the situation." And Goffman's (1983) most systematic statement about social situations refers to the "interaction order," which consists of "systems of enabling conventions, in the sense of ground rules for a game, the provisions of a traffic code, or the syntax of a language." The interaction order is an autonomous order of organization, in relation to both the broader society and the psychological properties of the actors.[6]

Although the interaction order consists of rules and conventions through which members of a setting or society achieve stability and mutual understanding, Goffman (1983) argues that they are not applied mechanically. Violations of social rules do not threaten the social "game" underway so much as they serve as resources for accomplishing the very projects that adherence itself involves, including the definition of self and the creation or maintenance of social meaning (Goffman 1971:61). For example, given that a rule exists against seeking out a stranger's eyes, doing so can be a means of making a pickup or making oneself known when meeting a new acquaintance for a drink or coffee. Similarly, given that staring at someone is an invasion of personhood, a stare can become the basis for a warranted negative sanction for misbehavior. Overall, interactional norms are not tight constraints on actions but are more like rough guidelines or "ground rules" (Goffman 1971) that permit actors to accomplish a variety of social projects, depending on how they align themselves with respect to those ground rules. In the normative order of clinical testing, subtle gazing, smiling, and pacing can be ways for a child to solicit feedback or for a clinician to inadvertently convey approval or disapproval of a candidate answer (Maynard and Marlaire 1992).

Goffman's theorizing and studies show how social situations can have an organization that is (a) independent of outside impositions, and (b) achieved through participants aligning their utterances and gestures to one another in systematic fashion. Just as people obtain a service by queuing properly, clinicians and children "do" testing together by way of a substrate of rule-like practices (i.e., for co-orientation and for elicitations and performances) assembled in temporal courses of action that include momentary—but highly ordered—adjustments in the implementation of test protocols (see chap. 4 and 5). Likewise, when clinicians assemble to report on their assessments and decide whether a child qualifies for an autism diagnosis, they do so by orienting tacit rules for doing diagnosis. As we will see, these rules include ways of organizing findings and impressions as discrete stories that are gradually assembled into a diagnostic narrative about the child (chap. 6). An implication is that just as in the local and embodied production of a service line or queue, the interactional work of testing and diagnosis is both unique and orderly for any situation of evaluation.

ETHNOMETHODOLOGY

Ethnomethodology (EM) takes an unconventional approach to analyzing what Goffman called the social situation. Where Goffman's work relaxed the theoretical hold that rules could have in explaining conduct, ethnomethodology has shown how rules could instead be treated as topics and features of the activities they are said to shape. That is, rules are produced in their detail within social actions rather than operating as outside causal or other forces. The analytic tactic is to examine rules empirically as *resources* for actors, who use them for various situated projects and ends of their own. It is not that behavior is unconstrained, disorderly, or arbitrary, but that rules, if they are operative at all, figure as part of actors' own *practices* of reasoning and methods of organizing a social setting.

As artful users of rules, then, actors often invoke them in an ex post facto, rhetorical manner to describe the morality of their conduct—or, as Garfinkel (1967) puts it, to make their conduct *accountable*. For example, jurors retrospectively invoke legal standards to explain how they arrived at a verdict, even when the route involved substantial commonsense and unstandardized reasoning (Garfinkel 1967:chapter 4). Ethnomethodologists classically have shown how residents at a halfway house use the "convict code" to account for disregarding officially prescribed ways of doing things (Wieder 1974) and how staff members at a social welfare agency get their "people processing" job done in part by departing from routine policies while still providing a sense of having conformed to them (Zimmerman 1970). To repeat, rules are *features* of actions rather than explanations for them and serve as resources with which actors continually assemble local order out of contingency.

To the degree that testing and diagnosing autism are rule-governed, this is because there are protocols to which clinicians orient, both in the testing situation itself and in assigning scores and aligning them to diagnostic criteria. However, as we will see, such protocols do not—indeed, cannot—strictly guide how interactions transpire, as clinicians must deal with any number of contingent occurrences in the course of interaction, including not only the unpredictability of children but also their own mistakes and variant implementations, as well as the vicissitudes of the instruments they use. They work to adhere to their instructions but sometimes must adapt or discount them in order to complete a test item and decide about diagnosis. For example, a child's response to an item may be ambiguous in terms of whether it qualifies as typical or atypical (see the case of Sara Brennan, discussed in chap. 7, and the clinicians' discussions about whether she showed appropriate eye contact and other conduct). Redoing the item has its limits (such as the amount of time available for completing a test), and yet decisions have to be made.

Our ethnomethodological orientation allows us to probe just how clinicians make their testing and diagnostic decisions, often in the face of high uncertainty, pressures to complete an evaluation in a timely fashion, and other obstacles. Rules and protocols do not solve these problems but remain as features of the very practices by which clinicians nevertheless manage their testing and diagnostic determinations in ways considered valid for all practical purposes.

CONVERSATION ANALYSIS

Alongside its concern with self-generating order in social situations, a unique aspect of ethnomethodological research is its concern with "indexical expressions" (Garfinkel 1967; Garfinkel and Sacks 1970), utterances whose meaning and understandability depend on the context or circumstances in which they appear. It is generally recognized that what linguists call deictic utterances, such as *this, that, here, there,* and so on, assume particular meanings according to their speech environment. Garfinkel (1967) developed this insight further, observing that the sense accorded to any utterance, gesture, or other action fundamentally depends on the circumstances and particularities of its production.

In conversation analysis (CA) much more than in EM, there is what can be called a "generalizing impulse" (Clayman, Heritage, and Maynard, forthcoming; Maynard and Clayman 2018) that seeks common features of social actions while also accommodating the details of specific instances of talk. In the field's most influential conversation analytic inquiry (Sacks, Schegloff, and Jefferson 1974:700), the cofounders of CA suggest that the organization of turn taking has both a "general abstractness and a local particularization potential." Accordingly, in one of his early published lectures, Sacks (1989[1964]) draws from a collection of greeting and identification sequences in telephone calls to a psychiatric hospital and describes how counselors (as call recipients) can tacitly ask for callers' names by first introducing themselves. At the same time, callers—people in distress who may wish to stay anonymous—can avoid self-identifying without explicitly refusing by asking for repair ("I can't hear you"). This results in a clarification sequence, rather than a self-identification, and allows the caller to effectively skip over the earlier request to self-identify. Assembling and analyzing collections of sequences such as turn taking or identification allows the analyst to establish *generic* methods for doing social actions, while also preserving the particularities of each specific case.

Goffman's notion of interaction order suggests the importance of such generic practices for our study. If there are generic (but locally ordered) aspects to how participants engage in autism assessment and diagnosis, then our findings should be relevant to other environments where these activities occur, particularly ones related to atypical interactions of various kinds (Antaki and Wilkinson 2012; Garcia 2012; Wilkinson, Rae, and Rasmussen 2020; Wootton 1999)—for example, those involving participants with aphasia, frontotemporal and other forms of dementia (Mates, Mikesell, and Smith 2013), learning disabilities, intellectual disabilities, schizophrenia, and other psychiatric conditions. That is, the methods and rules clinicians use to elicit and make sense of children's behavior in autism clinics may be employed in other clinical (and nonclinical) settings where atypical interactions occur, while adhering to different forms of accountability (i.e., different diagnostic categories and criteria).

Ethnomethodological Conversation Analysis: Six Aspects

In our conclusion (chap. 8), we take this generalizing impulse even further and consider our study's wider import—its implications for other disorders besides disability and for an understanding of the organization of everyday ("commonsense") interaction across many contexts. For now, we have defined our approach as one that draws on Goffman's ideas about the interaction order, ethnomethodology's concern with the practices that achieve everyday order—including its appearance as rule-related or protocol-infused—and conversation analysis and its approach to handling indexical or context-dependent words and gestures for their use in assembling social meanings. We complete this chapter by discussing methodological orientations in the field of CA, as it is also informed by ethnomethodology. We regard the practices of everyday talk in both ordinary and clinical settings as manifestations of commonsense competence, and we see discrepant performances of such competence as identifiable against this commonsense backdrop.

(1) UTTERANCES AS SOCIAL ACTIONS

In one of his early lectures on conversation, Sacks (1989[1964]) proposed that the most banal and familiar conversational utterances are social objects that *accomplish* actions and activities, without necessarily formulating those actions as such. Accordingly, CA attempts to describe and analyze a host of ordinary activities: informing, criticizing, insulting, complaining, advising, describing, requesting, apologizing, joking, greeting, and many more. These activities are rarely formulated by their initiators in so many words. We do not say, "This is a greeting: Hello!" We simply say, "Hello." Nor does the syntactic structure of an utterance often convey its force as an action. For example, we use interrogative forms to align with a speaker's complaint talk ("Oh, isn't he dreadful?"); declarative forms to make requests ("It's cold in here"); and imperatives to invite ("Come in").

In the medical interview, patients may perform the activity of asking the doctor for an explanation of medical symptoms through *declarative utterances*: "My stools lately have seemed dark, and I'm wondering if that's because I did start taking the vitamins with iron too, and I'm wondering if the iron in those vitamins could be doing it." As *social actions*, however, Gill (1998:356) calls these "speculative explanations"; they tacitly ask the doctor to confirm or disconfirm what the patient proposes to be the reason for a particular condition. In testing for ASD, a clinician may simply start an instrument's subtask, not by announcing she has questions and expects answers, but simply by saying, "What do you do when you're hungry?" (see chap. 4), which, without previous instruction of any kind, implicitly requires a relevant, verbalized solution to the problem of hunger.

(2) SEQUENCING

The production and understanding of an utterance as an action derives, as Schegloff (e.g., 1995:194) puts it, both from its *composition* and from its *position* in a sequence. Composition can include syntactic, semantic, lexical, phonological, intonational, articulatory, and other features, while position derives from features of the social context, especially an utterance's place in an organized sequence of talk. Conversation sequencing was explored in early papers on turn taking (Sacks, Schegloff, and Jefferson 1974) and on "adjacency pairs" (Schegloff and Sacks 1973). The latter are formed as two closely positioned vocal or nonvocal turns, such as (1) questions and (2) answers, or in the clinic, (1) a clinician blowing up a balloon and letting it flutter to the ground to elicit (2) a child's response, such as retrieving it for another round (see chap. 5).

In the clinical context, starting analysis with a focus on turn taking and adjacency pairs translates into a concern with everything from "how are you" questions and their replies to history-taking questions and answers during the medical exam, testing prompts and their responses, diagnostic announcements and their receipts, treatment proposals and their acceptance or rejection, and many other kinds of sequences. However, as chapter 6 shows, when clinicians assemble to discuss their testing results and decide whether to rule an autism diagnosis in or out, the relevant organization is not the adjacency pair but rather a narrative structure adapted from ordinary conversational practices (Jefferson 1978; Mandelbaum 2013) that allows for the person communicating their results to complete a *series* of turns, upon whose completion a recipient is to show some form of understanding or alignment to what has been said.

Any participant's communicative action is doubly contextual (Heritage 1984b:242). First, the action is *context shaped*, meaning that its contribution to mutual understanding derives in part from its relationship to the immediately preceding utterance or set of activities. An utterance during a test, such as "you eat," makes sense relative to a testing question or prompt that it follows, such as "What do you do when you're hungry?" As obvious as this seems, it is crucial because close examination of the answering utterance can reveal the exact way in which its speaker has parsed and analyzed the prompt. Second, conversational actions are *context renewing*. Every current utterance will itself form the primary framework for some next action in a sequence. When a child produces a response, it occasions actions that deal with and analyze the adequacy of that response. Moreover, sequencing reconditions (i.e., maintains, adjusts, or alters) any broader or more generally prevailing sense of context that is the object of the participants' orientations and actions—a property of interaction Garfinkel (1967:7–9) calls *reflexivity*.

The doubly contextual quality of utterances contributes to the larger interactional environment or overall activity (such as the organizational texture of the examination) within which these utterances make their step-by-step appearance. Clinicians may base their evaluations not only on an immediate response to a question or other stimulus item but also on the way local question-answer sequences exhibit the child's orientation to the overall testing activity (Maynard 2005).

(3) INTERACTIONAL DETAIL AS A GENERIC SITE OF ORDER AND ORGANIZATION

Research in CA has shown that interaction is deeply orderly everywhere. As Zimmerman (cf. Heritage 1984b:241; 1988:415) has put it, "No scale of detail, however fine, is exempt from interactional organization, and hence must be presumed to be orderly." Such a presumption is perhaps a bit strong; stated differently, the matter is that "any detail that is available to the interactants is *potentially* relevant for the researcher" (Clayman and Gill 2012:123, our emphasis). Either way, this implies an interest not just in participants' words or utterances but also in silences, overlapping talk, sound stretches, breathing, prosody, and so on. Hence, conversation analysts transcribe audio and video recordings to show as many of these features as possible in orthographic form, often with graphics as accompaniments (if possible), although the recordings themselves are the ultimate resource for analysis.

This fascination with detail is not some kind of pointillistic end in itself but rather a recognition of how participants orient to the pervasive question of "why that now" in talk-in-interaction. The *that* includes a level of granularity to which participants pay attention: a micropause, a hesitation, a stretching of sound, a brief gesture, a particle such as *uh* or *oh* or *well* and the like, along with larger units such as words, sentences, and paragraph-like entities such as narratives. "Pay attention" means that they take details into account in analyzing a coparticipant's action and in producing an intelligible response. Whatever the level of detail is, the practice it embodies (such as using a silence to indicate disapproval) may have a generic aspect, in that the practice is usable in a variety of interactional environments for doing the action it can convey. The import of this is not to disembody practices from further detail in those environments. Rather, it is to appreciate two matters. One is that analysis must be very detail-oriented, because this is how participants are oriented. The other is that identifying generic aspects of a practice may carry the analysis beyond the specifics of particular instances.

The analytic sensibility of CA may be difficult to appreciate because social science has a great tendency to be variationist (i.e., concerned with how phenomena diverge depending on the backgrounds of participants, the venues in which data are collected, or other distinctions). "But," as Schegloff (1986:147) has argued, "underlying that which varies, we can often find themes of interactional organization to which participants are oriented whatever their milieu, and these have no lesser analytic status" than what varies. In our study, the phenomena and practices we identify and analyze having to do with competence, diagnostic narrative, and the like, can be said to exhibit generic organizational properties that are independent of the sited nature of the data as well as the demographic or other identities of participants.

These practices implemented in interaction also reach beyond what could be construed as the limited scope of our study. Indeed, our data come primarily from one site, but over two widely spread time periods: CDDC in the mid-1980s and mid-2010s. In addition, we have audio recordings collected from a New York clinic in 1972.[7] Thus, the data span several decades, historical periods, and geographic locations, giving them a broad scope. As for the CDDC data collections, we used "convenience" sampling, with families being approached on-site about participating in the study. Both studies received approval from a university internal review board (IRB). In all cases, the parents provided informed consent for their child and themselves to be video recorded. The assent from any child over eleven years old was also obtained. Overall, our collection consists of sixty-one cases (thirteen cases in 1985 and forty-eight cases in 2011–15). The children's median ages were 5.6 (1985) and 4.5 (2011–15). All subjects from 1985 were white, as were the majority (87%) in the 2011–15 group, with the others being African American ($n = 3$), East Asian ($n = 2$), Hispanic ($n = 2$), and South Asian ($n = 1$). Two subjects from the 1985 data received a diagnosis of autism (both male); among the contemporary group, it was thirty of forty-eight (62.5%). Of the latter, twenty-six were male (87.6%) and four were female (13.3%).

Across periods and settings, we find the practices we have analyzed for "doing testing" per chapters 4 and 5 (cf. Maynard and Turowetz 2017b) and "doing diagnosis" per chapters 6 and 7 (cf. Maynard and Turowetz 2017a; Turowetz and Maynard 2017) to be general in the sense of transcending time periods, clinics, and backgrounds of children and families (cf. Maynard and Turowetz 2019)—even as diagnostic criteria, assessment protocols, and politics have changed. We would also add that recent research out of Great Britain, such as that of Hayes and colleagues (2020; 2021) and Hollin and Pilnick (2018), suggests the cross-cultural reach of our research. For these reasons, we expect our study of two clinics across three eras to have wide applicability, resonance, and implications.

(4) GROUNDING ANALYSIS IN PARTICIPANT ORIENTATIONS

An important methodological consequence flows from the concern with sequencing, actions, and details. Given how a turn that initiates an adjacency pair sequence is assembled to convey a social action (i.e., according to its composition), the next speaker will display an understanding of that talk and action in their turn (Sacks, Schegloff, and Jefferson 1974). This means that the original speaker can inspect the next turn for a coparticipant's analysis of what they have said. If the analysis displayed in that next turn does not align with the original speaker's own understanding, then *their next* turn can be devoted to correcting the matter. Accordingly, *repair* of all kinds of conversational or interactional trouble exhibits systematic sequential properties (Schegloff, Jefferson, and Sacks 1977), endowing conversation with in-built procedures for its maintenance as mutually understandable, and allowing for interaction to succeed.

Because interaction is a situated affair, it entails *local determination* by participants, who manage its course on a turn-by-turn basis. And because of the requirement that participants display their understanding on this local, turn-by-turn basis—a matter mentioned in chapter 1 with regard to John Robison's tendency to announce topics without regard to what someone else has said—*analysts have a "proof criterion" and "search procedure" for the analysis of any given turn—namely, seeing how recipients construct their knowledge of it.* That criterion pertains regardless of the particular practices by which a turn is assembled, and is used by participants and analysts alike to make sense of any given interaction.

(5) SINGLE CASES AND COLLECTIONS

CA aims to develop claims about systematic structural organization in interaction. Such claims are supported by substantial accumulations of instances of a practice, each of which the investigator examines as an individual case.

Ideally, the more cases on which an analysis can depend, the stronger the analytic claims will be.

In chapters 4 and 5, we work with collections of sequences drawn from interactions in which clinicians are assessing children for autism and related disabilities. Chapters 6 and 7, which investigate how clinicians use narrative methods for arriving at a diagnosis and communicating it to parents, rely on several dozen case conferences about children and informing interviews with parents from our collection. At the same time, however, our analysis of patterns across cases is complemented by single-case analyses. As sites of social order in their own right, single cases play a crucial role in CA research. Insofar as "social action done through talk is organized and orderly not, or not only, as a matter of rule or as a statistical regularity, but on a case by case, action by action, basis," it is possible to bring the resources of past work in CA to bear on single episodes and cases (Schegloff 1987a:101–2). Moreover, any claim about the organization of interaction should be discoverable in the details of each case in the analyst's collection: such organization is an intrinsic feature of interaction, of its achieved orderliness, and should be grounded in the sequential order properties of interaction rather than in statistical generalizations (e.g., averages or other measures) added to the data but not findable in any single case.

These features of conversation analysis theory and method imply a systematic approach to the organization of interaction that distinguishes it from studies that rely on educated intuition, sophisticated prior theorizing, less disciplined ethnographic inquiry, the systematic coding of utterances, or underspecified notions of context. Although depending on the study CA inquiries may make use of intuition, theory, ethnography, or coding, CA research draws on these other resources in an extremely disciplined way (Maynard 2003:chap. 3).

(6) ETHNOGRAPHIC COMPLEMENTARITY:
INTERVIEWS, MEDICAL RECORDS, AUTISM NARRATIVE

In the present study, we rely on comprehensive fieldwork that included ethnographic observation and interviewing, as well as the systematic collection of video recordings.[8] Our main ethnographic contributions derive from reviewing recordings with clinicians to enhance our understanding of the interactions with children or families and interviewing those clinicians when needing clarification of technical terms or their orientations implementing test protocols. For every child and family in our data, we engaged in extensive observation—at least two members of the research team (which varied from four to six members over the course of the study) sat in the observation parlor next to the room in which testing, diagnosing, and informing interviews were conducted, and took notes which became part of the database for each case. These notes have helped us to identify phenomena for later investigations conducted after the video recordings were converted to reviewable "movies" and transcribed. They also have been consulted to help us understand aspects of the recordings not explicated on the recordings themselves (such as where a usually present clinician or family member was when they were temporarily missing on the recording.) In addition to interviews and observations, we also obtained the sometimes-extensive medical records for most of the children in our mid-1980s and more recent studies (which took a separate protocol and IRB approval from the main study). We drew on these records, as will be seen, to track the overall "career" (as defined in chap. 1) of a given child—their diagnostic and therapeutic history prior to their appointments at the CDDC, and the treatment and other recommendations CDDC clinicians generated in written form to send to families after their visits.

We do not conduct interviews with parents. For the most part, we access their concerns through the medical records and, more importantly, their words and actions in their interactions with clinicians. Nor do we have interviews with the children being diagnosed (even if we could have), again because our focus is not on what they might say *about* their experience, in the clinic or elsewhere, but rather on *interactional* episodes as such. For present purposes, we are interested in parents' and children's views on autism only insofar as these become relevant and consequential during interactions in the clinic. If the participants do not articulate their views or formulate their experiences in the course of these interactions, however, we do not speculate about or otherwise incorporate them into our analysis. In tracking their *actions*, this is at least indirect evidence of participants' understanding or subjectivity with regard to experience.

This is not to say that the views of autism of parents, children, or other family members are unimportant. While they do not bear directly on how we analyze our data, our analysis of autism more generally includes selections from the considerable autism biographical and autobiographical literature, which Hacking (2009) describes as "autism narrative." These narratives also comprise ethnography of a certain sort, and they inform our understanding of the everyday and institutional experiences of people on the spectrum and their families. We should note that when we use the term *autism narrative*, we are excluding works of fiction, such as Mark Haddon's (2003) famous novel *The Curious Incident of the Dog in the Night-Time*. As we use the term, *autism narrative* refers strictly to biographical and autobiographical writings.[9]

We recognize that biography and autobiography are a unique genre and cannot be cross-checked in the way that, for example, a participant observer can verify subjects' accounts about life in some social world (Becker and Geer

1957). But we also know that traditional ethnographic interviews can be contaminated because of the relationship between researcher and subject (Charmaz 1996:35). Likewise, autism narrative is often collaboratively produced, as when an author's writings are edited by another person, and these relationships also could be problematic. However, Hacking (2009:1468) suggests that "it does not matter that in some cases the autist is not the sole author of the final words of the text" because the goal is for thick description, which is aided by renderings that are co-constructed and that are loyal to the dense and rich world of the autistic person. In addition, thick description may necessitate, particularly in some cases where the autistic person is severely impaired, a kind of translation because of the qualities that common sense detects among autistic persons: prescribed interests, limitations in expressiveness, and challenges related to social interaction, although some autistic writers, such as Temple Grandin and John Robison, are lucid in their autobiographical descriptions.

Fortunately, autism narrative preserves the integrity of the person's experience through gestalt-like portrayals of incidents that avoid reductionist intellectual or cognitive accounts about the autistic person. In other words, rather than providing generalized definitions or explanations, or following cognitive science in equating autism with deficits in "theory of mind" (Hacking 2009:1472), autism narrative can and does provide holistic pictures or mosaics of socially based encounters. In Hacking's (2009) view, they follow the leanings of the philosopher Wittgenstein and the gestalt psychologist Köhler, both of whom argued that we gain access to another person's experience by *seeing* their behavior *in relation to* the observable indications in a concrete setting, rather than having to make *inferences* about their inner life on the basis of those indications. Hacking gives the example of smiling: When we see someone smile, we do not *infer* that they are happy. We *see* their happiness as configured in how and what they present to us. Inferences are only required when we cannot make sense of what we are seeing or have reason to doubt our perception. To say that we need inferences to understand the other is a mistake of the sort that leads to hypotheses like theory of mind in the first place. Autism narrative teaches us how autistic people experience their world, and therefore makes their actions seeable and sensible for neurotypical readers.

The seeing provided by autism narrative is thick. It offers a perspective and vocabulary that grants us access to the uniqueness of the autistic person and their lifeworld, making it possible to establish intersubjective understanding where previously there may have been only mutual incomprehension. Given our effort in this book to capture the individuality and particularity of autism, biographical and autobiographical narrative and its mosaics are a most valuable resource.

All in all, we can say that while we rely primarily on audio and video recordings for our data, other resources such as interviews, observations, medical records, and autism narrative complement those data in ways that round out our investigation (cf. Maynard 2003:chap. 3).

The Use of Detailed Transcriptions for the Study of Social Interaction

We have emphasized the importance of detail for the CA enterprise. As Hepburn and Bolden (2013:57) state in their comprehensive review of transcription conventions, it is important to capture the "rich subtlety" of everyday talk and social interaction because participants themselves attend to this subtlety to mutually understand what is going on in their conduct together. Gail Jefferson, who became a central figure in CA, but before that worked as an undergraduate assistant for Harvey Sacks and developed the transcription system for CA, recognized that the seeming minutiae of interaction are, to borrow a phrase (Goffman 1967), "where the action is."

As we pursue our empirical inquiries in subsequent chapters, we often rely on the Jeffersonian transcription system. For readers, it is important to become acquainted with this system. Observing and using the transcription symbols, one can "hear in one's head" how the talk may have sounded and visualize how embodied actions may have transpired. However, if our analysis of an extract does not make use of particular details (emphasis or volume, for example) because the participants do not seem oriented to them, then for easier readability we use "regular orthography," or "normalized transcripts," as may be indicated in the header for the extract in question. So, dear reader, please carefully read the conventions described in the next pages of this chapter.

Appendix

AUDIO TRANSCRIBING CONVENTIONS[10]

1. Overlapping speech

```
A: Oh you do? R[eally   ]        Left-hand brackets mark a
B:              [Um hmmm]        point of overlap, while
                                right-hand brackets indicate
                                where overlapping talk ends.
```

2. Silences

```
A: I'm not use ta that.         Numbers in parentheses
   (1.4)                        indicate elapsed time in
B: Yeah me neither.             tenths of seconds.
```

3. Missing speech

```
A: Are they?
B: Yes because . . .
```

Ellipses indicate where part of an utterance is left out of the transcript.

4. Sound stretching

```
B: I did oka::y.
```

Colon(s) indicate that the prior sound is prolonged. More colons, more stretching.

5. Volume

```
A: That's where I REALLY
want to go.
```

Capital letters indicate increased volume.

6. Emphasis

```
A: I do not want it.
```

Underline indicates increased emphasis.

7. Breathing

```
A: You didn't have to worry
about having the .hh hhh
curtains closed.
```

The *h* indicates audible breathing. The more *h*'s the longer the breath. A period placed before it indicates inbreath; no period indicates outbreath.

8. Laugh tokens

```
A: Tha(h)t was really neat.
```

The *h* within a word or sound indicates explosive aspirations (e.g., laughter, breathlessness, etc.).

9. Explanatory material

```
A: Well ((cough)) I don't
know.
```

Materials in double parentheses indicate audible phenomena other than actual verbalization.

10. Candidate hearing

```
B: (Is that right?) (   )
```

Materials in single parentheses indicate that transcribers were not sure about spoken words. If no words are in parentheses, the talk was indecipherable.

11. Intonation

A: It was unbelievable. I ↑had
a three point six? I↓think.
B: You did.

A period indicates fall in tone, a comma indicates continuing intonation, a question mark indicates increased tone. Up arrows (↑) or down arrows (↓) indicate marked rising and falling shifts in intonation immediately prior to the rise or fall.

12. Sound cutoff

A: This- this is true

Dashes indicate an abrupt cutoff of sound.

13. Soft volume

A: °Yes.° That's true.

Material between degree signs is spoken more quietly than surrounding talk.

14. Latching

A: I am absolutely sure.=
B: =You are.

Equal signs indicate where there is no gap or interval between adjacent utterances.

A: This is one thing [that I=
B: [Yes?
A: =really want to do.

Equal signs also link different parts of a speaker's utterance when that utterance carries over to another transcript line.

15. Speech pacing

A: What is it?
B: >I ain't tellin< you

Part of an utterance delivered at a pace faster than surrounding talk is enclosed between greater-than and less-than signs.

Autistic Intelligence as Uncommon Sense

Born in India and diagnosed with severe autism, Tito Mukhopadhyay (2003) was nonverbal. To those around him, he engaged in odd-seeming behavior, giving the appearance of extreme withdrawal from the social world. Eventually, Mukhopadhyay became capable of reading and writing, emerging as an accomplished poet with a remarkable ability to convey insights from the world of autism. He has been featured in news stories, television shows, documentaries, and many other media through which he informs the public about his condition.

Mukhopadhyay's writings manifest forms of reasoning and understanding that are invisible to those of us immersed in the commonsense world and its taken-for-granted ways of being and behaving. In the following selection from his book *The Mind Tree*, Mukhopadhyay (2003) uses the third person ("the boy") in describing his experiences:

> I want to mention that once when the boy got hurt in the elbow, his mother had soothed his head, as the boy was not able to point the place where the pain was. (22)
>
> He felt that his body was scattered and it was difficult to gather it together. He saw himself as a hand or as a leg and would turn around to assemble his parts to the whole. He spun round and round to be faster than the fan. He felt so that way! He got the idea of spinning from the fan as he saw that its blades were otherwise separate joined together to a complete circle, when they turned in speed. The boy went to an ecstasy as he rotated himself faster and faster. If anybody tried to stop him he felt scattered again. (28)

Mukhopadhyay writes that he felt disjointed, as if his limbs were separate entities that he didn't recognize or control. When he hurt his elbow, he was unable to show his mother where he was injured. But watching a fan, he saw that separate parts could come together if they moved fast. And so he spun round and round like the fan and felt his parts fuse together as a whole. Apparently not understanding this, others "tried to stop him."

In reasoning and acting as he does, Mukhopadhyay embodies *autistic intelligence*, which is a method (or methods) of sensemaking involving distinctive, non-commonsense ways of using *first-order*—or *fundamental— competence*. Although all people sometimes use first-order competence in autistically intelligent ways, most do so less often and more selectively than Mukhopadhyay. First-order competence, in turn, is a building block for *second-order competence*, which includes tacit, taken-for-granted practices for assembling social actions into larger, routine social *activities* (Clayman and Gill 2012:124). These activities encompass everything from mundane greeting exchanges—the building blocks of which include such first-order competences as joint attention, mutual gaze alignment, turn-taking, questioning and answering, and so forth—to medical exams, courtroom proceedings, and clinical evaluations. A crucial feature of social activities is that they are structurally greater than the sum of their parts—grasping the parts is necessary but not sufficient for competent participation in the whole.

Someone with first-order competence would have the basic ability to participate in an environment of testing. For example, when someone says, "What is two plus two?" the recipient must be able to recognize their action as a question and respond with an answer. However, as a later example in this chapter illustrates, an individual may be able to participate mechanically in a series of question-answer sequences while producing wrong or even nonsensical answers. That individual may be incapable of showing, or may choose not to show, second-order and abstract competence—abstract in the sense of disentangling *what* is being asked from *how* actions and activities are being fashioned. For example, when someone responds to the question "What makes you feel happy?" by answering "chairs," as did one of the children we observed (see below), they have exhibited a capacity for first-order participation—the ability to engage in a question-answer (adjacency pair) sequence—but not the acumen for producing second-order responses. Abstract competence involves an interactional *structure* that depends on a nearly invisible scaffolding of ordinary practices to achieve its coherence. Attwood (1998:76) provides an instructive example: "A young man was asked by his father to make a pot of tea. Sometime later his father was concerned that he had not received his refreshment and asked his son, 'Where's the tea?' His son replied, 'In the pot, of course.' His son was unaware that the original request implied the preparation and presentation of a cup of tea for each person."

In following his father's request or directive to make tea, the son showed first-order competence by boiling water and steaming the tea. But he failed at second-order competence—what "the original request implied"—which is structural and abstract in the sense of moving beyond the literalness of talk to incorporate the tacit aspects of an utterance's action. "Please make a pot of tea" is a request that includes a variety of unstated but ordinarily understood performative components: boiling water, pouring the water over tea leaves, steeping for a few minutes, pouring into cups, serving the cups.

In this chapter, we not only further define and illustrate concepts that have to do with different forms of competence; we also explore how autistic intelligence is often subterranean with respect to the surface of the official, second-order structure of activities that it can enable. Such intelligence can also be used strategically in the sense of achieving one's goals irrespective of the larger or official purpose of ordinary social actions, which in an autism clinic like CDDC means participating with a clinician in a range of commonsense tasks assembled through the implementation of standardized instruments, including the Autism Diagnostic Observation Schedule (ADOS) and (in some cases) cognitive tests. Clinicians use these assessment tools alongside checklists, questionnaires, information from medical records, and direct interviews with parents and children to help establish diagnostic conclusions.

Diagnostic conclusions, it can be said, take autistic intelligence for granted, hardly paying it any attention, even though it forms a critical substrate for accomplishing the common actions and activities and the structure of tacit understandings that clinical instruments are designed to assess. In this chapter, we provide examples of how such intelligence not only facilitates second-order competence but can also impede its expression. We further develop this point about facilitation in chapter 5, which explores the varieties of autistic intelligence and shows that even in instances where several children miss out on the structure of a commonsense task, they do not do so in uniform ways but in idiosyncratic ones that regularly exhibit first-order competence.

Taken together, chapters 4 and 5 suggest that when a child errs on a task, the error reveals much more than an inadequate command of common sense. Within the turn-taking, sequential structure of the interaction, there is often valuable information about the child's way of making sense of their world. And so, in addition to describing aspects of the child's conduct that often are said to be autistic, we can inspect such conduct for its *intelligence*, which is all too easily missed or dismissed when persons with autism are assessed by the neurotypical criteria listed in the DSM and built into assessment tools like the ADOS and ADI-R.[1]

Rethinking "Autistic Intelligence" as First-Order Competence

Mukhopadhyay's recollections convey that even in so-called low-functioning forms of autism, there may be a cauldron of sensibility that manifests *autistic intelligence*. However, this term is not new. Leo Kanner, who originated the diagnosis of autism, and Hans Asperger, who identified the syndrome that bears his name, wrote about the autistic intelligence of the individuals they treated. *But they reserved that term only for the most obvious and superior forms of performance.* In his famous paper, "Autistic Disturbances of Affective Contact," Kanner (1943:247) writes, "The astounding vocabulary of the speaking children, the excellent memory for events of several years before, the phenomenal rote memory for poems and names, and the precise recollection of complex patterns and sequences, bespeak good intelligence in the sense in which this word is commonly used." Like Kanner, Asperger observed that the children in his clinic displayed odd gaze patterns,[2] stereotypic behavior, limited awareness of others, disturbances in social contact, and preoccupations with their own impulses. Yet he also notes that some of the children displayed special interests and aptitudes, originality, and independence of thought. Such "autistic intelligence," Asperger (1991[1944]:62, 70) suggests, encompasses distinctive talents in art appreciation, character judgment, and mathematical and other forms of intellectual achievement, and it could provide for success in various professions.

But what if forms of autistic intelligence[3] are both more mundane and broader than the limited versions that Kanner and Asperger espouse? Autistic intelligence is something we all have—after all, the Greek root of autism is "self." Such intelligence shows an orientation to one's own thoughts or associations, which is why *autist* as a noun and *autistic* as an adjective are appropriate words to use and suggest a contrast with *common* sense. Another way of putting it is that autism involves ego focus or self-attentiveness, whereby a person's actions are grounded in their own world and relevancies (Heritage 1998:295–96; Jefferson 1984:194).[4]

Common sense, by contrast to self-attentiveness, involves other-attentiveness, as a person pays attention to the social world around them and to the structure of tacit meanings that others impart through the use of utterances and embodied conduct. In chapter 1, we considered a selection from John Robison's (2007:20) autobiography, *Look Me in the Eye*, in which he reports a sudden insight at age nine—namely, that when a playmate directed his attention to something, he needed to reply with "an answer that made sense in the context of what he had said." Common sense as other-attentiveness means that a participant pays attention to another's world as a condition for bespeaking one's own.

That we all have both commonsense and autistic intelligence can be seen in such skills as humor, as when the late comic George Carlin (2011) joked about the common salutation "Have a nice day": "I had kind of an interesting morning this morning. I call it interesting for a good reason. You see I don't have a nice day anymore. Frankly, I don't bother with them. I feel as if I'm sort of beyond the nice day now; I feel as though I've had my share. Why not let someone else have a few? Why should I be hogging all the really nice ones? Of course, people still want me to have one. Everybody wants me to have one!" Carlin's bit resonates because he is piercing through the commonsense, other-directed salutation "Have a nice day." Such joking depends on willfully playing with concrete and literal understandings of words or phrases. Puns do the same thing (Sacks 1973), but when they are "unintended" (as they often are), it is simply a manifestation of autistic intelligence being deployed without one's awareness of doing so. This is a characteristic feature of autistic intelligence: its manifestation is neither a purposeful nor cognizant aspect of one's social action.[5]

Those of us swimming in the world of common sense find it funny when someone points out that the things we say to one another every day, such as "Have a nice day," are inane, rote, and impersonal. For those with more autistic intelligence, whose ways of thinking and acting center their own unique experience, *the effort goes the other way.* They must exert unusual effort to remember what others expect to hear. For John Robison, as noted in chapter 1, it was not until he was older that he came to realize what a proper (i.e., commonsense) response to someone's bad news should be. That autism diagnosis depends on the commonsense perspective is captured well in Mukhopadhyay's (2003:23) description of diagnosis:

> The boy went to the Institute where the clinical psychologist after studying him, told the parents that they had an 'autistic' SON.
>   "It is a state when the child is so withdrawn that he is unable to understand what is going on around him."
>   "I understand very well," said the spirit in the boy.

The psychologist offers a commonsense perspective that, while no doubt grounded in formal diagnostic procedure, misses an important component of Mukhopadhyay's experience. Here is Kanner (1943:242) many decades earlier, describing the group of children he examined at Johns Hopkins: "There is from the start an extreme autistic aloneness that, whenever possible, disregards, ignores, shuts out anything that comes to the child from the outside. Direct physical contact or such motion or noise as threatens to disrupt the aloneness is either treated 'as if it weren't there' or, if this is no longer sufficient, resented painfully as distressing interference."

Mukhopadhyay (2003:29) succinctly and insightfully sums up the deficit model embodied in these descriptions: "That projected the boy as a total weird personality and instead of getting respect for his 'haves', he gets the curious looks or 'sympathies' from the strangers." If his fascinations are uncommon and generate curiosity from those who are rooted in the commonsense world, Mukhopadhyay lacks neither inner mindfulness nor awareness of that outside curiosity. Similarly, Grandin (1995:44) reports that, at age three, "Although I could understand everything people said, my responses were limited."[6] Autobiographical reflections like these indicate that even if children with autism are unable to fully participate in the commonsense world, they can nonetheless deploy autistic intelligence in pursuit of activities that they find interesting, comforting, or pleasurable, all the while remaining indifferent to—but far from ignorant of—the fact that others often view their actions as something of a spectacle.

Both Mukhopadhyay's diagnosing therapist in the early 2000s and Kanner in his 1943 writings about autism disregard the possibility that someone like Mukhopadhyay can be fully aware of their own sense of limitation but also— and extremely important—their need to be respected for their "haves," rather than what can be imputed as their "have-nots." As Mukhopadhyay (2003:27) puts it, "People love to take special interests in the 'cannots' and not the 'cans.'" In Mukhopadhyay's case, one of those "haves" or "cans" is an acute awareness of the sorts of interventions that could be helpful to him. He describes how he was able to recruit onlookers or caregivers to help him achieve immediate goals, for example by pointing or gesturing when he needed hands-on physical guidance, something that his mother was able to provide.[7] When she held his shoulder, Mukhopadhyay (2003:48) could feel the presence not only of her hand but also of his own hand as linked to the shoulder: "I have concrete proof that to start with any new activity, it is important for the autistics like the boy, to be held at that part of the body, which does the work as the 'relating' ability develops slowly through practice. Then it can be faded out as the person gets the habit of that particular work." And, in the epilogue to this story, Mukhopadhyay (2003:89) reports, "Today, the fragmented self of hand and body parts which I once saw myself as, have unified to a living 'me', striving for a complete 'me.'" His body had become a commonsense body.

First-Order, Fundamental vs. Second-Order, Structural Competence

To better understand the overall capacities of children, we need two terms: first-order competence and second-order competence. First-order or fundamental competence refers to practices of talk and embodied action that are reasoned and skillful in their own right and that sometimes (but not always) permit orderly engagement with another participant. Second-order or structural competence refers to ways that tacit understandings layer first-order practices to render forms of talk and embodied conduct fully other-oriented and collaborative.

Because social life is made up of everyday and institutional activities, participants must be able to use first-order practices in ways that enable distinct activity frameworks. Such frameworks include pretend play, athletic competitions, classroom learning, and occupational endeavors, all of them organized in and through interactional sequences. Participating in such frameworks requires a grasp of their gestalt contexture (Prizant 1982): the purpose and meaning of the whole activity, which is greater than the sum of its parts (Maynard 2005). In other words, the sequences that make up the activity require tacit embellishment by the participants, who must be able to distinguish the proverbial forest for its trees. In the autism clinic, this means that participants must have a command of the basic sequences, like questioning and answering, or directing and responding, and relate them to larger frameworks of activity, such as demonstrating knowledge of "what to do in different situations" (see below regarding a test for this) or how one brushes one's teeth (see chap. 5). These frameworks are what Heritage and Atkinson (1984:13) describe as the "structures of social action," which are like gestalts—the holistic purpose for which the sequential parts are being produced.

THE RELATIONSHIP BETWEEN FIRST- AND SECOND-ORDER COMPETENCE

Most—but not all—of the children we observed at CDDC exhibited first-order competence during examination: their practices, whether verbal, gestural, or otherwise, were sensible and assessable in the immediate interactional environment. However, not all of the children were able to use first-order competence in ways that achieved success (by test criteria) at the second-order, structural level. It wasn't that these children were withdrawn or *in*active. Rather, they pursued other and often competing activities, such as idiosyncratic forms of play, self-oriented storytelling, or somatic manipulations beyond the realm of testing as such. In doing so, they used first-order competence in autistically intelligent ways.

We aim to show how putative failures of second-order competence, whether they involve refusing to perform at all or simply getting an answer wrong, can nonetheless indicate other competences and forms of intelligence. Clinicians may misconstrue these fundamental skills or miss them entirely because of the demands placed on them by the protocols they administer. Indeed, even when a child fails a test item, that failure reveals more than inadequate common sense; it also exhibits an orderliness that can provide valuable insight into the child's methods for making their sense of the world. Accordingly, within the autistic elements of the child's conduct (i.e., its atypical, self-attentive character) there lies an intelligence that we want to highlight, one that is all too easily missed or dismissed when autistic children (or adults, for that matter) are evaluated by neurotypical criteria.

To use terminology already present in the autism literature, "talent in autism comes in many forms." One well-documented form is the ability to "recogniz[e] repeating patterns in stimuli" (Baron-Cohen et al. 2009:1377). This talent, which may derive from sensory hypersensitivity, can manifest as obsessive attention to detail (Baron-Cohen et al. 2009:1381) and is an example of first-order competence. Yet because they can interfere with other activities, this and other talents are often treated as deficits. That such talent constitutes ability and not (only) disability is something that has not fully made its way into official forms of diagnosis and treatment. Given the need for evaluating children, the time involved, and the challenges of bringing first-order or fundamental competence to the surface of the testing environment, this lacuna is understandable. Though our research cannot rectify the needs, time constraints, or challenges associated with appreciating autistic intelligence more broadly, it may help lay a path toward that end, and toward capturing the individuality of any particular child.

WHY THE DISTINCTION BETWEEN FIRST- AND SECOND-ORDER COMPETENCE MATTERS

The availability of information about a child's particular intelligence means two things. First, in the clinic, the common sense embedded in the assessment process can be thrown into finer relief. As Blackman (2005:139) observes from her own experience of autism: "It may be that the social deficits which are the cornerstone of an autism spectrum diagnosis tell us far more about the person who made them markers for such a diagnosis than about the child whom he observes. I realise that social life and affections are essential for being human, but I still wonder whether the 'me' factor is properly understood. That is, the whole testing procedure is somehow actually constructed on whether the tester observed the person to socialise in a way the tester understood to be socialisation." To us, it is not only about what examiners understand but also *how the instruments they administer encode common sense*. Because these instruments are conduits for what a wider society takes for granted, children who do something different from what the assessment asks for provide an avenue into understanding the structure of ordinary common sense.

Second, probing or reflecting on the differentness a child brings to the assessment may mean adjusting or aligning to the world of the child. To the degree that it is possible to appreciate and relate to that world, in the clinic and elsewhere, clinicians, educators, family members, and others will be better equipped to teach, treat, and make sense with the child, expanding their own environments of common sense and their taken-for-granted ways of thinking, acting within and designing those environments in the process. As mentioned earlier, we discuss in our concluding chapter (8) what our research means for the shaping of such *prosthetic* environments.

In the next sections of this chapter, we illustrate in more depth the distinction between first- and second-order competence. We analyze how first-order competence operates and how a child may apparently fail to display it during an examination. Finally, we unearth first-order competence from a subterranean level that is all too often overlooked or even mistaken for incompetence.

Showing Fundamental Competence but Inadequate Structural Knowledge

School officials referred Ronnie Martin, four years and ten months old, to the CDDC in 1985 because of concerns about "decreased eye contact and flat affect." He was described as being "more excited over how a door opens rather than in contact with his peers," having "limited attention span and difficulty playing with peers, often appearing to be in his own little world." This "appearing in his own world" may have been manifested in Ronnie's performance on a subtest of the Brigance Diagnostic Inventory of Early Development (1978). In our terms, the performance is a good example of how testing can attempt to call for the use of commonsense knowledge.

The subtest is called "Knows What to Do in Different Situations," a remarkable if inadvertent definition of commonsense knowledge, and the skill being tested is described this way: "Gives appropriate responses for different situations" (Brigance 1978:172). While the clinician reads test items from a booklet on the table in front of her and scores answers in the same booklet, she presents the test items orally to the child, who holds his hands together on the table or positions them in other ways rather than using them to assemble or place objects, as they may be required to do for other tests (see fig. 4.1).

For some questions on this subtest, Ronnie answers correctly by showing second-order competence, which in this case requires abstracted reasoning. That is, second-order competence frequently involves what Margaret Donaldson (1978) calls "disembedded" knowledge: an exhibit of aptitude removed

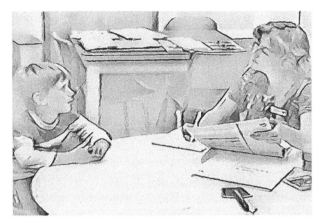

FIGURE 4.1

from the ordinary "flow of events" and local "situations" that surround and contextualize everyday experience. Thus, a task on an examination is abstract if it is removed from "all basic human purposes and feelings and endeavors" (Donaldson 1978:17)—"encapsulated" or "isolated from the rest of experience" (Donaldson 1978:78).[8]

To "What do you do when you're sleepy?" Ronnie replies, "Go to bed." However, in answer to "What do you do when you're cold?" (extract 4.1 and fig. 4.1), which is meant to generate a generic solution that is independent of any specific individual or context (Maynard and Marlaire 1992:516), he incorporates a particular referent into his answer:

TRANSCRIPT 4.1: CASE J: BRIGANCE INVENTORY (NORMALIZED)

```
1   Amy:    Whatyado when you're cold.
2   Ron:    Go in the house, when me and Jimmy are cold.
3   Amy:    Arright, what if you're in the house and you're still cold, whatya
4           do.
5   Ron:    Stay in.
6           (0.5 second silence)
7   Amy:    Okay.
```

At line 2, Ronnie cites an experience he had (or would have) with a specific other person—presumably a friend or playmate. As Donaldson (1978:78) has remarked, "Now it is of the essence of these kinds of problem that you are required to stick strictly to the given. . . . Thus if you are given a problem about two boys called Pete and Tommy you are not supposed to introduce information about any real Pete or Tommy who happens to be known to you!" Alas, instead of adhering to the more limited premises of the question—a "theo-retical" situation (Maynard 2005:209) to be experienced by anyone—Ronnie personalizes his answer, departing from a generic solution to the problem and referring to a limited experience in time (when he is with "Jimmy") and space (near "the house") using a definite article ("the") that circumscribes a possible shelter.

By asking another version of the question (lines 3–4), Amy not only re-jects Ronnie's answer but more strongly suggests the need for an abstract or disembedded response by replacing the question's initial *when* formulation with *if*, a canonical marker of a hypothetical. Note too that in asking a follow-up question, Amy is operating within the parameters of test protocol. The manual (Brigance 1978:172) instructs examiners: "Wait for the child's re-sponse. If the child's response is questionable, incomplete, or evasive . . . make additional requests or ask follow-up questions such as these: 'Tell me more; Can you tell me more? What else can we do?'" However, in answering the subsequent version of the question, Ronnie's response (line 5) retains an im-plied reference to "the house"—presumably his own—and thereby remains at the level of embedded rather than disembedded thought. (During a pause at line 6, and when she acknowledges the answer at line 7, Amy is writing on her score sheet, which can be seen in fig. 4.1).

Ronnie's exhibit of embedded thought—his use of experience-based asso-ciations evoked by the question rather than the sort of disembedded interpre-tation that would count as correct by test criteria (Maynard 2005)—shows, in our terms, fundamental, first-order competence but inadequate second-order or structural competence. Although Ronnie does orient to and participate in the social activity of testing, it is as he deploys a form of "associative" rea-soning (cf. Frith 2003:120) that does not meet the test's structural criteria for "knowing what to do," which require a more theoretical-disembedded ori-entation to the questions. As a result, Ronnie's overall test score is depressed, and he is eventually diagnosed with an autism-related disorder. As we will see in chapter 6, indeed, clinicians treat the associative logic shown in his answer as evidence of a concrete-thinking style that is symptomatic of autism.

FAILURE TO DISPLAY ADEQUATE
SECOND-ORDER COMPETENCE

In Donaldson's (1978:77–81) terms, Ronnie's answer to the question about be-ing cold is lodged in "human sense" instead of strictly adhering to the struc-tural or tacit premises of the question by removing considerations of any actual context, such as being outside a house and with a friend. A correct answer at the structural level would be something like "Put on a jacket." Although his answer does recapitulate the premise of the question, "When . . . cold," such that if the answer is not as disembedded as it should be, it nonetheless displays a "tie" or connection to what is asked.[9] In both answering the question and tying back to it, his answer displays two forms of fundamental or first-order competence, even if it is structurally inadequate with its omission of the task's and the item's tacit requirements.[10]

WHEN FIRST-ORDER COMPETENCE IS (SEEMINGLY) ABSENT

On the "what do you do when" Brigance test's question about being cold, Ronnie exhibits fundamental, first-order competence that shows his participation in the "interactional substrate" of testing (Maynard and Marlaire 1992). Although he does not fully demonstrate second-order structural competence, he displays an orientation to the testing environment and the questions being asked. In some cases, however, children may appear not to deploy first-order competence at all. That is, at least from the interlocutor's point of view—be they a clinician, parent, educator, or someone else—the child does not, or cannot, answer questions, respond appropriately to directives, or otherwise engage in fundamental joint actions necessary for social activities. Indeed, sometimes an immersion in first-order competence can inhibit the display of second-order competence, as when a child like Tito Mukhopadhyay repeats an action over and over again, seemingly oblivious to copresent others. However, it is still a matter of fundamental, first-order competence and autistic intelligence when we realize that such behaviors may provide internal coherence and meaning for the one exhibiting the behavior, such as calming hyper-responsive or exacerbated activity of the sympathetic nervous system (Hirstein, Iversen, and Ramachandran 2001).[11]

In the example below, though, it is not the child's retreating or self-stimulating with which a psychologist whom we call Dr. Peggy Emerson is dealing. She is administering the Differential Abilities Scale II, or DAS-II, (Elliott 1990) to Marcus Davidson, a four-year-old boy. Per Dumont, Willis, and Elliott (2009:1), the DAS-II "was developed with a primary focus on specific cognitive abilities rather than on general 'intelligence.'" Marcus, who was already receiving speech therapy and was on a waiting list for occupational therapy, was referred to the CDDC because of difficulties at school and because there were previous indications (including from his pediatrician) that he could be on the autism spectrum. During a "picture similarities" task, Peg is attempting to get Marcus to match a picture of a foot on a small card to one of four items shown

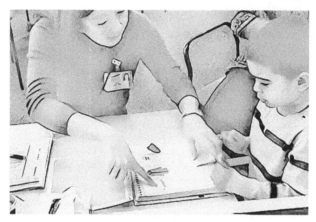

FIGURE 4.2A. Lines 5–6

in the testing manual (a robe, coat, stocking, and hat, referenced below with the word "image"). The Picture Similarities test is one of several on the DAS-II that tests for nonverbal reasoning—officially, per Dumont et al. (2009:160), "the ability to discover the underlying characteristic (e.g., rule, concept, principle, process, trend, class membership) related to a specific problem."

Try as she might, Peg cannot obtain the required "matching," or, more specifically, pointing behavior from Marcus, much less the correct answer. In the midst of her efforts, as we will see (line 24 in extract 4.2 below), Peg formulates what he "didn't" do. But while it is true that he has not complied with her directives, the episode is dense with other kinds of efforts—forms of intelligence and competence—on the part of Marcus that we will analyze.

In her right hand, and with curled fingers around it (fig. 4.2a), Peg holds a small toy,[12] which has a role in what happens during the further interaction with Marcus. Our transcript (4.2, later in this section) starts as Marcus may have already been told to match the foot picture on the card in front of him with the proper image (stocking).[13] While tapping the foot picture (line 1), Marcus, in a high-pitched voice, is saying what sounds like "choo" (line 2 below), but which could be announcing the word "shoe." After Peg produces a small smile and brief head nod (line 3), she says, "thank you" (line 4), which suggests closure to the sequence. After this, Marcus issues another "choo" (line 5) at an even higher pitch than the previous one. Here, he may be treating her nonvocal nod and smile, along with her "okay," as an approval or other positive assessment. In any case, Marcus's line 5 utterance appears responsive to the entirety of Peg's embodied and vocalized movements. Peg then solicits (lines 6–7) Marcus's orientation to the test item proper. With her left hand, she removes the card from under Marcus's hand, and he responds with tapping motions as she indicates with her right index finger the images from which he is to choose the match. Her wh-question (line 6) includes a turn-final address term—a way to "personalize" an inquiry (Lerner 2013). She also produces a pointing gesture (lines 7–8), a "look" admonition (line 9),[14] and moves her index finger across each of the images (line 10), thereby directing Marcus to place the picture near the image with which it could be paired (fig. 4.2a).

TRANSCRIPT 4.2 CASE 9 PSY:1

```
1              (1.2) ((Marcus tapping on picture of shoe))
2    Mar:      ↑Choo (0.5) ↑Choo::!
3              (1.3) ((Marcus gazes at Peg; Peg nods, smiles))
4    Peg:      Thank you:
5    Mar:      ↑↑Choo[::! ((tapping the card))
6    Peg:           [Where does it go buddy.
7    Peg:           [((takes card with l. hand, puts r. index finger on image))
8              (.)
9    Peg:      Look.
10             (1.4) ((Peg taps on each of the four images))
11   Peg:      Sh[ow me. (0.2) ((replaces card to Marcus's area)) ↑Where's it] go.
12   Mar:        [ ↑Wooo:: ((rests head onto left arm))        ↑wooo::    ]
13   Mar:      ↑Woo::::::::::::::oo. ((head resting, taps forefinger on card))
14             (1.2) ((M head still resting))
15   Peg:      Do ya want ↑this? ((Peg holds a small toy in front of Marcus))
16             (2.4) ((Peg withdraws toy then brings back partially; Marcus lifts head))
17   Peg:      ((brings toy back, in front of Marcus, points to foot picture))
18   Mar:      [((Reaching arm and hand toward toy))]
19   Peg:      [((points to foot picture)) Show me, ] ((head nod)) yes.
20   Mar:      Mm[::. ((withdraws arm)) ]
21   Peg:        [Show me where it goes.]
22   Mar:      ((Tapping on test booklet))  To mee::
23   Mar:      [To mee::
24             [((Twice, Marcus reaches out and back to Peg-held toy))
25             (1.8) ((Marcus takes picture card, reaches, and hands it to Peg))
26   Peg:      ((Taking card from Marcus)) [ ↑ ↑You did not ↑sho::w!
27   Peg:                                 [((returning card to Marcus))
28             (0.2)
29   Peg:      Put it,
30             (0.8)
31   Peg:      Put it where it goes. [((drags finger across images on page))
32   Mar:                           [((taps on foot picture with r. hand))
33   Peg:      [Where does it ↓go.] ((completes the dragging))
34   Mar:      [(Whe::re::::: it) ] ↓go. ((swipes left hand across page))
35             (1.5)
36   Peg:      Where does it ↑goh::oh. ((begins writing in test booklet))
37   Mar:      ((Yawn))
```

Marcus may have difficulty understanding Peg's wh-prefaced "interrogative"-type directive (Goodwin and Cekaite 2013), due to the directive's syntax: studies have shown that children with autism have more difficulty answering wh-questions than do typically developing children (Daar, Negrelli, and Dixon 2015). Here, Marcus has to coordinate the wh-word with both the noun that follows ("it")—a "pro-term" (Sacks 1992:163) that is vague about its referent—and the attached copula pro-verb form ("go"), which also lacks semantic concreteness (Bloom, Merkin, and Wootten 1982:1087).

Subsequently, Peg returns the picture to a position in front of Marcus (line 11) and issues a further, "bald" directive (Goodwin and Cekaite 2013:200) to "show me"—and recycles her earlier question without altering the problematic syntax. Marcus responds by leaning his head on the table and re-engaging his tapping motion as he produces "woo"-type vocalizations (lines 12–14). Peg watches Marcus during the silence at line 14, then performs a shift of "footing" (Goffman 1979, Goodwin 2007) that moves away from the matching task as such, but in a way that could affect its completion. With her right hand, she offers Marcus the toy that she has been holding (line 15), but takes it away (line 16), and brings it back part way, as she uses her left hand to point to the foot picture (line 17). Marcus reaches for the toy (line 18) even as Peg is pointing to the foot picture (line 19), after which she acknowledges this reach with a very quick nod of the head and clipped "yes" token (end of line 19).

Next, Marcus produces an "m" sound (line 20), and he pulls his arm back. Almost simultaneously, Peg produces an expanded directive (line 21), but Marcus taps on the booklet (line 22), which may well constitute a nonvocalized form of requesting (Dickerson, Stribling, and Rae 2007) as that is accompanied by a vocal form, "To me" (line 22), with its stretching on *me*. At line 23, Marcus repeats the vocalized request, quickly reaching for the toy twice (line 24, fig. 4.2b), and pointing toward himself as he retracts the gesture.[15] As he reaches out for the toy, we see Peg directing her gaze toward the test booklet (fig. 4.2b).

Failing to get the toy, Marcus plucks the foot picture-card and *offers* it to Peg (line 25), and she responds by taking it (line 26). His offer seems to implicate an exchange, as if handing over the picture card would result in his obtaining the toy. However, as Peg returns the card, she retains the toy, and formulates (as earlier mentioned) what he *didn't* do (line 26), a complaint-type utterance (Schegloff 2007:75) in that it notices an absence. She subsequently asks for remedy (lines 29, 31), once again phrased in terms of putting the picture card "where it goes." In sing-song fashion, she produces yet another "where-it-goes" directive (line 33), which ends with marked downward intonation. In

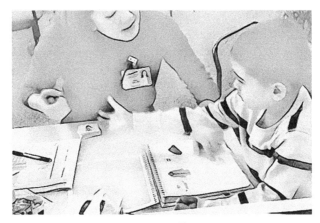

FIGURE 4.2B. Line 18

overlap with her utterance, Marcus appears to repeat the "where" directive in truncated form (line 34), employing a parallel intonation contour. He taps on the page with his right hand, and also seems to mimic her "dragging" gesture with his rapid, left-handed "swiping" movement across the images.

Of crucial importance here are Peg's interpretations of Marcus's conduct. By complaining that he did not "show" any image that would match with the foot picture, she is marking the absence of a response—*any* response—to her directives. Her interpretation positions Marcus as neglecting to show the first-order competence to complete a sequence. Indeed, by neither attempting to match the picture of the stocking to the correct image in the test booklet, nor acknowledging the test itself as a domain of activity, Marcus is not displaying first-order competence for *testing* as such. That is, in pursuit of other actions, and in contrast to how Ronnie was oriented to the Brigance "what do you do when" testing environment (fig. 4.1 and transcript 4.1), he is not interacting in a way that would allow the clinician to determine his capacity for second-order competence. Put differently, his apparent efforts at soliciting the toy eschew the minimum level of co-orientation and cooperation with Peg required to participate in the official activity of the session.

Later, when discussing the test with Marcus's mother, Peg says, "His participation and effort were pretty low . . . he really didn't want to necessarily perform what I was asking him to do." As a result, she explains, she was unable to obtain a "fair estimate" or "valid indicator" of his skills in the intellectual realm.[16] Notice the interpretation here: Marcus is said to *not want* to perform. Analytically, such a statement is consistent with ethnomethodological analyses (Garfinkel 1967:48) of commonsense reasoning (see chap. 1). Like everyday participants confronted with apparent failures at commonsense tasks, clinicians treat such conduct as specifically *motivated* conduct and invoke *psychological* factors to explain it. In our view, this ignores the possibility of an interactional rather than psychological or cognitive phenotype at the root of ostensibly autistic behavior—here, Marcus's self-attentive preoccupation with the toy object being held by Peg.

SUBTERRANEAN FIRST-ORDER COMPETENCE

Peg's assessment of Marcus as "not motivated" to participate, such that she was unable to make a reliable estimate of his skills, may be the end of the clinical story. But it is not the end of the interactional one. Although Marcus did not exhibit the kind of first-order competence necessary for an official assessment, close analysis of his actions reveals other forms of such competence and autistic intelligence.

First, if Marcus is saying a version of "shoe" at lines 2 and 5, he may well be making a match between the picture of a foot and something that goes on it—as the image of the sock indeed does. As we suggested above, he is announcing that match. Second, when Peg tries to entice him with the small toy wheel and withdraws it from his grasp (lines 15–17), he reaches out (line 18) and requests the object in an embodied way, before retracting his arm when it is clear that he is unable to grasp it (line 20). Third, his "To mee::" utterances (lines 22–23) could be heard as forms of vocal requesting, accompanying further attempts at reaching for the toy (line 23). He may also be exerting effort at line 25 to achieve an exchange of the card for the toy.

Announcing is an interactional skill, as are the reaching, requesting, and exchange actions, in that these gestural practices implicate both the party doing the gesture and the addressee or recipient of the action (Goodwin 2003b:225). There is no evidence that Peg discerns these efforts: they are momentary, and in the case of the vocalizations, not well-spoken grammatically or prosodically. Peg also has her gaze directed elsewhere than toward Marcus's pointing and gesturing in a way that can ignore those moves. His efforts, in other words, mostly are not within Peg's "domain of scrutiny" (Goodwin 2003b:221; cf. Hindmarsh and Heath 2000).[17] Finally, when Marcus (at line 34) appears to repeat Peg's ". . . where it goes" utterance, he exhibits a hearing of her talk, even if it takes the form of an echo or mimic (he also appears to echo or mimic her gestures at line 34). All of these various practices on Marcus's part are what we call *subterranean* first-order competence: subterranean because they are mostly (or perhaps *only*) visible through careful observation, but otherwise *below* the official testing activities and their commonsense structuring underway during the interaction.

If we can say that our EMCA approach puts interaction under a microscope, it does so to make visible the fine details and structures of social action that are often beyond the threshold of visibility to participants. Indeed, clinicians cannot, as a practical matter, attend to all the particulars that our transcripts capture and perform activities such as testing at the same time. Garfinkel's (2002:152–153) example of clapping hands along with a metronome is relevant here: it is not possible, Garfinkel observes, to "make time"—keep the beat—and "mark time"—count the metronome's clicks—simultaneously without losing the beat. Doing the activity properly, in other words, means erasing the lived work of its production, which occurs at a tacit level of methodic endeavor. However, as we explore in the conclusion to this chapter, by analytically recovering features of that work, it may be possible to bring awareness of especially salient details into professional practice, and thereby integrate them into the professional's domain of scrutiny.

Strategic Use of First-Order Competence

Whereas Marcus did not display the type of first-order competence that would make assessing the correctness of his answers possible—at least from the clinician's perspective—our next example is one in which such evaluation *is* possible. However, the child fails at the second-order, structural level. Tanner Johnson was six years and five months old when, according to his medical record, his family doctor referred him to CDDC, citing "concerns of a pervasive developmental disorder." During an intake session, the boy's parents reported that his kindergarten teacher was concerned that he was inattentive, avoided group activities ("circle time"), and had general difficulty answering questions.

Such difficulty emerges in a particular way in a section of the ADOS concerning emotions. According to the exam manual (Lord et al. 2012:116–17), the goal of this section is "to observe both the content of what the participant says and also the degree to which the child or adolescent who is verbally fluent can use language to talk about more abstract topics, particularly those associated with emotions"; the emotions module, also according to the exam manual, engages an area of behavior known to be "a challenge for many people" and highly problematic for individuals with autism. From the growing genre of autism narrative (e.g., Nazeer 2006; Robison 2007), we know that

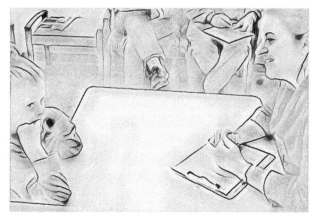

FIGURE 4.3

people with autism do experience the full range of human emotions, but have trouble conveying them with much subtlety or precision and understanding the affective expressions of others (Attwood 1998:56; Frith 2003;110–11; Losh 2006). To put the matter in social psychological terms, people with autism often have difficulty with "emotion management," with "feeling rules"— knowing when and how to express an emotion (Hochschild 1983)—and with awareness of others' emotions. Hence, the emotion questions on the ADOS provide something of a unique access to the phenomenon of first-order competence. Are there identifiable practices by which a child who has difficulty answering a question about emotions in a disembedded-structural way nevertheless engages with the clinician in other tangible, fundamentally competent ways?

In the interaction (fig. 4.3 above), Tanner and psychologist Dr. Ellen Miller are sitting across from each other at a table. At line 1 (extract 4.3A) below, Ellen poses the first in a series of scripted ADOS questions about emotions. In the manual, the question reads, "What do you like doing that makes you feel happy and cheerful?" Following a pause (line 2) and further hesitation (line 3), Tanner answers, "Chairs." During the pause, he has shifted his gaze momentarily to a mirror on his right (see fig. 4.3), in which he can view his parents' reflections.[18] As can be seen at the top of figure 4.3, the parents are side by side on a sofa that is formed by two conjoined chairs, and it seems Tanner is using this image to fashion his answer. (He may also be utilizing his own kinesthetic chair-sitting experience, but his glance at line 2, and subsequent quickly produced answer at line 3, suggest that it is the visual resource on which he draws.)

TRANSCRIPT 4.3A: CASE 42: PSYEMOQ:1:52

```
 1  Ell:    Hey, (.) so Tanner, what makes you feel happy?
 2                  (0.5) ((Tanner glances to mirror on right, fig. 4.3))
 3  Tan:    Uh hih uh:: chairs.
 4                  (0.4)
 5  Ell:    ((smiling and smile voice)) Chairs make you feel happy.
 6                  (0.3)
 7  Tan:    We did everything on this number.
 8  Ell:    No:t ↑ye:t. (.) .hhh hh (.) What kinds of things do you like to do
 9          that make you feel happy and excited.
10                  (4.3)
11  Tan:    Uh:m, ta:bles.
12                  (0.3)
13  Ell:    T(h)ables. Okay. Arright. .hhh
14                  (0.7)
15  Ell:    Wha:t kinds of things, (0.4) make you fee:l s:care::d.
16                  (5.2) ((Tanner glances toward the left where there is a
17                          dispenser of antibacterial lotion on the wall))
18  Tan:    Hand sanitizer.
19                  (0.4)
20  Ell:    Ha:nd sanitizer, right, okay! Guess what, we're going to do
21          something else, okay.
```

Tanner is using the physical features of the examination room to produce answers, at least in the sense of supplying a vocal object in the second turn of a testing sequence. So he displays fundamental, first-order competence and autistic intelligence, but not second-order, structural competence. (An example of the latter would be an answer such as "mostly like playing," the response by one of the children in our data and for whom autism was ruled out.) Tanner's answers illustrate Latour's (1987) point that nonhuman agents ("actants"), including rooms and other physical spaces, are not passive containers for action but active media that can be recruited by other agents (e.g., human actors) as they assemble social actions and objects. It is as if by blending his own vocalizations with locally available material-visual resources, Tanner "emplaces" the examination room (Gieryn 2000) in his answers. As Grandin (1995) famously has said, individuals with autism often are "thinking in pictures."

At line 5, with a smile and "smile voice" (Tartter 1980), Ellen repeats Tanner's answer ("chairs") along with the phrase that initiated the question ("make you feel happy"). Besides acknowledging his response, Ellen may be prompting him to elaborate by way of a "partial questioning repeat" (Robinson 2012), a form of repair that tacitly suggests her difficulty in understanding what Tanner is naming as a source of happiness. Rather than elaborating topically, however, Tanner treats her utterance as approving his answer by proposing, "We did everything on this number" (line 7), again showing an orientation to the testing sequence, and in particular implicating its closure. Indeed, throughout the ADOS, Tanner closely tracks when he and Ellen finish their tasks and urges quick movement through the test items. Announcements like the one at line 7, deployed as a procedure for advancing the test to completion, exhibit his first-order competence, but not in a way that shows second-order, test-relevant competence; indeed, he is more oriented to *getting through* or completing the test than *doing or performing* for the test in a second-order structural sense per se.

Ellen disconfirms Tanner's "we did everything" announcement ("Not yet," line 8) and then asks a revised version of her question, formulating it in action terms (lines 8, 9: what he would "like to do" related to feeling "happy and excited"). During a lengthy pause (line 10), Tanner shifts his gaze to the table on which his elbows rest and then moves his forearms to the table, bouncing his hands as the forearms reach it. This suggests an embodied nomination of the table, which he then designates vocally ("Uhm, tables," line 11) in answer to Ellen's question. Again, his answer exhibits first-order competence, though it is not correct or relevant by test criteria. We can also note that this answer ("tables") forms a pair-relationship with his previous answer ("chairs"), which may show sensitivity to the "poetics" (Jefferson 1996) of talk—it exhibits autistic intelligence: sound and category associations that arise, seemingly unbidden, in spoken language. Ellen registers his answer by repeating it (line 13). Although such repeat of his answer could be asking, at least indirectly, for a better answer, Ellen's laugh particle and accompanying smile voice treat the answer lightly, and she immediately produces sequence-closing acknowledgments ("okay, arright," line 13).

Ellen then asks about another emotion, "feeling scared" (line 15), and after gazing in the direction of a container of antibacterial lotion on the wall to his left, Tanner produces yet another intelligible—but irrelevant—response, "hand sanitizer" (line 18). Ellen registers this (line 20), then announces that they are going to move on to another activity (lines 20–21). Although she has not been able to elicit any emotion descriptions from Tanner, Ellen ends the activity at this point. The test manual provides for this possibility in stating, "It is not intended as a test of cognitive function, so if it is very difficult for the participant, you should note that and move on to the next probe" (Lord et al. 2012:117).

EMBEDDED KNOWLEDGE

By the second-order, structural criteria of the test, Tanner's answers are incorrect. Although he is able to produce answers that are intelligible and at least minimally fitted to Ellen's questions in terms of sequencing and grammar, his responses do not constitute competent performances according to ADOS structural criteria. This could partly reflect the known difficulty persons with ASD have in comprehending and expressing emotions. Tanner's overall score on the ADOS came out at twenty-one, well above the age-normed cutoff of nine that qualifies a child for the autism diagnosis. On the basis of this score, as well as the results of the Autism Diagnostic Interview–Revised (ADI-R), standardized behavior checklists, and other information, the clinicians diagnosed Tanner with ASD.

If Tanner's performance on the questions about emotions may appear nonsensical from a commonsense point of view, there are nonetheless other matters to consider beyond his apparent inability to name what makes him feel happy, excited, or scared. First, we can observe that Tanner's answers show first-order competence and autistic intelligence in that they are sequentially relevant and appropriately placed: they answer a question, exhibiting "practical logic" that is no mean skill in its own right (Ochs and Solomon 2004:155) while artfully making use of tactile, visual, and embodied aspects of the local environment. Second, Tanner is far from resisting or appearing oblivious to the course of action that the clinician initiates, as in the example involving Marcus. In fact, as noted, he is strongly oriented to getting through the ADOS questions and to monitoring their progress (e.g., line 7) or exerting efforts to control the activity. Finally, Tanner's first-order competence at filling answer slots with different verbalizations may be seen as a clever adaptation in how he uses resources that have a coherence in their own right. Each answer draws from visual resources in the immediate environment. Indeed, the fact that difficult questions about emotions do not cause him to withdraw suggests a resourcefulness that could prove relevant for helping him participate in regular social environments. We consider this resourcefulness in greater detail next.

FIRST-ORDER COMPETENCE AND COMMON SENSE

Tanner's use of first-order competence is strategic. At the outset, he begins tracking the progress of the assessment and enumerating the tasks he has completed along the way. For example, when Ellen puts a "first thing" on the table for Tanner to do—"a puzzle," as she says—Tanner begins assembling the pieces according to the markings on a design sheet in front of him. Midway through its assembly, he says, "Okay, this is puzzle one," and Ellen agrees with him. After completing the puzzle, Ellen proposes, "It's time for us to do something else together," and Tanner responds, "One was a puzzle." Again, Ellen agrees, "That's right activity number one was a puzzle." She collaborates in the tracking that Tanner is doing, and after almost every task, he proposes its completion in numeric terms. Thus, following the puzzle task, Ellen works to engage Tanner in make-believe play using a collection of small toys and action figures. As they finish such things as "putting out a fire" and "driving an ambulance," Tanner announces, "We completed number two." Then, as they put the toys away in a plastic bag, Tanner says, "Now we'll get out number three," and Ellen once again agrees, "Now we'll get out number three, that's right."

Tanner's ability to answer questions and track the progression of the ADOS exam "out loud" is a form of first-order competence and autistic intelligence that facilitates exam completion independently of his level of second-order competence. It also illustrates his ability to assemble and participate cooperatively in testing as a coherent activity. However, as the tasks become more challenging for Tanner, this very form of competence seems to work toward movement out of tasks (e.g., the questions above regarding emotions) rather than engaging their substance. Indeed, as the ADOS exam progresses toward its end, Ellen solicits a display of what the ADOS manual calls "joint attention," encouraging Tanner to attend to a remote-controlled toy rabbit. However, Tanner only partly orients to the rabbit, and after he puts down the remote control, Ellen proposes, "[Let's] see what else we've got." Then:

TRANSCRIPT 4.3B: CASE 42:

```
Tanner:  We did all everything on this number.
Ellen:   Yeah we did.
Tanner:  Number one check, number two check, number three
Ellen:   Check!
```

The exam is brought to a close shortly after this.

LINGUISTIC ASPECTS OF INSTRUMENT DESIGN AND IMPLEMENTATION

Tanner's capacity for tracking and monitoring the ADOS activities may be his way of establishing a sense of control or coherence in his environment (Frith 2003:158; cf. Grinker 2007:185), even as he disattends the larger purpose to which his activity is to be oriented.[19] It is a fascinating phenomenon to watch, and Ellen seemed to delight in Tanner's preoccupation with advancing through the exam. Although this manifestation of autistic intelligence may not always interfere with the performance of second-order competence, there are times when it does, in that Tanner may use this skill to shut down an activity prematurely when there are ways it could be pursued on terms more tailored to his abilities. That Tanner can answer emotion questions at all—providing an "answer," even as it misses its mark relative to the disembedded content of the question—suggests the possibility that something is amiss in the questions' verbal presentations. For example, they seem to lack precision by design, and as Stickle, Duck, and Maynard (2017) observe, their linguistic formatting can be difficult for recipients to parse coherently. Moreover, our data show variation in the way that clinicians ask the ADOS emotion questions. In transcript 4.3a above, Ellen says, "Hey, so Tanner, what makes you feel happy?" In another of our cases, from 2014 (number 41), the psychologist renders the question as, "What do you like to do that makes you feel happy?" More research is needed on whether and how these different question formats may affect a child's response.[20] In Tanner's case, it is worth considering whether it would be possible, within the constraints imposed by standardization, to provide different ways of formulating or embellishing the questions about emotions.

Conclusion

Kamran Nazeer was four years old when he started in a special school for autistic children in New York City in 1982. As an adult, Nazeer (2006) wrote an intriguing book called *Send in the Idiots: Stories from the Other Side of Autism* about what happened to four former classmates whom he contacted and interviewed twenty years after they attended the school. Although one of the classmates, Andre, grew up to be a brilliant computer scientist, he also had a tendency to use puppets to handle the contingencies of conversational interaction. Nazeer (2006:23) points out that it is not the *complexity* of spoken language that is a problem for autistic individuals like Andre, who understands the words perfectly well, but rather its *flexibility*: words or phrases can have more than one meaning, and Andre finds that lack of consistency frustrating. In our ethnomethodological terms (Garfinkel 1967:29), we would say that words in conversational interaction are indexical, in that their meaning depends on local particulars that can change rapidly: a term or clause can be used literally, ironically, metaphorically, narratively, or in any number of other ways, and the usage can shift over the course of a single conversation. Bar-Hillel (1954) notes how the meaning of a statement such as "I am hungry" fully depends on who says it and when. The force of the utterance also depends on whether it is being said ironically, complainingly, illustratively, or in any number of ways that the setting of its use helps to determine.

In ordinary conversation, we find not only the voices of the individual participants (Bakhtin 1981), but also each person's myriad stances toward the actions being performed. One may first be explaining, then complaining, then punning or teasing, or complaining *and* teasing. For both speaker and recipient, keeping things coherent in the midst of such flow is difficult under the best of circumstances, and it was simply beyond Andre's capacity. So even as Andre pursued his career as a computer scientist, whenever he was a participant in informal conversation (and in a canonical exhibit of autistic intelligence), he used his puppets to handle the different stances or voices needed to manage its flow (Nazeer 2006:24):

> So when he didn't fully understand what someone else had said, or when he couldn't properly express himself or when it was going to take too long to work out how to do so, he literally stopped being himself, shed the obligations of the role that he was already in, and took a new role. Using the puppets, he could also, for example, be ironic. When he wanted to say something ironic, he gave that line to one of the puppets. This way he wasn't saying something that wasn't literally true or contradicting something that he had said earlier: the puppet was doing it.[21]

The enormous flexibility required to participate in a social activity, even one as tightly organized as testing, places demands on second-order competence that can be challenging for those with autism. We see this in Ronnie's incorrect answer to the "What do you do when you're cold?" question, an answer that was not so much wrong as oriented to the question in what Sacks (1989[1964]) has called a "constructive" or concrete manner. However, it was designed to be heard as a "composite" requiring a certain kind of answer: categorical, disembedded, and hypothetical (see note 6 and Maynard 2005). The composite force of the question is tacit, and the examinee is expected to recognize what is being asked for. But although he may not have grasped the tacit expectation behind the question, Ronnie's ploy of drawing on personal experience and relating it to the question in tangible ways does exhibit autistic intelligence. Likewise, when Marcus avoided Peg's directives to place the picture of a sock on the appropriate test-booklet image, and when she shifted her stance to entice him with a small toy, he effortfully worked to attain the object. This suggests an ability to track an embodied course of action, rather than an orientation to the matching task before him as such. Perhaps the matching task required an aptitude for thinking in pictures, which Temple Grandin (2006:28–29) has come to see as only one kind of autistic intelligence. Understanding the relation between participation in the matching task and the toy reward (i.e., how, if he would match the picture of the foot to the stocking, he would then be compensated with the toy) required an altogether different kind of skill and flexibility, one that may have been impeded because of the abstractions involved in the clinician's directives. If indeed he was unable to perform the structural matching task, it was still the case that he showed considerable fundamental competence in seeking the toy that Peg held in her hand.

Tanner's uncommon sense took the form of co-organizing exam sequences and tracking, even hastening, the progress of the overall assessment. These actions, too, are manifestations of first-order skill. Mechanical though his answers may be in terms of filling a sequential "slot," these skills also suggest avenues for inquiry into what Tanner may need to learn—and be taught—for him to become more flexible in using ordinary language to express his experiences. They may also suggest what may need to be modified in a verbally oriented curriculum (or other social environment) to draw out his knowledge about emotions or other states and experiences. Whether it is possible to teach an autistic person how to handle the flexibility of speech—to deal with the indexical properties of talk and action in ways that go beyond the "constructive" and concrete—remains an open question.

In the meantime, within the context of the ADOS, first-order abilities are easily glossed over or interpreted as instances of the rigid, stereotyped behaviors associated with autism. As a result, they are seen to indicate the *absence* of competence, rather than its *presence*. Put differently, first-order abilities may exist at a kind of subterranean level, as we saw in the case of Marcus. Likewise, underneath Tanner's "failure" to display second-order competence is a set of other appreciable skills—in sequencing, timing, and using environmental affordances as resources for "answering" questions, among others—that approach invisibility when viewed through the tacitly employed lens of common sense.

If subterranean competencies are obscure in relation to ordinary common sense, they are also outside the purview of what we might call clinical common sense—what *any* clinician can be expected to know as a matter of course—an idea that recalls Foucault's (1973:60–61, 166–67) notion of the "clinical gaze" in Western medicine. Since it first developed in Enlightenment Europe, this gaze has focused on naming disorders rather than treating patients as whole persons. As such, it misses or ignores whatever is not in its domain of possible diagnostic knowledge. We can think of the ethnomethodological approach as an *alternate* to the clinical gaze, having to do with what Garfinkel (1996:9) calls the what-more aspects of common sense that are not seeable from the clinical perspective. In the autism clinic, the what-mores are the taken-for-granted, alternate practices that undergird official assessment activities. Seeing these practices for the ways they both enable assessment and occlude important aspects of children's conduct requires a specifically *interactional* gaze. In chapter 1, we referred to the "language of autism" as one that orients to communication and action in unique ways relative to the social environments of common sense in which it is deployed. To learn this language, it is necessary to get beneath the surface and probe the myriad subterranean competencies that, all too often, are indistinguishable to ordinary and clinical gazes alike.

Varieties of Autistic Intelligence

Diagnosis highlights what members of a category have in common. Apply-ing a diagnosis like autism to an individual child means suppressing their particularities and selectively stressing the attributes they share with other autistic children. In the process, generic deficits are stressed while first-order competence and autistic intelligence, to the extent that they are visible at all to common sense, become even more subterranean than before. This is because documenting a diagnosis means collapsing individuality and idiosyncrasies possibly visible during testing into synoptic qualities aligned to definitions of disorder. In contrast, the analysis of autistic intelligence is important because it identifies and preserves what is specific to the person, and what makes them unique as opposed to representative of a generic category. At the same time, though, such analysis may reveal a paradox that inhabits autism assess-ment: first-order competence underlies the second-order skills required by the assessment (such as producing an acceptable response to a question, "so-cial press," or other clinical initiation), but can also interfere with the display of those very same skills. This paradox, in turn, calls attention to the sheer variety in forms of autistic intelligence that children exhibit, in the clinic and elsewhere.

The present chapter begins with a case that exemplifies the paradox—the way that one kind of competence may undermine another kind. This will lead us to a more general consideration of how manifestations of autistic in-telligence are not idiosyncratic elements of the assessment process but per-vasive features in it. Just as autism biography and autobiography suggest the pervasiveness of such manifestations in everyday settings, we can see how, in the clinic, they are present in many if not most of the tasks children are asked to perform. Indeed, they are especially visible in instances where the child has difficulty with a task. Whereas the ADOS tends to homogenize such troubles by reducing them to a numerical rating, we find that no two children experience the same difficulty, and that the precise character of the difficulty or trouble can provide a point of entry into the child's own world. In other words, even as a child may officially be scored as having a deficit in their performance of a particular task, the sensemaking methods that led to the faulty performance can become visible by close attention to detailed features of the interaction. Our stance continues to be that such sensemaking methods, although overlooked diagnostically, can provide information about the child as an individual and the sorts of modifications to the social environment that would maximize quality of life for the child and others in that environment (as we further explore in chap. 8).

How First-Order Competence May Interfere with Second-Order Skills

Lyn Hadden was five years and ten months old when referred to CDDC in 1985 because of concerns about her development. According to her medical records, Lyn's parents and teachers reported that she was not progressing in school "as expected," would "daydream," had "difficulty expressing herself," and could get "frustrated easily." Eventually, after seeing a speech and language specialist, a psychologist, an audiologist, and a special education clinician, Lyn was found to have normal hearing and intelligence (math and reading were at grade level), but with some delays in the areas of sequencing, processing, and comprehending language. The clinicians concluded that Lyn had mild learning disabilities and recommended that she be evaluated again at a later date. She was not assessed for infantile autism or pervasive developmental disorder (PDD), the two autism-related categories available in the then-current version of the DSM (APA 1980). For that very reason, her case illustrates the generality of the phenomenon we are describing—the way first-order competence can obstruct second-order competence whether or not a person is identified as autistic.

Our example comes from Lyn's performance on the "blending" subtest of the Woodcock-Johnson (1977) cognitive exam, which was administered by special education clinician Dee Smith. The test involves the clinician breaking up words into phonetic components and saying them to the child, who is asked to merge the sounds into the appropriate word. Following test protocol, Dee began by reading a series of two-syllable words from the test booklet, each of which she broke into separate components. Lyn correctly blended the first few words ("win—dow" [window]; "muh—ther" [mother]; "tay—ble" [table]; and "can—dee" [candy]), all of which represented two-syllable words. Here, she seamlessly displayed second-order competence, effectively rendering the first-order competence that underlay her structural performance invisible.

However, when Dee next reads out the components of a one-syllable word ("ro—dah" [road]), Lyn blends them into something like "rhoda" instead of the required form. Even when Dee prompts her twice more, she continues to repeat "rhoda." Given her success with the previous five items, this seems unusual. But analytically, we can see and hear how Lyn tracks the *local history* of two-syllable words Dee has been reading to her. This is a first-order skill. We know from Sacks (cf. Maynard and Marlaire 1992:726) that in interaction, the "position of an item on a list is relevant to hearing what that item is," meaning that participants hear prior and current items as connected. Because the previous sound components in Dee's prompts all blended into two-syllable words, Lyn may also have been relying on the "poetics" of talk, which includes sound patterns and other aspects of prosody (Jefferson 1996), to identify a rhythmic model for solving the second-order problem. That model, which combines paired sound bursts into two-syllable words, worked for previous test items but leads to failure when the two-syllable pattern is disrupted by a one-syllable word.[1] Thus, it seems that Lyn deploys first-order competence in a way that interferes with her ability to display the second-order competence the test requires. Yet we can also observe that although she does not make sense in the way that the test expects, what she is doing is not nonsensical. It is methodical and competent in its own right, even if it produces an incorrect answer in this case. Importantly, her fundamental competence could possibly be used to illuminate her language difficulties, and then design more effective ways to work with her.

The fact that the paradoxical relationship between first- and second-order competence can show up in the assessment of a child who was not being evaluated for autism, and who in today's terms would be regarded as neurotypical, suggests a prototype for the way many children perform during testing. While their fundamental skills *enable* participation in the social activity of testing, for example by helping them recognize a test question as a question and produce an answer in the appropriate slot, such skills can also *disable* the very second-order performance they otherwise facilitate. We will see examples of this in the next section, which focuses on a boy we call Tony Smith. Our analysis will demonstrate how his displays of first-order competence are not just happenstance but occurrences exhibited across a variety of tests and other tasks. We then explore the kinds of autistic intelligence displayed by other children in response to a task on the ADOS. For Tony and these children, displays of autistic intelligence are pervasive and valuable sources of information about their particular characteristics and learning styles.

Commonsense Testing

Tony Smith was seven years and nine months old when school officials referred him to CDDC in 1985. According to his medical record, Tony's teachers reported "autistic-like" behaviors, neurological problems, and other difficulties and felt that a "whole picture" evaluation would be helpful in determining an appropriate class placement for him. His parents shared these concerns, and agreed with the school's referral for evaluation at the CDDC. To assess the matter, clinicians employed the then-operative third edition of the Diagnostic and Statistical Manual of Mental Disorders (APA 1980), which, for autism-related disorders, listed sixteen areas of impairment across three broad categories: "qualitative impairment in reciprocal social interaction," "qualitative impairment in verbal and nonverbal communication and in imaginative activity," and "markedly restricted repertoire of activities and interests."

In the 1980s, CDDC frequently assigned large teams of specialists to assess a child (today the teams are usually much smaller). In Tony's case, the specialists included a pediatric psychiatrist, pediatrician, social worker, special education clinician, speech and language pathologist, and occupational therapist, all of whom assessed Tony and interviewed his parents. They eventually diagnosed Tony with autism.[2]

Tony displayed a variety of first-order competencies across multiple tests. These competencies, however, received little or no notice. For the most part, they remained subterranean. Furthermore, when clinicians did notice them, it was usually in the form of a brief anecdote highlighting some positive aspect of Tony's behavior. We call this highlighting practice *anecdotal optimism*. Like the other practices we have been examining, anecdotal optimism is present in both our historical (1980s) and contemporary (2010s) data, as we will see later in the chapter when we once again consider the case of Dan Chapman. Overall, we suggest that while anecdotal optimism can have beneficial effects, it can also obscure or misinterpret first-order competencies.

The first example with Tony involves the Brigance subtest "Knows What to Do in Different Situations," which we saw Ronnie Martin doing in chapter 4. Recall that the skill being tested is described as "Gives appropriate responses for different situations" (Brigance 1978:172), a clear exhibit of how assessment can involve matters of common sense. Like Ronnie, Tony initially displayed disembedded knowledge, answering "What do you when you're hungry?" by saying, "You eat," and responding to "What do you do when you're sleepy?" with "You rest." However, when Laura Sims, the special education professional administering the test, asked, "What do you do when you're cold?" he ended up saying, "And then you get frozen."

It is possible to view Tony's answer as an instance of the sort of associational, literal thinking to which autistic individuals may be prone (Frith
2003:120–22). Examples abound in the literature. Grandin (1995:32) observes,
"For example, an autistic child might say the word 'dog' when he wants to go
outside. The word 'dog' is associated with going outside." About her grown
autistic daughter Jessy, Park (2001:41) reports, "So we read from the morning
paper: the company is downsizing. 'A certain number of people are going
to be cut.' '*Cut?!!*' The astonishment in her voice makes it plain: the autistic
literalism survives." While such literal and associational thinking are skills
in their own right, they can interfere with the display of second-order competence. On the Brigance subtest, Tony seems to be running question-and-
answer content together, as suggested by his "*and then*" formulation and its
implication that "getting frozen" is the consequence of being cold.[3] If so, he
is not competently orienting to the larger activity framework of testing—a
commonsense matter—which requires bounding off each question-answer
sequence from those that come before and after. Nevertheless, inspecting the
series of question-answer sequences in which "and then you get frozen" culminates, we find evidence of a skilled activity: building a narrative from the
test questions and their answers. In this narrative, by way of the pronoun or
categorical *pro-term* "you" (Sacks 1992a:342), someone is hungry, then eats,
then becomes sleepy, then rests (or falls asleep), then gets cold, and finally
becomes "frozen." That Tony produces such a narrative (and at least one other
one having to do with going in a dark room, watching TV, and falling asleep)
suggests that he is a creative, imaginative, and skilled storyteller with the
ability to construct a coherent chronicle from otherwise unrelated question-
answer pairs. This is a form of first-order competence that the test elicits but
does not recognize; indeed, within the framework of the test, it appears as
incompetence, as the *absence* of understanding the rules for participating in
the social activity of testing.[4] As a result, the examiner is prone to overlook
the competencies that are *present* in answers like Tony's.

To be more specific: although Tony sometimes fails to participate (or participate adequately) in Laura's commonsense world, *she also fails to participate in his different world.* Margaret Donaldson, whose concept of "decentering" we discussed in chapter 4, relates a story about a teacher who told Laurie
Lee,[5] then a young boy in his first-grade classroom, to "wait for the present"
after she called his name to check attendance. At the end of the day, Laurie
went home angry and dispirited. When his mother asked him what the matter was, he complained, "I sat there all day but I never got it"—the *present.*
Donaldson (1978:17) remarks, "The obvious first way to look at this episode
is to say that the child did not understand the adult. Yet it is clear on a very

little reflection that the adult also failed, at a deeper level, in understanding the child—in placing himself imaginatively at the child's point of view." Of course, the design and instructions—protocols—for administering the Brigance instrument do not encourage such decentering.

Even if—or perhaps because—the clinician does not decenter, the sense that Tony is or is not making remains a joint achievement produced (1) in conjunction with the design of the test instrument, particularly the order and structure of its questions, *and* (2) the cues the clinician inadvertently gives off by asking the questions in variable ways (Maynard 2005). First, the juxtaposition of questions and answers about hunger, tiredness, and coldness may elicit associations like the ones Tony displays, which illustrate how tests can intermingle with a participant's *un*common sensemaking practices. To coin a word for this feature, we suggest that testing instruments have an *interactive* component, which is to say that they are, in the terminology of Latour (1987), like "actants," which we discussed in chapter 4 (see also chap. 6). As Grandin (1995:27) remarks, visual thinking means "difficulty stopping endless associations." A single input can trigger another, and then another, with the different pieces of information combining in ways that have autistic coherence for the individual but not necessarily for those engaged in everyday commonsense reasoning, or as that reasoning is installed in psychological assessment. Test items can cue such associations for a child.

Second, in addition to their interactive component, Tony's answers have an *interactional* component. Laura's talk and gesturing may signal Tony in ways that tacitly encourage his narrative constructions during the "What do you do when" test, partly in response to the subtle linguistic manipulations in Tony's answers (Maynard and Turowetz 2017b). For example, at first she marks a boundary between her questions. After Tony answers "You eat" to the question about hunger, she says "okay" before asking about being "sleepy." However, after Tony says "You rest," she invokes the next question *without* any boundary marker. Instead, she immediately says, "What do you when you're cold?" The quickness may help to animate his associations. Additionally, following Tony's own use of a connective after the question about being "cold"—"*and* then you get frozen"—Laura uses that connective in her prompt, "And then, okay what else?" Connectives are prototypical ways of building a story—as well as maintaining other across-turn linkages (see note 6 and Heritage and Sorjonen 1994); such a device could encourage the construction of coherent storylike components from what are supposed to be disparate, disconnected question-answer pairs.

The tacit contributions of the clinician to the assessment process are similar to what happens in animal laboratories when experimenters attempt to prepare rats or other specimens for specific procedures. The "naturalistic ani-mal" must be actively transformed into the "analytic animal" that appears in published reports, which involves discounting its "subjective" qualities and making it countable for scientific purposes (Lynch 1988). In the process, how-ever, the experimenter's preparatory work disappears from view. In Tony's case, to elicit correct and accountable answers, the clinician is working not so much with his imputed subjective qualities but rather with his observable conduct. That such effort could actually undermine the goal of answering correctly is outside the clinician's awareness, in much the same way that a metronome escapes the awareness of the musician working with it (see chap. 4 and Garfinkel 2002). In consequence, both the child's first-order competen-cies and the practices that occasion them are not visible in the clinician's final evaluation report.[6]

In sum, Tony's failure at second-order, structural competence may be related to the very first-order competencies that reveal themselves on close inspection and that the clinician and test coproduce but do not officially reg-ister. As discussed in chapter 4, these competencies are subterranean. Tony's methods for making sense of the test questions are not shared by Laura or the creators of the Brigance, and they are easily overlooked or dismissed as incompetence—in other words, he is seen to fail at performing the structural task. It is as if autistic intelligence and its uncommon sense are hidden in plain sight. Appreciating that intelligence requires moving out of the clinical gaze and into an interactional one.

DOES TONY KNOW WHAT IS REAL?

A second example of Tony's autistic use of first-order competence emerges when Laura is giving him a subtest from the Psychoeducational Profile (Schop-ler and Reichler 1979). On this subtest, the child is shown pictures of two similar objects and asked to explain how they differ (Turowetz 2015b). The objects are distinguished in terms of general concepts such as height, size, and shape. For example, presented with a picture of a tall boy standing next to a short one, a child needs to distinguish them in terms of height. In one part of the test, Laura shows Tony a picture of two cups, one empty and the other full. Laura asks, "Which one is empty?" and Tony points to the correct one, after which Laura says, "If this one is empty, what is this one?" (pointing to the one that is pictured as full). Tony's answer is "Pour in."

Insofar as "Pour in" is not a test-relevant answer, or one that could dem-onstrate Tony's grasp of an abstract concept (at least per the test's definition; cf. Piaget 1952), it constitutes a failure of second-order competence. But neither

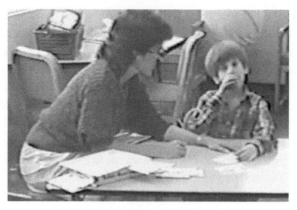

FIGURE 5.1. Tony pretends to sip.

is the answer unintelligible (or "from outer space," as it were). Tony goes on to ask if he and Laura could drink from the cup. This could be an effort to initiate pretend play, raising the possibility that his "Pour in" comment was not meant as a disembedded "answer" but a first-order directive for Laura to take her turn drinking from the cup picture. Then, as Tony takes an imaginary sip from the cup (see fig. 5.1), Laura responds, "It doesn't come off—it's only pretend."

During the test and in a subsequent conversation with her colleagues, Laura interprets Tony's question "Can you drink it?" and his sipping gesture as confusing a *real* cup with an *image* of a cup. She proposes that Tony may not be able to distinguish reality from image, although the clinicians finally decide that Tony's questions about drinking from the cup were "problem-solving" strategies. However, neither interpretation—that he cannot distinguish reality or that he is problem-solving—nor the possibility that Tony was initiating pretend play, makes their way into the official diagnosis or reportage about Tony, and the clinicians' assessment is that he is operating below age level on tasks like these in a way that fits with his autism diagnosis (Turowetz 2015b). Seeing that Tony's efforts could be play-initiations requires an interactional gaze rather than a clinical one.

WHOSE ACTIVITY IS GOING TO PREVAIL?

In a third example of first-order competence, Tony was asked to assemble the six rectangular pieces of a puzzle into the image of a cow (fig. 5.2). Like the previous example, this task is part of the Psychoeducational Profile (Schopler and Reichler 1979). After a previous puzzle task, and starting rather abruptly with "You try this puzzle for me," Laura issues a series of *directives* (e.g., "Can you make a picture of a cow?"; cf. Goodwin 2006) that encode varying degrees of entitlement—markers of her right to compel Tony to participate in the second-order activity of assembling the puzzle (Curl and Drew 2008). Tony never succeeds at this task.[7]

Although he may fail at the structural task of assembling the picture as such, Tony pursues a variety of differently competent activities, such as manipulating the puzzle pieces, lining them up, and lifting a piece as if it were a hinged door. He also issues "counter-directives" (cf. Schegloff 2007b:16–18) by telling Laura to "watch" and then quickly moving the pieces around in ways that she could monitor (see chap. 8). In this way, he works to enlist Laura in his activity instead of participating in hers. When Laura offers help, Tony says, "No don't help me!" with increased volume and pitch. For a while, Laura complies with Tony's own admonitions, then again attempts to elicit his cooperation in assembling the puzzle before finally giving up and transitioning to another task.

And so, because Tony does not at all seem oriented to doing the test and assembling the cow picture, he fails to display second-order competence. Instead, he is self-attentively immersed in his own activity. In a sense, Tony is planted in a three-dimensional and tactile world through touching, holding, and seeing such matters as setting the puzzle edges in line. Laura, by contrast, is proposing a local but collaborative world in which the corporeality of experience is subordinate to talk-based instructions and the assembly of a two-dimensional picture. This tension between two- and three-dimensional activities persists throughout the episode, and it parallels another tension between orienting to an externally imposed plan and—as a feature of what we

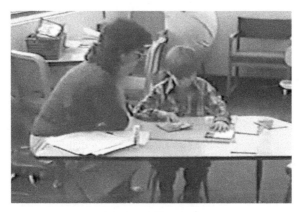

FIGURE 5.2. Cow puzzle

discussed earlier about the interactivity of the test instrument—to the palpable availability of the puzzle pieces themselves.

Clinicians refer to the episode involving the cow puzzle in later discussions among themselves and with Tony's family, which allows us to define the matter of anecdotal optimism. This is a pattern by which a clinician (or parent) reports on the child's action, assesses it positively, and provides a benign psychological interpretation of it. Accordingly, in the informing interview with Tony's parents, Molly Gardner, the psychiatrist and team lead on the case, asked the other clinicians if they had an example of "concepts" on which Tony was "currently working." Laura, who administered the Psychoeducational Profile cow puzzle test item, volunteered an account referring to the episode, saying, "A while ago, he wanted help with everything. And now, when you want to offer help, he's sort of rejecting." She remarks that although this could be interpreted as "contrary behavior," she sees it in a more positive light: it was really a "struggle" with "being a little more independent." Molly concurred, adding, "And it goes along with the emergence of his showing pride in being able to do things."

The clinicians' anecdotal optimism formulates a *psychological* version of Tony's behavior, while the *interactional* competence he exhibited—being able to compete with Laura for which activity would transpire with the puzzle pieces—is neglected. So too is the possibility of exploring the implications of his skill at appropriating aspects of the testing environment—its "affordances" (Gibson 1986)—or at least those of this particular subtest, for his own purposes. He devises a unique set of tasks for the puzzle pieces, and he is able, at least briefly, to involve his adult interlocutor in these tasks, if only as a participant observer. Moreover, in a pattern of interactional conduct that has been documented in other research, and that we will show in chapter 8, when Laura aligns to Tony's initiatives, *then* he also cooperates with hers.

Our point in exploring three instances of Tony Smith's first-order competence is to show both how prevalent *and* how heterogeneous it can be, even for a single individual. In our data, forms of autistic intelligence appear regularly and pervasively across testing and subtesting environments for any given child. Moreover, recalling the paradox we introduced at the beginning of this chapter, the practices of first-order competence that can enable the display of second-order or structural competence in testing may be the very ones that interfere with exhibiting such competence (and its association with second-order typical development). Because they reflect matters that are taken to be indicative of autism—associative thinking in the "What do you do when" environment; ambiguous social initiatives with the picture of an empty cup; or seemingly obsessive preoccupations with the pieces of a puzzle—such behaviors may have diagnostic relevance. However, they also have other dimensions that can only be called (as we have been calling them) intelligent. Yet the particular forms by which this intelligence is expressed seldom show up in the diagnostic profiles that are shared with parents, schools, or others in arenas where the child will be participating.

Compared to stories about a child's *general tendencies*, those about the *instances* in which autistic intelligence is exhibited, such as the examples above involving Tony Smith, are rare. We explore this imbalance in chapter 6, and further demonstrate how anecdotal optimism only highlights psychological or humorous features of the behavior, rather than drawing insights about the child's fundamental competence, autistic intelligence, and uncommon sense, which represent significant points of entry into the child's world and methods of sensemaking.

Autistic Intelligence as a Child's Distinctive Expression

It may be tempting to think that autistic intelligence is homogenous across the spectrum. Because autistic children share a diagnosis, it is easy to make the mistake of assuming that they will display the same kinds of what we are calling first-order, fundamental competence, often at the expense of second-order, structural skill. The interactional facts, however, tell a different story. In considering how Tony's first-order competence may be excavated from beneath the surface of testing, we illustrated the varied forms such competence can take, even in the same child. This section of the chapter, by examining the various ways in which children on the autism spectrum "fail" at an ADOS activity called the Demonstration Task, demonstrates further that autistic intelligence is heterogenous and indicative of particularized competencies.

We document a range of first-order competencies exhibited by a set of children as they adjust to the second-order demands of the ADOS, and the ways those competencies can interfere with their ability to meet such demands. To put the matter of heterogeneity differently, whereas success on the ADOS tends to be rather uniform, failures are unique: no two children fail in the same way, and *how* they fail can offer valuable information about their ways of sensemaking. The analytic strategy is to inspect the failures for their orderliness, thereby discerning the uncommon sense that remains invisible when the child is rated on the basis of what they *did not do*—for example, show joint attention, make eye contact, or engage in back-and-forth conversation—rather than on what they did and how they did it.

As they make uncommon sense of their environment, children exhibit individual skills and propensities that both affect, and are affected by, their interactions with other agents, including not just their clinical interlocutors, but also assessment tools and their design features. Though excavating these skills from the subterranean level may not affect a child's eventual diagnosis per se, we suggest once more that knowing of their existence can lend to working with the child and adapting to their particularities, as well as helping them adapt to those of the neurotypical world.[8]

THE DEMONSTRATION TASK

The Demonstration Task is an activity on the ADOS-2 that is designed to assess "the participant's ability to communicate about a familiar series of actions using gesture or mime with accompanying language" (Lord et al. 2012:113).[9] The test manual instructs the clinician to say, using appropriate demonstrative gestures and motions, "Let's pretend that this is the sink, this is the hot water, and this is the cold water," and then, "pretend to draw the toothbrush." Next, the clinician should state, "Now I want you to show me and tell me how to brush my teeth. Start right at the beginning. You've just come into the bathroom to brush your teeth. What do you do now?" In our analysis, we look at four cases where children—three of whom eventually received an autism diagnosis—responded to the Demonstration Task in atypical ways. Of particular interest here are the heterogeneous forms of first-order competence the children exhibit and its relationship to the second-order activity they are being asked to perform.

DEMONSTRATION TASK EXAMPLE 1: DAN

Recall that at the time of his evaluation, Dan Chapman was nine years old and in the third grade at school and that he was referred to the CDDC because of his "significant behavioral challenges," a history of aggressive and disruptive behavior at school, difficulty with two-way conversations, and other matters. After Dr. Jennifer Erickson explained what they would be doing, and then rather awkwardly asked Dan if he wanted his mom "in the room for this" (chap. 3), she went ahead to administer the ADOS. This included the Demonstration Task, which she initiated in the scripted way by laying out the imaginary sink and objects and using a variety of "directive" forms, asking Dan to "show me and tell me how you brush your teeth." As she does this,

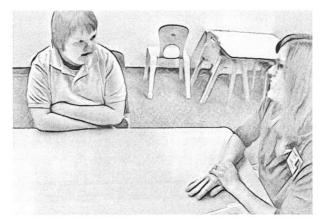

FIGURE 5.3A

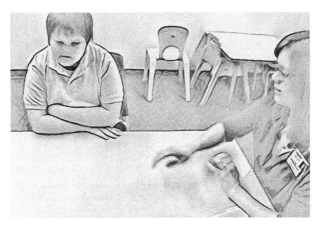

FIGURE 5.3B

Dan trains his gaze on Jennifer, only looking away as he begins to shake his head horizontally in an indication of refusal (see fig. 5.3a, 5.3b).[10]

After the initial directives and Dan's consistent refusals, Jennifer follows the test protocol that specifies how to handle noncompliance. She is to show how to drive a car. But as she goes through the steps involved ("I put the key in the ignition, turn it on"), Dan still shakes his head laterally in a show of resistance. There is an exception at one point, when he claims to have already learned about driving a car. Jennifer says, "You do?" but after Dan nods affirmatively, she returns to her car-driving demonstration. As she resumes her demonstration, Dan again resists, which he signals with two lateral movements of his head. Upon completing the demonstration, Jennifer takes the next step in the protocol, which is to ask Dan to "show me and tell me how you'd wash your face." In serially responding to this and another subsequent series of such directives, Dan shakes his head six more times. Finally, he gets up from the chair, leaves the table at which he was sitting, and kneels in the corner of the room (behind a chair) close to where his mother is sitting, as Jennifer says, "You don't wanna try that one? Okay." In all, Dan has refused participation quietly but firmly more than a dozen times across multiple efforts on Jennifer's part to elicit a demonstration.

Although Jennifer eventually reengaged Dan in testing, they never did complete the Demonstration Task. In our next chapter (6), we will see how Jennifer and colleagues made sense of Dan's withdrawal behavior, which Jennifer will describe as "his most atypical response"—but without reference to the interactional particulars that occasioned it. We will also see how, in discussing the episode, she shows anecdotal optimism.

DEMONSTRATION TASK EXAMPLE 2: JUSTIN

According to his medical records, ten-year-old Justin Campbell was referred to CDDC because school personnel had "observed some borderline signs of ASD," including "social communication difficulties." His parents reported that Justin "had a one track mind," that it was difficult to get him to follow directions, and that he "tends to be anxious" and worry more than is warranted. Both the school and the parents were concerned about his "difficult interaction with peers." At CDDC, a psychiatrist, Dr. Elizabeth Smithson, who diagnosed Justin with ASD, did so with the provision that an anxiety disorder, which may have been interfering with his execution of tasks on the ADOS, needed to be ruled out.

Elizabeth begins the task in a unique way. After finding out that Justin has three younger siblings, she says, "Okay, so pretend that your seven-month-old sister, pretend that she is now two. Okay, and you are gonna teach her, pretend I'm her, you're gonna teach ME how ta brush my teeth, okay?" (We have given the pseudonym "Anna" to Justin's sister.) Then she produces the directive below:

5.4 CASE 44. DEMO:1 (NORMALIZED)

```
Eliz: So pretend that this is the sink (.) here's the cold water, here's the
      hot water, here's the water spout, here's a toothbrush, here's some
      toothpaste and here's a glass of water. So you come into the bathroom
      and what do you do?
Just: (Take the hand that Anna wants (0.3) hh put some (    ) on and then gel
      and put the toothpaste on then put water on. Brush.
Eliz: Okay, okay, very good, very good.
```

Justin's performance of the Demonstration Task is the tersest one in our collection. Figure 5.4 shows how he holds his head with his left hand and arm

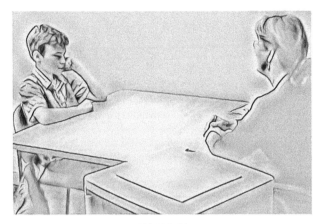

FIGURE 5.4

while gazing down at the table for the entire time. He uses no gestures. Often, according to protocol, a clinician will prompt the child for gestures, but in this case, Elizabeth elects not to do that.

The performance or nonperformance of the Demonstration Task on the ADOS can affect scoring in two ways. First, for the task itself, there is a half-page section of the booklet that poses the following questions:

(1) Does the child represent familiar actions in gesture?
   -If so, how does he or she do this?
   -Does the child use his or her body to represent an object (e.g., a finger for a toothbrush) or mime the use of a pretend object?
(2) Evaluate the child's report of a routine event and the pragmatics of teaching a sequence of actions.

On this page, for Justin, the psychiatrist simply wrote, "0 gesture."

In another section of the ADOS, there is a list of "Language and Communication Skills" that clinicians are to evaluate during the entire course of the examination. These include, for example, whether there is echolalia or frequent repetition of previous speech, stereotyped or unique uses of words or phrases, and, pertinent to the Demonstration Task, item "A9. Descriptive, Conventional, Instrumental, or Information Gestures" (fig. 5.5). For this item, on Module 2 of the ADOS, clinicians are instructed to include behaviors that occur during the Demonstration Task. As figure 5.5 shows, the lower the rating, the better a child does in terms of gesture use; conversely, a higher rating indicates limited gesturing. In Justin's case, Elizabeth put a 3, suggesting that Justin is lacking in this skill.

A9. Descriptive, Conventional, Instrumental, or Informational Gestures

The focus of this item is on descriptive gestures that enact or represent an object or event (such as acting out rinsing a toothbrush or showing how a roller coaster curves through the air). Gestures that are conventional (e.g., clapping for "well done"), informational, or instrumental (e.g., pointing, shrugging, head nodding, or head shaking) receive partial credit. When coding, exclude emphatic gestures (e.g., "beats" accompanying speech); include behaviors that occur during the "Demonstration Task" and throughout the ADOS-2 evaluation. The emphasis is on how the participant uses gestures before he or she is prompted or asked to do so, or gestures that the participant adds as he or she responds to a requested description (e.g., pretending to spit after demonstrating how to use a toothbrush, as requested). Pointing is included here as an instrumental gesture, as it is not coded separately in Module 3. Grabbing and reaching are not coded here.

 0 = Spontaneous use of several descriptive gestures. These gestures may be typical or idiosyncratic, but must be communicative. May also use conventional or instrumental gestures.

1 = Some spontaneous use of descriptive gestures, but exaggerated or limited in range and/or contexts (e.g., occur only during "Demonstration Task"), OR frequent use of conventional or instrumental gestures, but rare or no use of descriptive gestures.

2 = Some spontaneous use of informational, conventional, or instrumental gestures, but rare or no use of descriptive gestures.

3 = No or very limited spontaneous use of conventional, instrumental, informational, or descriptive gestures.

8 = N/A (e.g., limited by physical disability).

FIGURE 5.5. Scoring the demonstration task

DEMONSTRATION TASK EXAMPLE 3: SARA

Sara Brennan came to CDDC when she was three years old. Her case turned out to be diagnostically ambiguous, and for that reason it illustrates the difficulties that clinicians face with children who seem to fall on the borderline between developing "typically" and having ASD. To appreciate these challenges and put further flesh to the body of working tasks that autism testing and diagnosis involves, we return to Sara's case in chapter 7.

Sara's family doctor initiated the request for an evaluation at CDDC for "developmental delay and concern for social interaction." Previously, Sara was found to have language and gross motor delays, and she had received remedial services through a "birth-to-three" intervention program. When the family was seen at CDDC, the team evaluating Sara consisted of a developmental pediatrician, who interviewed the parents, and a psychologist, who administered the ADOS. A speech and language clinician (whom we call Aaron Schultz) sat in and observed the ADOS to assess Sara's language, since he could not conduct a separate evaluation because of scheduling conflicts.[11] However, as we will see, his role was crucial in helping to determine her diagnosis.

Sara's performance during the Demonstration Task was very different from others we witnessed. Per the ADOS instructions, the psychologist, Dr. Ruth McCain, lays out the imaginary sink, faucets, toothbrush, and cup, and gives Sara the instruction, "I want you to show and tell me how to brush my teeth." In response, Sara gets up from her chair and starts walking across the room, as Ruth then says, "Wait! How do you do brush your teeth?" But Sara is seeking, and brings back, a box of tissues that sits atop an end table near the sofa where her parents are seated. As Sara returns to the exam table, Ruth says, "Oh you needed tissues?" Sara then sets the tissue box down and pretends to sneeze, engaging in a small jump as she does so. Ruth responds, "How do you brush your teeth? Show me," and Sara "sneezes" again, simultaneously and once more jumping up from her seat and grabbing a tissue that she puts to her nose (fig. 5.6). Ruth then proposes, "Oh you're pretending to sneeze?" and adds a display of recognition, "Ohhhhhhh." She tells Sara to "go throw it away," and Sara discards the tissue in a small trash can nearby.

Subsequently, following ADOS protocols, Ruth tries a different tack, retrieving a towel and a box with soap from the accompanying bag of implements and asking Sara to "show and tell me how you wash your face." This time, Sara takes the soap out of the box and appears to mime face washing,

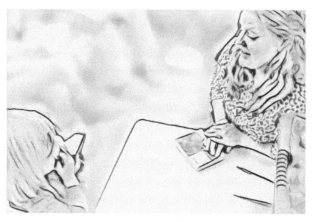

FIGURE 5.6

but after Ruth asks her, "Can you tell me too what you're doing?" Sara only continues to mime. Then the following transpires:

TRANSCRIPT 5.6: CASE 34: DEMO:2 (NORMALIZED)

```
Ruth:    ((points to Sara's hands)) What'ya doing?
Sara:    Wash my hands.
Ruth:    ((vertical head shake)) You're washing your hands.
Sara:    Yep.
Ruth:    M'kay.
Sara:    Done.
Ruth:    All done? Then what?
Sara:    We done.
Ruth:    You're all done.
```

After this, and after Sara asks about Ruth's phone, Ruth moves to another ADOS activity.

We do not have the ADOS scoring for Sara, but because she does not gesture much, even on the face-washing task, and does not produce vocal descriptions, it is likely that item A7 (fig. 5.5) would have been a 2 or 3. We do know that Ruth and the developmental pediatrician who saw Sara at CDDC wrote in their medical summary that Sara had "Deficits in nonverbal communicative behaviors used for social interaction; ranging from poorly integrated verbal and nonverbal communication, through abnormalities in eye contact and body-language." This characterization, it is also noted, is drawn from and quotes the DSM-5 criteria for ASD. In the summary, Ruth also made a separate and succinct remark about Sara: "[She] has more success when language is removed," while the speech and language specialist who observed Sara diagnosed "Significant expressive language disorder and childhood apraxia of speech" (apraxia denotes a motor speech disorder).

DEMONSTRATION TASK EXAMPLE 4: MAX

Max Bailey was five years and four months old at the time of his evaluation. Although Max was not diagnosed with autism (as we discuss in chap. 7), his case sheds light on the others we discuss, all of which involve the diagnosis.

Dr. Ellen Miller, the psychologist, has given Max a test of cognitive ability (the Differential Abilities Scales–II) before starting the ADOS. As part of the ADOS, she engages him in a series of tasks culminating in a pretend birthday party for a toy baby. She then goes immediately into the Demonstration Task. As she puts away the props from the previous task, Ellen announces that she and Max "need to play a pretend game" in which "I need you to be the teacher and teach me how to brush my teeth." On the table, she then identifies a sink, toothpaste, toothbrush, and water and asks, "Can you show me and tell me how do I brush my teeth? What do I do?" Max repeats part of Ellen's question, saying "Brush your teeth?" and Ellen confirms his understanding with "Yeah," followed by a directive to "show me" (line 1 below). Max opens his mouth in a smile formation, and moving his head from side to side, he moves his hand—in a kind of fist formation that can indicate holding a toothbrush—back and forth across his mouth (line 2) to mime brushing (see fig. 5.7).

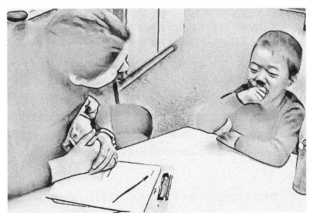

FIGURE 5.7

As Max does this movement (line 2), he simultaneously makes a hissing noise, possibly simulating the sound of running water or the toothbrush moving across his teeth.

TRANSCRIPT 5.7: CASE 18: DEMO:1

```
 1  Ell:    Yeah. (0.4) You do it (.) You show me how it works.
 2  Max:    SH:: ((Max motions like he is rubbing his hand over his face))
 3  Ell:    Uh huh:,
 4          ((Max puts his fist up to his mouth; Ellen nods))
 5  Max:    Ah:::!
 6  Ell:    Okay now what do you do you go ((mimics brushing and sound)) and
 7          then what.
 8  Max:    ((puts fist to mouth)) PH:::t
 9  Ell:    And then what do you do after that.
10          (.)
11  Max:    Blihht!
12  Ell:    SPIT! GOOD JOB, good jo:(h)b. .hh ex:ce:llent okay.
```

Ellen responds with a continuer ("Uh huh," line 3) that encourages elaboration, and Max makes a fist and raises it to his mouth (line 4), as if to mime drinking water. As he does this, Ellen affirms Max's gesture by nodding vertically (also line 4). After moving his fist away from his mouth, Max produces a sharp exhale (line 5). Ellen prompts Max to supply the next action in the sequence (lines 6–7), and he puts his fist to his mouth again and exhales sharply (line 8). Ellen next prompts him to produce a subsequent ("after that") action (line 9), and Max makes a vocalization that sounds like a combination of the word "spit" and the acoustics of actually spitting (line 11) as he bends over the imaginary sink. Finally, Ellen registers his answer with a characterization of what he has done ("SPIT!") and positive assessment (line 12).

Compared with Justin, Max uses more gestures and makes more eye contact. He shows positive affect (e.g., smiling) and seems engaged in the activity. Furthermore, while his use of language is minimal, he does use words in competent ways, such as requesting clarification (by repeating part of Ellen's instructions) and answering a question (demonstrating "spit"). At the same time, however, Ellen scaffolds or buttresses his demonstration when she prompts him for missing items and elaborations in the task, which suggests a performance that is not fully adequate by ADOS standards.[12]

First-Order Competence in the ADOS Demonstration Task

In none of our four examples did the child perform the Demonstration Task in the way ADOS defines as fully, structurally correct. According to test criteria, a competent demonstration involves the coordination of explanatory talk and gesture, as well as interactional engagement and embodied orientation to the clinician giving the test. Thus, while all of the children exhibited *some* second-order competence—even Sara eventually participated in the face-washing demonstration—none of them completely satisfied the test's definition of a structurally competent performance that would include both vocal and gestural, embodied expressions. (When we underwent ADOS training at CDDC in 2015, which we further describe below, we saw video footage of a full-fledged performance by a typically developing twelve-year-old, who performed competently on all dimensions.) According to the DSM (APA 2013) and ADOS criteria, undertakings like the Demonstration Task showed each of these children to have "clinically significant, persistent deficits in social communication and interactions, as manifested by . . . the following:"[13]

a. Marked deficits in nonverbal and verbal communication used for social interaction
b. Lack of social reciprocity

These characteristics ring true even for Max, for whom the clinicians eventually ruled out the autism diagnosis (chap. 7), which—alongside the example of Lyn and the "blending" subtest—show how more typically developing children can manifest traits that are otherwise consistent with autism. For the three children doing the Demonstration Task who come to share the autism diagnosis, that label conceals the diversity of their performances by assimilating them to a set of homogeneous criteria. This matter of how children perform in diverse ways on the ostensibly same task once again brings forward the individuality of any given child.

"IF YOU KNOW ONE CHILD WITH AUTISM, YOU KNOW ONE CHILD WITH AUTISM"

From our most recent CDDC collection of 49 cases, we have a subcollection of twelve in which the ADOS Demonstration Task was administered. For two of the children (including Max), autism was ruled out as a diagnosis, while for the other ten (including Dan, Justin, and Sara), clinicians arrived at an ASD diagnosis. Although above, we examined just four out of this dozen, it can be said that every child in this subcollection performed the task in particular—and sometimes interestingly idiosyncratic—ways.

As the familiar saying goes, this could simply reflect the fact that "everybody is different." However, we have an angle on the matter coming from our ethnomethodological perspective (Garfinkel and Wieder 1992). Each social situation is marked with its singularity, uniqueness, "just-thisness," or haecceity, which exists not in the solitariness of the child's own "performance" taken as his or her own manifestation, but rather in the relation between what is asked of or prompted from the child, on the one hand, and the way the child makes sense of this initiation, on the other. Such singularity could not be otherwise, and it is why the truism in the subtitle for this section of the chapter about "knowing one child with autism" resonates with lived experience: while autistic intelligence can be said to exhibit common features across the spectrum that provide for its coherence as a social phenomenon, each person has unique methods for making sense autistically and in interaction with their social environment. Accordingly, the singularity of the autistic person is a particular and situated accomplishment. For the environments in which the person resides, rather than (only) asking the person to take on the trappings of tacit understandings that pervade ordinary everyday life, the commonsense world can be tailored more closely to the person. Surely, if the family of Greta Thunberg, and the larger world of agencies and individuals concerned with climate change, can adjust to and accommodate her experiences and reasoning, then our smaller scale communities, schools, and families have the capacity for making similar adjustments to common sense, however pervasive and otherwise solid it seems to be.

Can autism diagnosis help in such endeavors? Potentially, though practitioners would need to address a number of challenges currently built into the diagnostic process, including its conception of autism in terms of deficits, the often subtle contributions of clinicians and their assessment tools to children's behavior in the clinic, and the way the ADOS and other instruments may inadvertently affect a child's behavior, while also structuring the clinician's perception of that behavior. We address these issues in the remainder of the chapter.

ASD AS DEFICIT

It is a well-known fact, obvious on the surface of DSM statements of diagnostic criteria, that the rating systems for the ADOS and other assessment tools for autism are deficit oriented. Of course, this is not different from diagnostic processes involving any seeming bodily or mental anomaly, where "even if we assume that virtually all *symptoms* exist on a spectrum, there is a point at which symptoms suddenly break from expected patterns" and a "threshold" is crossed (Schnittker 2017:220). Clinicians specializing in mental illness or disability are not different, in this respect, from their colleagues who diagnose and treat organic disease, and whose concern is with pathological deviations from biological health. Furthermore, across the range of illnesses, diagnosis occurs through a process known as "subtractive abstraction" (Abbott 1988; Cassirer 1953[1923]; Foucault 1973; Martin 2011; Mirowsky and Ross 1989). As Abbott (1988:40–41) writes, "Diagnosis not only seeks the right professional category for a client, but also removes the client's extraneous qualities" (cf. Mirowsky and Ross 1989:12). In the case of developmental disorders, clinicians need to document how a child is *disabled*. As a result, clinical discussions about diagnosis, medical records, and treatment recommendations may make it seem as if children diagnosed with ASD are homogeneous carriers of marked deficits who are similarly—if not uniformly—lacking in typical traits. All three of the children with ASD in our examples of the Demonstration Task could be said— and were said—to be so "marked" by means of diagnostic descriptions that obscured the details of their actual, real-time performances.

Among the details that each child's diagnosis subtracts (their age, gender, family background, geographic residence, and others) are the specific forms of first-order competence and autistic intelligence they display during testing, as well as the ways they use those competencies to participate—even if unsuccessfully—in second-order activities. Thus, in resisting Jennifer's attempts to engage him, Dan was extremely patient before finally disengaging from the task. Justin was succinct but precise in his verbal descriptions, and Sara was energetic and playful as she enacted her interpretations of the task. Her curious response to the "show me and tell me" directive may exhibit what Wootton (2002:151) has described as a mode of involvement where a child has diminished regard for local matters and instead leans on knowledge that they bring to an event. That is, perhaps Sara has recently learned or participated in an instructional or other practice involving the pretense of sneezing and using a tissue and so orients the ADOS "pretend" directive in terms of that more familiar routine. And in our example of a more typically developing child, who nevertheless was scored unfavorably on the Demonstration Task, Max shows that he possesses the skills for both showing and telling how to brush one's teeth, even if he does not coordinate them in the way the assessment requires.

Yet these first-order competences, and the distinct ways children draw on them for second-order performances under what can be described as arbitrary, test-furnished conditions, may provide avenues for the development of skill sets. Could Dan's claim of knowledge about learning to drive be exploited by asking him to give a verbal and embodied explanation of driving? Could Justin expand on his correct but brusque verbal output? Could we find out where Sara's orientation to the brushing-teeth request was acquired and how it became transformed into a sneezing routine to see what would improve her understanding of a quite different directive? Could Max's effective but nonvocal portrayal of brushing his teeth be accompanied by better verbal output?

Could such considerations, in their specificity, inform the recommendations that clinicians, after diagnosing a child or even ruling out a diagnosis, provide for family members, school personnel, and others who deal with a particular child, as opposed to the generic one in diagnostic manuals and nomenclatures?

Even more, could the behaviors a child exhibits in these contexts provide information about adjustments that commonsense actors could make in more everyday contexts? The most dramatic possibility relates to Dan's patient-seeming responses to the more than a dozen entreaties to demonstrate brushing his teeth. Although Jennifer was persistent in directing him to do the task, she showed restraint in many ways, simply changing the syntax of her directives and at no point intensifying them in a more demanding way. Dan's ultimate withdrawal was complementarily quiet and restrained, suggesting that he has a set of skills for avoiding uncomfortable circumstances and that there may be more to the interactional stories about what are described in his medical record as "meltdowns," incidents that "have required seclusion and/or restraint procedures," and tendencies to "escalate" at school.[14]

Interaction and Interactivity

We have said that the assessment process is both interactional and interactive. How might some slight alteration in the way clinicians present tasks to a child affect their performance? Consider what clinicians often—but far from always—say before asking for the tooth-brushing demonstration: In the episode with Dan Chapman, recall how Jennifer stated, "So the next thing I'd like to do is kinda silly." Similarly, with a 13-year-old boy, who was not diagnosed with autism (case 28), Jennifer said, "So I want you to show me and tell me how to brush my teeth," then continued, "I'm from another planet okay? And I don't know how to brush my teeth. All right, it's pretty silly." Such characterizations, while aiming to lighten the upcoming task,[15] may elicit varied reactions depending on the age of the examinee. Hollin and Pilnick (2018:1221) document an instance with an adult with ASD who was tested with the ADOS:

```
Dee:  Next thing (0.9) this one you might feel a bit silly doing it mm
      hmm, but can you imagine (.) that I::'m just a:: small child and
      erm (.) Well (.) I'm a small child and I don't know how to: make a
      cup of tea. Can you show and tell me how to make a cup of tea, if
      say the kettle is he::re, the mug's he:re, tea bag is here. Can you
      show and tell me?
      (3.7)
Joe:  Hhh:: (.) no (.) no I [can't]
Dee:                        [No  ] (.) why's that?
Joe:  Cause I can't imagine you to be a ch(h)ild
```

Joe has difficulty with imagining the clinician to be a child, a category that is fitted to feeling "a bit silly." When a nine-year-old boy like Dan is supposed to do something "silly," could that also be a disincentive? At a more subtle level, what other cues might a clinician inadvertently provide that affect how a child performs? For instance, in example 2, Elizabeth asked for Justin's performance, not in the standard way ("pretend that I don't know how to brush my teeth"), but in a somewhat confusing fashion by first eliciting information about his siblings; then asking Justin to do the task for his younger (seven-month-old) sister by pretending that she is "two"; then asking him to pretend that she, the clinician Elizabeth, is the sister; and finally, directing Justin to "teach ME how to brush my teeth." Given that Justin suffers from anxiety, this may have been an effort to put him more at ease. But could this awkward-seeming presentation, which differs from the script substantially, have had the opposite effect?

We have also seen that the interactive features of the test instrument affect a child's performance. The Demonstration Task interweaves a complex set of imaginative and performative elements: the need to "see" a sink and other implements that the clinician draws on the table with her finger (minimally, as the ADOS instructs her); the differently formulated proposal to "pretend" that "I don't know how to brush my teeth"; the requirement to give a verbal account of the task at the same time one is miming it; and so on. Just which of these features—or others—might make the task difficult or misleading for a given child?

The ADOS as a Way of Seeing (and Not Seeing)

When clinicians administer the ADOS, they take its interactive (instrument-related) and interactional (participatory) features for granted, in the sense that such features occupy the tacit background relative to the focal issue of whether a child is showing structural competence—whether they are providing correct or incorrect answers or engaging in appropriate or inappropriate social conduct relative to the "presses" that the ADOS administrator implements. Indeed, an important part of becoming a competent examiner is learning to see children's behavior in instrument-relevant terms, code the behavior into correct categories, and accurately score its patterning. For example, where a layperson might simply see a child raising their hand, clinicians learn to see such actions as potential communicative gestures and discriminate them from noncommunicative gestures: Is the child facing the clinician or another person? Is the child making "eye contact," or gazing into the "middle distance"? Does the child return the gaze of the clinician or parent? Is the child using language in conjunction with the gesture? And so on.

Developing this evaluative skill set takes time and effort. We learned this directly when, as mentioned earlier, we participated in an ADOS-training seminar. It was a three-day course designed to introduce novices to the rudiments of ADOS administration, although more experienced practitioners also attended. As part of the training, we watched video footage of two children being evaluated on the ADOS, one of them autistic, the other neurotypical. After viewing the first tape (of the child with autism), we each coded the behavior, jotting notes in designated areas of the scoring sheet as we went along. Then we broke into groups to discuss our decisions and scores. While everyone agreed that the boy in the video was autistic, there was much disagreement about how to score individual items: for example, after the clinician called his name, was the child gazing at her when he glanced in her direction? Or was he merely responding to what he perceived as a noise, rather than to a summons that the clinician produced? How could we know? We also commiserated about how difficult it was to juggle the logistics of testing: administering activities, paying attention to the child while recording observations and scores, deciding whether something (e.g., the aforementioned raised hand) counts as an assessment-relevant observation, and so forth. We then repeated the process for the second video (of a typically developing child).

Later, during a general question-and-answer session, we heard one veteran clinician, a developmental pediatrician, describe her experience with the ADOS over the recent years of its implementation in the clinic. She explained that at first she was skeptical of the ADOS. It struck her as hopelessly subjective, and she resented having to convert her clinical impressions, honed through years of working with autistic children and using different instruments, into quantitative indices associated with ADOS protocols. However, she went on to say that as she used the protocol more and the scoring process became familiar, she grew to appreciate and approve of it. Although she still had doubts about categorizing and scoring specific behaviors, she had grown comfortable with the instrument as a whole and confident about the objectivity of its results.

In effect, this clinician described the path practitioners follow as they become competent ADOS-users—or users of any other clinical instrument, for that matter. They become adept at administering the instrument in ways they and other professionals consider valid and reliable, or professionally competent. However, in focusing on instrument-relevant behaviors, clinicians may see children's first-order competences as deficits (where they notice them at all), diminish their relevance to an overall diagnostic picture, and explain them in psychological terms along the lines of what we have called anecdotal optimism. Consequently, they may remain unaware of matters that a close analysis of interaction can reveal, and may miss matters of consequence for the child's postclinical career.

In our presentations to clinicians, we admit to having the luxury of being researchers who can view (and review), transcribe, and analyze our recordings, putting us in a much different position than those making in situ judgments and shouldering enormous professional responsibilities. We could hardly expect that our interaction order, our ethnomethodological and conversation analytic form of inquiry, would be shared—although it probes the foundation of what any kind of endeavor, professional or otherwise, requires in terms of tacit background expectations and practices. As we have stated earlier (and see below), our theoretical and methodological enterprise recognizes that professional work always involves a set of foregrounded tasks whose accomplishment requires a primary orientation to the mandates and goals of the institutional or organizational context. A feature of this work is necessary disattention to the taken-for-granted interactional substrate that makes following those mandates and achieving those goals possible.

Still, clinicians have generously allowed that our findings are significant and interesting, while emphasizing their own lack of training about interaction as well as the very real pressures they experience to minimize the time spent with any given child or case. As we explain in chapter 1, the CDDC had a six-month-long waiting list for children seeking an autism evaluation, and clinicians were under pressure to perform assessments at a faster pace while not compromising their professionalism. To be more attentive to individual manifestations of autistic intelligence in the ways a child deals with ADOS or other tasks would require skills clinicians have not been taught, instructions about testing that currently make no reference to first- and second-order competence, and time that is already in short supply and that shows signs of becoming even more limited in the near future.

Conclusion

Were a fuller picture of a child needed or wanted for diagnosis, is there a way to elevate or center the background features of test performances? The challenges are clearly formidable. Diagnosing autism is an arduous and complicated task that involves the use of standardized criteria and instruments—such as schedules, tests, and questionnaires—in combination with a child's medical history, results from a physical examination, and presenting symptoms. Moreover, a child's evaluation at a clinic like CDDC is but one step, albeit a crucial one, in a patient career that develops contingently through time

(Balogh, Miller, and Ball 2015). For the purposes of generating a valid, accurate, and reliable outcome, the diagnostic process requires what we (Maynard and Turowetz 2019), following others mentioned above, have called
subtractive abstraction, in which information about concrete individuals and
their behavioral complications gets sacrificed in the quest for a standardized
diagnosis.

However, there is another kind of abstraction, which instead of removing
information preserves it in a more holistic, gestalt-like fashion. Such a picture
is abstract in a different sense: it provides texture and meaning to the details that distinguish a multifaceted "figure" from the "ground" that provides
its backdrop. In chapter 3, we anticipated such a possibility by way of Hacking's discussion of the thick description and holism that autism narrative—
biographies and autobiographies of autistic persons—can provide. For the
realm of diagnosis, however (and looking forward to chap. 6), we consider *instantiation stories*, which narrate singular instances of conduct on the part of
the child that say what *this* child has done at *that* specific time and place.[16] Such
stories are holistic in their preservation of at least some concrete information
about a child who otherwise too easily disappears into a diagnostic category.

When comparing the actions of children across activities and questions,
directives, or other actions within them, autistic intelligence is unique and
particular to any given child, and thus is extremely varied. Moreover, it is not
confined to only one kind of instrument that implements an official assessment for a child. Autistic intelligence is also not exclusive to what, following the literature, we might call level of functioning. That is, "low-" as well
as "high-" functioning children with autism deploy such intelligence (Seedhouse, Stribling, and Rae 2007). For example, Auburn and Pollock's (2013)
study of a child with severe autism shows how capable he is of initiating episodes of laughter, drawing on intimate knowledge of his coparticipants to
establish instances of sharing and teasing. And although we may see autistic
intelligence across the spectrum as belonging to the child as an individual,
it is also interactional and interactive. Autistic intelligence is not a thing the
child possesses, so much as it is a way of orienting actions in interaction with
relevant others.

When working to develop a child's capacity for second-order performances
and expressions of disembedded forms of knowledge, these relevant others—
copresent family members, teachers, and clinicians—may need to direct more
attention to that child's autistic intelligence. In a phrase, and to echo Mukhopadhyay's (2003) words, first-order competence and autistic intelligence are
about the child's "cans" rather than "cannots," their "haves" rather than "have-
nots." At the same time, when practitioners of common sense, whether in the

clinic or more ordinary social environments, reflect on breaches to common sense, it is possible to render those breaches as forms of reasoning in their own right. Earlier we discussed what has been called the language of autism. Using that phrase, the task is to incorporate the language of autism into ordinary, jointly held and taken-for-granted methods and practices, as did Sue Lehr in adapting Ben's "hit me" demand at the bottom of an escalator to a playful discourse in which she used a "tilt" command and gesture to calm him down (chap. 1). Rather than staying with rigid commonsense ideas regarding "behavior in public places" (Goffman 1963), she expanded her repertoire of practices and incorporated them into ordinary conduct.

Doing Diagnosis: Narrative Structure

In the last chapter, we described one way in which Dan Chapman violated the commonsense order of testing. After several unsuccessful attempts by psychologist Jennifer Erickson to engage him in the Demonstration Task, nine-year-old Dan stood up from the table where they were seated, walked to a corner of the room, knelt down behind a chair, and refused to continue with the task. To a commonsense observer, Dan's refusal to perform such a simple undertaking with no explanation or vocal protest may seem nonsensical. Although Jennifer was eventually able to reengage Dan in testing, she never did get him to demonstrate how he brushes his teeth or to offer an account for his refusal. In this chapter, we will see how Jennifer and her colleagues used storytelling and narrative to transform episodes like this one into aspects of Dan's diagnosis.

We have three goals in this chapter, which focuses on how clinicians decide on a diagnosis. Drawing from the study of testing and diagnosis, our general point is that the problems in interaction that children diagnosed with autism experience do not belong to the child alone. Interactional troubles result from a mutual failure at sensemaking: the child does not share methods of understanding belonging to the adult (whether clinician or other), *but neither does the adult share those of the child.* By entering the child's world and learning their methods of reasoning, clinicians and other adults can begin to incorporate the child's *uncommon* sense into their own practices of *commonsense* reasoning, including the provision of diagnostic conclusions.

First, we identify a phenomenon that we call the *narrative organization of diagnosis.* This phrase describes how clinicians, based on their testing, use narrative as a method for making sense of children's behavior, arriving at a diagnosis, and communicating the results to families. We also show how family

members participate in the narrative process, aligning with or, less often, resisting what the clinicians are proposing.

Second, we show how narrative organization is exhibited in the way clinicians diagnosed two children with autism in different historical eras. One
case involves Dan Chapman, who was diagnosed in 2014. The other one involves Ronnie Martin, who received an autism-related diagnosis in 1985 and
whose performance on the "What do you do when" subtest from the Brigance
Inventory was documented in chapter 4. In both periods, the narrative organization of diagnosis is clearly exhibited, which suggests that it has been a
stable feature of the interaction order of the clinic over time—even as nomenclatures, legal mandates, clinical discourses, and other features of the society
have fluctuated (Maynard and Turowetz 2019). Ronnie's case also illustrates
how clinicians use a narrative practice we call "category attribution" to fit a
child's particular features to generic diagnostic criteria.

Third, as previous chapters have partly anticipated, we explore how a
wider consideration of narrative methods may lend to appreciation of the
individuality of any given child who receives a diagnosis of autism. In particular, we ask whether it is possible to diagnose in a way that neither ignores
the child's unique sensemaking methods nor assimilates them to generic diagnostic criteria. This expansive kind of diagnosis may be difficult, but not
impossible, under the current medical model of autism, which stresses personal deficit. It may involve reconceptualizing autism along the lines of an
interactional phenotype.

Overall, the chapter follows clinicians across eras and cases as they collaboratively make sense of assessment results and observations and, if the evidence so indicates, reach a diagnosis of autism. As they discuss and deliberate
a case, clinicians do more than simply add up its particulars. They constitute
those particulars as relevant and consequential features of *this* case, so that
the particulars become indices of the case and the case confers meaning on
the particulars. Accordingly, the question of *what* clinicians make of a case is
inseparable from *how, in interaction with one another, they make the case*. In
our analysis, as we have said and plan to show, that "how" consists of narrative
methods of reasoning. These methods organize discussions not only among
clinicians but between clinicians and family members, who need to be able to
make sense of the clinicians' conclusions and their means of arriving at them.

Narratives, Stories, and the Achievement of Diagnosis

Storytelling is a pervasive feature of social interaction. In everyday life, people notice and tell stories about experiences of potential interest to members

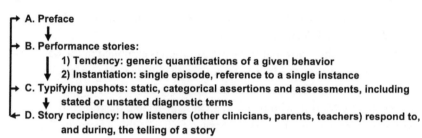

A. Preface

B. Performance stories:
    1) Tendency: generic quantifications of a given behavior
    2) Instantiation: single episode, reference to a single instance
C. Typifying upshots: static, categorical assertions and assessments, including
    stated or unstated diagnostic terms
D. Story recipiency: how listeners (other clinicians, parents, teachers) respond to,
    and during, the telling of a story

FIGURE 6.1. Diagnostic narrative

of their community (Sacks 1984).[1] In the clinic, professionals adapt this mundane competence for telling stories and building narratives to the business of diagnosis, using it to organize observations and reports about patients (Maynard and Turowetz 2017a; Maynard and Turowetz 2019; Turowetz 2015a; Turowetz and Maynard 2017).[2] An important aspect of the clinician's professional competence is the ability to recognize what Sacks (1992b:218) calls "storyable characteristics." For clinicians, storyable characteristics are those with diagnostic significance; they may be drawn from direct observation and testing in the clinic or from third-party reports (i.e., by parents or teachers) about a child's behavior.

Clinicians produce stories as part of an overall narrative structure that pervades what is often called a "pre-staffing" or "case conference," where after having seen a child for testing or other purposes, clinicians gather and talk, telling stories about what they have found. Scholarly literature on stories and narratives, going back to Labov and Waletzky's (1967) classic study, tends to conflate the terms we are using, as if *story* and *narrative* were nearly synonymous. In our research, however, we distinguish these two terms. Narrative structure consists of a sequence, which can stand alone or be linked to a previous or succeeding narrative, wherein stories serve as evidence on behalf of an overall diagnostic claim.

The narrative sequence for diagnosis is shown in figure 6.1. The sequence includes four elements: a narrative preface, performance stories, typifying upshots, and story recipiency.

The narrative preface (A) initiates a narrative sequence and directs the listener's attention to relevant features of the forthcoming story or stories.

Performance stories (B) are central to the narrative sequence and describe a child's performance on one or multiple occasions, according to two major types: tendency stories and instantiation stories. Both types provide evidence for or against diagnosis, but they do so in different ways.

Tendency stories (B1) combine multiple instances of a behavior into a single claim about the child's propensity to do something. They are similar to what Ainsworth-Vaughn (1998:151) and Riessman (1991) call "habitual" stories, and they are marked by (a) modal verbs (*will, would, can, could, may, might*) that suggest a disposition toward certain behaviors (cf. Bruner 1986:26; Edwards 2006); (b) adjectives that encode capacities (e.g., "She is *able* to do x"); (c) quantifiers (e.g., *all, some, every, a lot, always, never*) that specify the scope and frequency of a behavior; (d) *when-* and *if*-adverbial clauses that connect specific occasions or conditions with a behavior by locating it in particular places or times (e.g., "*when* he's stressed, he does a lot of x"); (e) dynamic verb phrases—often with gerund-type suffixes that indicate an ongoing action sequence (e.g., "she is/was *struggling*"), as opposed to one that is static or closed (e.g., "he *struggles* with x"); and (f) impressionistic verbs such as *seem, appear,* and *look,* which characterize assessments of conduct as likely or probable (e.g., "she *looks like* she's doing a ritual"). Given their focus on quantity and magnitude, tendency stories have a built-in flexibility that allows speakers to modify the strength of a claim depending on how recipients respond. For example, in the face of resistance, a speaker may pursue recipient alignment by downgrading a statement like "he does *a lot* of x" to "he does *some x*." This allows the speaker to retreat from an initially strong version of a claim to a weaker or more ambiguous one.

Instantiation stories (B2) relate a single episode of the child's conduct as it occurred at a specific time or place. These stories are regularly marked by spatial and temporal formulations (e.g., *there, here, before, after*), are organized chronologically (e.g., "x happened, *then* y happened"), and are introduced with *instantaneity markers*—phrases such as *for example* and *like* that project a telling about a specific instance of behavior or conduct (cf. Wiscons 2020).

Typifying upshots (C) constitute a third narrative component. These are static assertions, usually based on preceding stories, which make assessments of behavior that carry tacit or explicit diagnostic implications. For example, at the end of a story, a clinician might say of the child, "s/he *is x*" or "s/he *has x*," positing x as a fixed attribute the child possesses.

Notice that the narrative components differ in terms of the amount of detail they include about any concrete event or behavior. Whereas instantiation stories are about specific occasions, tendency stories generalize over multiple occasions, and typifying upshots do not refer to any occasion or set of occasions but to a property of the child extrapolated from an indeterminate number of occasions. The latter two components are closest to diagnostic criteria in terms of their generality—a point that will be important for our comparison of story types and the kinds of knowledge they produce.

In addition to the (A), (B), and (C) narrative components produced by the teller, (D) manifestations of *recipiency* are a crucial feature of the narrative sequence—how those listening to a story exhibit their understanding of it (Goodwin 1984; Jefferson 1978; Lerner 1992). The arrows originating from point D in figure 6.1 are meant to indicate that displays of recipiency occur throughout a telling, and not just at its conclusion, although post-conclusion is the position where more expansive comments by recipients occur. It is also where another clinician—or the current teller—may launch the next narrative sequence or story type (tendency or instantiation). In showing agreeing or disagreeing alignment to what has been told, recipients contribute to the overall diagnostic narrative.

Narrating Diagnosis: Ronnie Martin in 1985

The distinction between tendency and instantiation stories is an important one because these stories generate contrasting kinds of knowledge about a child. Tendency stories are generic, whereas instantiation stories are particular. Of the two story types, tendency stories are by far the more frequent, occurring about 80 percent of the time (Maynard and Turowetz 2017a), whether as part of pre-informing meetings (case conferences) among clinicians or in informing interviews with parents (who also may provide diagnostically relevant stories and contribute to narrative sequences). This predominance matters for the picture of the child that clinicians ultimately produce, because while both story types abstract from the original clinician-child interaction, they do so differently: tendency stories subtract details from the original interaction so as to subsume them under more general descriptions (e.g., distinct instances of repeated speech are collected and glossed as "echolalia"), whereas instantiation stories preserve details of the original interaction in ways that provide for formal understanding (Abbott 1988:103) of actual conduct, but with fuller texture and specificity (Martin 2011:194). Instantiation stories, in other words, are more holistic in their preservation of the original occasion, even though they share with tendency stories the practice of foregrounding the child and backgrounding the clinician and test (Maynard and Turowetz 2019). Briefly put, tendency stories bring the child's *generic features* into focus, while instantiation stories can make the child's *particularities* available for inspection.[3]

We can explore this matter by way of the Ronnie Martin case, which, as we noted in chapter 4, is from the 1980s, before the upsurge in the rate of autism diagnoses in the United States. Besides allowing us to probe the distinct forms of knowledge produced through tendency and instantiation stories, examination of this case demonstrates the generic way in which narrative structure inhabits clinical diagnosis. In comparing more contemporary data (such as that involving Dan Chapman, to be examined next in this chapter) to that from the 1970s and 1980s, we find that the methods for doing diagnosis have not changed over time, at least in the clinics with which our study is concerned. These methods constitute what we are calling the interaction order of the clinic. What *has* changed are the criteria and instruments clinicians use for diagnosis, and the body of psychiatric knowledge on which these tools are based. Amid such changes, however, clinicians have continued to employ a stable set of practices to produce their findings, applying new criteria and assessment tools through methods of sensemaking endogenous to the interaction order of the clinic.

In other words, in examining medical-diagnostic clinics such as CDDC, we find a generality to diagnostic practice in the face of terminological, cultural, and other changes across time (Maynard and Turowetz 2019), a matter for further consideration in our concluding chapter. Finally, the Ronnie Martin case allows us to explore an additional feature of diagnostic narrative that we call *category attribution*, a practice through which clinicians fit individual children to generic diagnostic categories.

DIAGNOSING RONNIE DURING THE PRE-STAFFING: CLINICAL DISCUSSIONS

When we introduced Ronnie Martin in chapter 4, we noted that he was four years old at the time of his assessment at CDDC, which took place in 1985. Along with many strengths, Ronnie showed behavior patterns that could be interpreted as signs of autism. In an earlier example, we saw Ronnie treat a hypothetical question more literally than the test allowed, producing an answer that involved his friend "Jimmy." The issue of literalism came up when the team of clinicians who evaluated Ronnie met for a pre-staffing conference about his case. The team included a psychologist, psychiatrist, pediatrician, special education specialist, occupational therapist, and speech pathologist, all of whom had conducted individual assessments of Ronnie over a two-day period.[4]

The pre-staffing meeting is so named because it is prior to the "staffing," which is the informing interview where clinicians share their findings with families. In Goffman's (1959b) terminology, it is a "backstage" region where team members can determine a diagnosis before going "front stage" to communicate it to the family. The clinicians who evaluated Ronnie gradually assembled a narrative that supported a diagnosis of atypical pervasive developmental disorder (APDD), a category that was listed alongside infantile autism under the umbrella of pervasive developmental disorders in the then-operative DSM-III (APA 1980). As they discussed Ronnie informally, the clinicians alternated between using the official APDD diagnosis and the term *autism* itself. Today, Ronnie would be seen as having autism spectrum disorder.

Initial Discussion about the School's View

The pre-staffing case conference for Ronnie began with the clinicians discussing the school's referral, suggesting that the school had "in effect" (not officially) already made a diagnosis of autism but that the family was "gonna have a lot of problems with the label."[5] The clinicians had also sensed such "problems," and throughout their discussions, they anticipated that the parents would be resistant to an autism diagnosis.

Special Education Report

After these preliminary discussions, Dr. Debbie Olson, the special education clinician, begins to share her findings. She starts by addressing Dr. Bill Pender, the psychologist and team leader on Ronnie's case, with a preface about the "readiness tests" she does with four- and five-year-olds, saying that Ronnie performed "at age level" (lines 1–3 below). This will touch off a round of narratives focused on the theme of Ronnie's literalism, a characteristic commonly associated with autism.

TRANSCRIPT 6.1A: CASE J: PRESTF2:1:1

```
 1  Debbie:  Anyways Bill ↑every↓thing I did with him on the: (0.2) rea:diness
 2           types of things that I do with four fi:- ↓five year olds? .h
 3           [He] ↓did all at age level.
 4  Bill:    [Mm]
 5  Bill:    Yeah.° (0.3) .hh yeah=
 6  Debbie:  =It's jus:t (uh)- (.) from talk↓ing to the ↑tea:↓chers it sounds
 7           like when he has to take those skills and ↑apply: it=
 8  Bill:    =Mm hmm=
 9  Debbie:  =to something, that's where he [falls ] ↓down and he doesn't=
10  ?:                                      [Mm hmm]
11  Debbie:  =have the generali[zation ] skills, and-
12  Bill:                      [Mm hmm]
```

Debbie is suggesting that Ronnie's scores are typical for a member of his age group. However, after Bill responds with "Yeah" tokens (line 5), Debbie adds a qualification: according to Ronnie's teachers (line 6), "when he has to take those skills and apply" them (lines 6–7), he "falls down" (line 9). This is a tendency story that culminates in a typifying upshot: "he doesn't have the generalization skills" (lines 9, 11).

Instantiation Story and Upshot: "He's Very Literal"

Following an immediate inbreath that projects a further turn at talk (6.1b, line 13 below), Debbie supports her claim that Ronnie lacks generalization skills by citing a specific instance of literalism. She begins with a story preface ("Did they tell you about," lines 13–14). Bill marks this as informative (with his "oh" at line 15 [Heritage 1984a]), and Debbie moves into the story proper (lines 16–17), which describes an educational film about child abuse, its message, and Ronnie's interpretation of that message.

TRANSCRIPT 6.1B: CASE J: PRESTF2:1:14

```
13   Debbie:  .hhh Did they >tell you about< how they showed a (0.6) a: child
14            abu[se ↑mo:vie] and that (0.5)=
15   Bill:       [O::h     ]
16   Debbie:  =and that he wasn't supposed to: y- (.) you're s'pposed to say
17            no: (.) ↑run ↓away and tell two friends.
18                (0.4)
19   Bill:    Mm hmm=
20   Debbie:  =Well: ↑he: ↓viewed his dad telling him to pick up his toys as
21            ch[ild abu]se, [(0.2) and] so he told his dad, ↑I can say no=
22   Bill:      [(   )]  [          ]
23   ?:                      [hhh hhh ]
24   Debbie:  =and I'm going to run ↓away and [tell two friends. (0.6)]
25   All:                                     [((General laughter))   ]
26   Debbie:  [You know? And he <could:n't distinguish>]=
27   All:     [((laughter))                           ]
28   Debbie:  [that it [$wasn't really child ] abuse$
29   Bill:    [hih heh huh That's funny .hh ]
30   Debbie:  It's [interesting ] that-=
31   Bill:         [That's good.]
32   Debbie:  =He's ↑very lit↓eral, [(y'know)]
33   Claud:                         [Yeah,   ] that comes out.
```

Describing the focal action of the story, Debbie recounts how Ronnie reacted to his father disciplining him by repeating what he had been told at school (lines 20–21, 24). The story elicits overlapping laughter from others in the room (lines 25, 27), as Debbie proposes the upshot that Ronnie could not "distinguish" his father's actions from "child abuse" (lines 26, 28). After Bill produces appreciative commentary on the story (lines 29, 31), Debbie suggests a further upshot: Ronnie is "very literal" (line 32), a point she emphasizes with vocal stress and rising-falling intonation. As Debbie completes her turn with "y'know," Dr. Claudia Evans (speech and language) aligns (line 33) with an agreeing upshot, "Yeah, that comes out." As it turns out, her utterance also operates as a preface to her own narrative sequence.

Added Typifying and Tendency Stories: "Yeah, That Comes Out"

Having illustrated narrative practices by drawing on Debbie's presentation, we will summarize Claudia's succeeding narrative. Referencing her speech and language exam, Claudia produces a tendency story based on her own observations of Ronnie and her knowledge of his family. Claudia says, "The only way" that Ronnie is "able to pick up other ways" of playing with toys is when "his little sister" does "other things." As with everyday "second stories" (Sacks 1989[1964]; Siromaa 2012) or story rounds (Ryave 1978), Claudia's story is thematically aligned to and elaborates on the prior one, contributing to an emergent narrative arc whose tacit upshot is that Ronnie learns by imitation. Next, Bill produces a narrative in which he reports a teacher's assessment that Ronnie does not do "creatively . . . new things with toys." He adds, however, that according to the teacher (in a tendency story), if they "show" Ronnie how to do such things as use a puppet, "then he can sort of imitate it," whereupon Debbie produces a typifying upshot, "He's a real good person for imitating and modelling," that aligns with this story and the overall narrative in progress.[6]

As the deliberation of Ronnie's case continues, a psychiatric resident reports that Dr. Molly Gardner (the supervising psychiatrist, who was not at the pre-staffing because of a scheduling conflict) had mentioned APDD and autism to the parents. Then the occupational therapist gives her findings. Each clinician systematically alternates between tendency and instantiation stories in support of upshots that, in turn, are aligned to APDD/autism as a diagnosis. Finally, as the pre-staffing comes to a close, Bill raises the issue of how the family is "coping" with the potential diagnosis. Debbie says, "I think they're really afraid that he's gonna be labeled," an assertion with which the other clinicians agree and which suggests an anticipatory stance regarding how to deliver the diagnosis: delicately. When we examine the news delivery below, we shall see such delicacy being enacted.

CATEGORY ATTRIBUTION AS A FEATURE OF NARRATIVE

In reporting their findings to Ronnie's parents, Samantha and Joe Martin, clinicians engage in a practice we call "category attribution" (Turowetz and Maynard 2016:618–22). This practice suggests a particular relationship between the child and representative members of a given category, with the implication that the child belongs (or does not belong) to that category. Because membership categories are "inference rich" (Sacks 1992a:40), clinicians may leave it to listeners (e.g., parents) to draw explicit conclusions about the child's relationship to the categories in play.

Category attribution regularly follows, or is featured in, tendency or instantiation stories about a child. Afterward, clinicians and story recipients may produce an upshot that *re-narrates* the initial story (about the individual child) in terms of the attributed category. Accordingly, the category attribution typically forms the middle part of a three-part sequence:

1. Claim about the child
2. Category attribution
3. Re-narration of (1) in terms of (2)

This sequence is collaboratively produced, in that it requires at least minimal displays of acknowledgment from recipients, and clinicians pursue such acknowledgment if recipients withhold it. Of course, acknowledgment does not necessarily imply agreement; aligning in the production of a sequence is not, in itself, evidence of affiliation (Stivers 2008).

We can distinguish two kinds of category attributions: First, there are those that suggest a particular child is *similar* to incumbents of a given category. Thus, in the course of discussing a child's abilities, a clinician may claim that "he is doing some things like *other kids his age.*" Second are those that suggest a child is *different* from members of a given category. For example, a clinician might distinguish what a child did during an assessment from what "*most kids*" do.[7] In both versions, the clinician tacitly proposes something about the child in relation to the category.

Delivering the Diagnosis

After two days of testing, the Martins sat down with the clinicians to hear their conclusions about Ronnie (see fig. 6.2; Ronnie's father and mother are at the left center, with clinicians and school personnel on either side). Joe and Samantha Martin had been through a lot: aside from ongoing troubles with Ronnie, their daughter (Ronnie's younger sister) had a history of health problems, and the clinicians raised concerns during the pre-staffing that she might also be suffering from developmental delays (though they resolved not to mention this to the parents). The clinicians agreed that the parents were in a fragile place, and they broached the diagnosis carefully.

The clinicians participating in the staffing included Molly Gardner, psychiatrist (who arrived late because she was involved with another case); Bill Pender, psychologist; Claudia Evans, speech and language pathologist; Dana

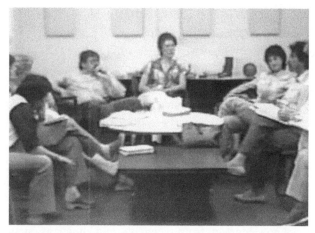

FIGURE 6.2. Psychologist Bill Pender (*right*) delivering diagnostic news to Mr. and Mrs. Martin (*center*). To Bill's right is Claudia Evans, speech and language, and in the left foreground, leaning forward, is the psychiatrist, Molly Gardner. Other clinicians and school personnel are arrayed next to these parties.

Reardon, an occupational therapist; and Debbie Olson, the special education clinician. Two of Ronnie's teachers were also in attendance.

As they did in the pre-staffing, the clinicians conveyed their findings in a narrative manner. They opened the staffing by sharing the results from their evaluations, with the parents regularly responding with tokens of acknowledgment or acceptance. In some instances, the parents also supplied "second" stories that drew on their own experiences with Ronnie to reinforce or refine themes from the clinicians' stories. Still, having anticipated parental resistance to the specific category of APDD or autism, the clinicians displayed caution. As the clinicians moved closer to articulating a diagnosis, the parents started to exhibit resistance, asking more questions and hesitating before responding.

Initial Category Attribution

The extended discussion that culminates in the delivery of Ronnie's diagnosis begins with the strip of talk in transcript 6.1c below. At lines 1–4, following a formulation about a "frustrating" thing, Bill produces the first part of the category attribution sequence, using a tendency story to advance his claim that Ronnie "does a lot of thinking" in "associative" or "concrete" or "literal" ways. Then, at lines 4–6, he produces an upshot ("what that means"), which contrasts what Ronnie "has" (memory) with what he lacks (knowledge about "how to apply it"). Following a generalizing preface ("a lot of times," line 6),

Bill refers to "examples" he has heard from parents that are "dramatic" (lines 6, 7) and proceeds to describe how a generic child (i.e., "the child," line 8) may interpret instructions about how to cross the street (lines 9–14). This is part two of the category attribution sequence—the category attribution itself. He then produces the third part of the sequence, returning to Ronnie specifically and including him among such children (lines 11–12) before elaborating on what children like him "will" do when crossing the street (lines 13–14).

TRANSCRIPT 6.1C: CASE J: 67–68 IN STF_III

```
 1  Bill:    I think >one of the things< that gets frustrating is that he-
 2           he does (.) uhm (.) a lo:t of th:inking tha- that variously
 3           can be called associative thinki:ng or concr:ete thinki:ng or
 4           l:iteral thinking (.) What that means is (.) ah (0.5) >ya know
 5           again where he< has the memory but doesn't know how to apply
 6           it. >You know< And a lot of times we'll hear examples from
 7           parents where ah (.) °↓this is a little p- dramatic but .hh
 8           u::h° something like where they- the ↑child has learned at
 9           home or in the school to .hh ah stop (1.0) and look both ways
10           before you cross the street. And to repeat ↑that even out loud
11           to yourself until you got it down. .h Well so:metimes >kids like<
12           ↓Ronnie will ↑do ↓that=will get to the co:rner, they'll sto:p?
13           (0.5) they'll look both wa:ys? (.) and >then walk into the
14           middle of the street when the cars are coming.<
15  Joe:     [Mm: hm.]=
16  Saman:   [Mm: hm.]=
17  Bill:    =See. [.hh .hh
18  Saman:         [Yeah
19  Bill:    But he can't (.) get (.) past the literal thinking where they're
20           ↑following your instructions.
21  Saman:   Mm:[hm ((nodding))
22  Joe:        [Right ((nodding)
```

The story elicits overlapping acknowledgment tokens from Ronnie's parents (lines 15–16), allowing Bill to go on and formulate a further upshot about Ronnie (lines 18, 19–20). With its emphasis on "literal," the formulation proposes how recipients should interpret the prior depiction in reference to Ronnie ("he," line 19); the parents respond with markers of acknowledgment or agreement (lines 21–22).

Implicating Autism

Next, Bill provides a further illustration of Ronnie's "associative" or "concrete" or "literal" thinking, this time from his own evaluation. This forms the first part of a new category attribution sequence that elaborates the prior one. Bill tells an instantiation story (not on our transcripts here) in which Ronnie responds to a question about "what's missing" from a picture of a rabbit with one ear by saying, "Egg, bunny, egg." Bill continues, "You can see where it comes from, but it is not logical thinking," whereupon, after telling the parents (and the teachers who also attended the staffing), "That's the big problem that you're all facing," he moves to the second phase of the category attribution sequence (lines 1–3 below) via a claim about "a group of kids" in whom these behaviors are seen, explaining that they are "not all that common," which is why the family is at the clinic.

TRANSCRIPT 6.1D: CASE J: STFII:48

```
 1  Bill:   Now we see that in kids. i- ina- ina- ina group of kids. It's not
 2          all that common. (0.6) Y'know (or-i) o:bviously or you wouldn't
 3          be here. .hh Ah i- it also goes with a lo:t of what Doctor
 4          Gardner may have talked- (.) to you about. (0.4) An which I
 5          noticed too. (0.4) Givin ye- jist a (.) qu:ick (.) list of
 6          things. .hh A::h of th:ings that are (.) that er look (.)
 7          unu::sual. But we se::e (.) they tend to go together. Some kids
 8          show all these (errors) (.) Ah the language is- is dela:yed (.)
 9          and unu:sual? it were (there) (.) echola:lic (.) repe:ating
10          things: or the si:ng so:ng  (.)  ((door sound)) or the too literal-
```

Bill suggests that what the psychiatrist, Dr. Gardner, and he (lines 3–5) have noticed about the behaviors ("list of things," lines 5–7) is that they "look un-usual" and "tend to go together" (line 7). The list already foreshadows a di-agnosis of autism, in that it describes some of the symptoms specified in the then-current DSM-III (APA 1980), including "gross deficits in language devel-opment," "peculiar speech patterns such as immediate and delayed echolalia," "abnormal speech melody" (APA 1980:87), and concrete thinking. Given the "group of kids" reference at the beginning of this excerpt, Bill's list in lines 76–78 performs an implicit category attribution which invites the inference that Ronnie belongs to this group.[8]

Moving toward an Autism Attribution

At line 10 (above), Molly Gardner enters the room ("door sound"), and Bill briefly interrupts his talk to acknowledge her. After returning to a narrative about Ronnie specifically (not shown) and listing a number of his behaviors from when he was younger, Bill produces the upshot: "all these tend to go together" and "when you see all these things together . . . there is a label for it." Rather than providing the label, however, he extends the upshot by describing category-bound behaviors (below, lines 1–6). After a silence (line 7), which, on the part of the parents, can show resistance to this description, Bill begins a further turn (line 8) that may implicate a re-narration that fits Ronnie to the category being described. However, Ronnie's mother, who had been dabbing her eyes with a tissue, interjects with an utterance (lines 9–10) that proposes to qualify, and possibly challenge, the implication that her son fits the pattern Bill is describing. She displays disalignment with Bill's talk through (what sounds like) her turn-initial "well" token and invocation of a category, "certain people," that is marked as contrastive ("though"). In doing so, she displays an understanding that a similarity-type category attribution had been underway, and suggests resistance to that attribution:

TRANSCRIPT 6.1E: CASE J: STFII:50

```
 1  Bill:   There are a group of k:ids who have a h:a:rd ti- they- they
 2          seem t- be more in their own world. (1.0) They y'know they
 3          kinna do their o:wn th:ing. An that's sometimes not always but
 4          sometimes shows up even early in childhood where they- .hh they
 5          seem to prefer to be alone a little bit mo:re (0.5) and they
 6          do̲n't like getting involved with other people quite as much.
 7          (1.5)
 8  Bill:   A:h .hhh WHAtever th[e histor-
 9  Saman:                      [(Well I think there are) ce:rtain people
10          though
11          (0.8)
12  Bill:   Mh yeah
13  Molly:  Yeah [I would think that that's wh:a:t: uh: where we were-=
14  Saman:       [(   ) a̲n̲y̲b̲o̲d̲y̲
15  Molly:  =what we were we[re talking about
16  Saman:                  [((blowing nose))
17  Molly:  Where we:: (.) what we had talked some about this morning .hhh
18          wa::s: (.) u::m: hh (1.0) that (.) uhm (1.0) what I̲ think is
19          important is to understand something about (.) what we think
20          is a probable underlying mechanism.
```

After a silence (line 11) and Bill's hesitating acknowledgment (line 12), Molly (lines 13, 15, 17) invokes a discussion she and the clinicians had had earlier, and proposes (lines 18–20) that there is probably an "underlying mechanism" causing Ronnie's troubles. Molly may be interpreting Samantha's teary appearance and resistive behavior as calling for assuagement or palliation, rather than progression toward the category attribution that can be anticipated from the trajectory of Bill's previous utterances.

During further description of Ronnie's symptoms (talk not shown), Molly draws a connection between those symptoms and "some kind of brain damage." The Martins seem taken aback by this term, and the clinicians then work to exit from the discussion. Bill displays a kind of agnosticism regarding brain damage, concluding with a dissimilarity-type category attribution (our emphasis): "there's something about how the connections are working [that] isn't allowing him to make sense of the world *in a way that a normal child might.*" From this point, Bill, Molly, and Debbie put an optimistic frame on the situation with various formulations about Ronnie's "positive things," such as "good language," "pre-academic skills," and "showing affection" (for details, see Maynard and Turowetz 2017a:261–64).

The Diagnostic Moment[9]

Although clinicians have aligned certain of Ronnie's tendencies or particular behaviors to normative developmental benchmarks, overall they have stressed how different he is from typical children. Ultimately, Bill delivers the diagnosis by referring to Molly and quoting her as using "a term called pervasive atypical developmental disorder"[10] (lines 1–2 below), for which he offers a tendency story ("what we really mean . . . is he shows many of the signs," lines 3–4). He then invokes the diagnosis (line 4) by way of anonymous quotation (it's what "other people call autism").[11]

TRANSCRIPT 6.1F: CASE J: STFIII:67

```
1   Bill:   .hh When doctor Gardner ((Bill gestures toward Molly)) uses a
2           term called >pervasive atypical developmental dis↓order,¹²< .hh
3           >what by- < I think what we really mean by that is he shows
4           m:any of the signs (0.9) that other people call autism
5           (0.4)
6   Bill:   But maybe not all of the signs and maybe to a (.) somewhat
7           milder degree.
8           (0.6) ((Samantha nods slightly))
```

The parents are silent (line 5), and Bill makes strategic use of a feature of tendency stories we mentioned earlier: in quantifying behavior, these stories can be used—as Bill does at lines 6–7—to retreat from initially stronger forms of the evidence they provide on behalf of diagnosis. That is, speakers can adjust the magnitude of a quantity (e.g., "not all") or make it more ambiguous (e.g., "somewhat milder") in pursuit of recipient alignment. This works to occasion a small nod from Samantha (line 8).

After the delivery of diagnosis, the parents, with Joe leading the way, orient to the practicalities of the diagnosis: what can be done, how it will be paid for, and the like. Bill assures them by saying: "One of the reasons that we think labels can be helpful, not just to put a tag on a kid, but when you use a label like atypical developmental disorder or autism, it's what we call a developmental disability. And because of that there are state regulations and local boards that are required, you know, to pick up the tab on certain kinds of services, and they may be willing to pay perhaps for all of the kind of things that we've been bantering about the last few minutes" (Case J STF_III:74).

The need for and availability of services is often the topic on which these informing interviews end.[13] This raises an issue that our research cannot address directly: What happens after diagnosis? Do families get the services that are indicated? Answering questions like these depends on future research that would investigate what we, following Goffman (1959a) on the "moral career," have called the postclinical phase of an autism career. In the conclusion to this chapter, and staying with the clinical phase of this career, we address a different issue, one concerning the matter of how instantiation stories relate to autistic intelligence.

Diagnosing Dan Chapman

Dan Chapman has been the child we have followed most consistently through this book. We have earlier (chap. 1) offered observations about his diagnosis and how it was told to his mother, Betsy. Now we can provide more detail with regard to the narrative organization of its determination and presentation. After she had administered the Autism Diagnostic Observation Schedule (ADOS), Dr. Jennifer Erickson first proposed a diagnosis for Dan during a meeting with the pediatrician, Dr. Leah Grant. Leah had met with Dan and his mother earlier in the day, interviewing Betsy Chapman and Dan together and asking about Dan's difficulties at home and school. As we saw in chapter 1, Leah and Betsy discussed a number of issues, including Dan's repetitive behaviors, need for order, extended mono-topical talk, and extreme difficulties at school. Their conversation raised concerns about autism, and so Leah had already formed a preliminary impression of Dan by the time of her later meeting with Jennifer. Leah opens the meeting with a question (below, lines 1–2) that elicits a story preface from Jennifer, who proposes that "an ASD diagnosis fits" (line 3). In overlap with "fits" (line 3), Leah shows recipiency, aligning to and agreeing with Jennifer's statement. Jennifer then reports that Dan "actually came up a little higher on the ADOS than I thought he would" (lines 5–6).

TRANSCRIPT 6.2: CASE 24: PRESTF:1

```
1  Leah:   And- and whu- what are your thoughts? Or what duh- what did
2          you find? With your: testing.
3  Jen:    I think- I mean I think an ASD diagnosis [(.) fits.      So      ]=
```

```
 4  Leah:                                  [It's appropriate. Yeah]=
 5  Jen:     =he: um: he ↑actually came up a ↑little ↑higher on the: ADOS than I
 6            thought he would just because he did so many nice things?
 7            [Like he was very polite:: and responsive:, and um::
 8  Leah:     [Oh good.
 9            (.)
10  Jen:     =tch anyway so .h so he- he came up with a thirteen. Um: and the
11            cutoff was a nine. So (.) he was (.) solidly .hh um:: in that (.)
12            range. He:: there was one point where he:: shut down briefly and
13            mom said actually that- that he was like completely done? For th-
14            like she kind of made that gesture ((Hand across neck)) [to me uh:=
15  Leah:                                                              [((Laughs))
16  Jen:     =but he ↑came back.
```

Jennifer's "actually" (Clift 2001) and "I thought" (Jefferson 1974) formulations at lines 5–6 mark a contrast between what she expected and what she observed, while her quantification ("a little higher") indexes behavioral tendencies that were not consistent with an autism diagnosis. She then supplies examples of such tendencies, proposing as a tendency story component in line 6 that Dan "did so many nice things" (note the vague quantifier "so many") and that he "was very polite and responsive" (line 7, typification). However, Jennifer qualifies the matter by sandwiching these positive remarks between the previous quantification, "higher on the ADOS" (line 5), and her subsequent portrayal of Dan's score as thirteen in relation to the "cutoff" of nine in lines 10–11 (as a reminder: the higher the score, the more it implicates autism). This subsequent portrayal, moreover, is introduced with hesitations (at lines 7, 9–10) and a marker of disconnection, "anyway" (cf. Drew 2005:76), that brackets off the positive assessments and continues to elaborate an autism diagnosis.

Having already proposed in her narrative preface the upshot that Dan has autism (line 3), Jennifer ties back to that preface at lines 11–12 by observing how his score was "solidly in that range." She then elaborates her narrative with a story, introduced by the instantaneity marker "there was one point." This is a post-upshot instantiation story about the Demonstration Task (lines 12–14), and Leah receipts the story—specifically the component where Jennifer mimics Mrs. Chapman's "cut off" gesture—with laughter (line 15).

PSYCHOLOGIZING AUTISM

A distinctive feature of diagnostic narratives is their portrayal of three key "actants" in the testing process: the child, the clinician, and the test instrument. As we noted in chapter 4, *actant* is the term that Latour (1987; 1993) coined to denote anything in a social setting that has agency by affecting what goes on in the setting. Though it may be obvious that clinicians and children have agency, objects such as tests can also be said to have agency, not only because professionals use them to assess and diagnose children but because they prescribe "accountably" correct procedures—they relate to protocols and other definitions for doing assessments and drawing conclusions. Thus, we can say that test protocols in use enable and constrain the social activity of testing.

Although we do not follow the considerable critical literature on the notion of actants, we think it is a useful concept for exploring an important facet of diagnostic narrative, namely that the child is the central figure in clinical stories, whereas the clinician and test remain in the background. This figure-ground relationship directs the story recipient's attention to what the child is doing and tacitly (or otherwise) suggests that their behavior embodies autism. Meanwhile, the clinician and test are constituted as unmarked, taken-for-granted elements of the story's background, an effect storytellers achieve through such practices as naming the test or task without further elaboration (e.g., "On *the Demonstration Task*, he . . .") and reporting their administrative work (e.g., "*I gave* test *x*," "*I asked* if she could give another example of *y*") while otherwise glossing their interactions with the child. Portrayed in this way, the clinician and test furnish the staging and props for the child's performances but do not contribute to them in any meaningful way. For example, notice how in extract 6.2, Jennifer's story makes only the briefest mention of the ADOS (lines 5–6) and her role in administering it (which is implied but not described explicitly), whereas Dan is the subject of most of her utterances. This matters, because in focusing on the child's actions, clinicians' stories elide the interactional and interactive setting in which those actions occurred.

Slightly later than the discussion in extract 6.2, the two clinicians (Leah, Jennifer) and an intern (Leslie) revisited Dan's performance on the Demonstration Task. Jennifer says that Dan's "most atypical response was that one time when he . . . got up and he walked away to the corner." For anyone familiar with autism, the very word *atypical* carries diagnostic connotations, as earlier APA Diagnostic and Statistical Manuals used this term (in combination with others) for definitional purposes. And clinicians regularly treat lack of responsiveness (such as Dan's walking "away") as an "interactional manifestation of autism" (Hollin and Pilnick 2018:1226). As Jennifer finishes speaking, Leslie enters with a candidate explanation for Dan's behavior. She suggests that he "didn't like" the question he was asked, and, confirming Jennifer's account, "he just got up and walked," which she then assesses as "frustrating." Her explanation suggests a motive for Dan's behavior: not *liking* what he was being asked to do. Jennifer responds by saying, "It was a hard question," and Leslie continues, "You said to do something and he just didn't want to do it." A few more seconds go by, and Jennifer, looking up from her notes, says, "It was just . . . he felt put on the spot . . . and so he just got up and walked away into the corner." That is, differing slightly from Leslie's account, Jennifer suggests that it is what Dan *felt*, rather than what he *liked* or *wanted*, that explains his disengagement from the test activity. Though the details may differ, we can observe that these accounts share an appeal to *psychological* factors or motivational dispositions to explain behavior. Indeed, Leslie's "just" formulation in her comment that Dan "just got up and walked away" is a "maximal" descriptor (Drew 1992:487) which suggests that there was nothing more to this action, as if it resulted directly and only from Dan's psychological state. In short, these accounts reduce complex social interactions to processes within the individual.

PROFESSIONAL COMPETENCE AND STANDARDIZATION

If it can be said that the clinicians explain Dan's actions by reducing them to manifestations of internal states—that is, by psychologizing them—we have two further points. First, and briefly, in chapter 5, we saw that Dan's actions related to the Demonstration Task were coproduced as a series of directive-refusal pairs. In this way, Dan's "shutting down" is neither abrupt nor sudden, nor is it a context-free direct outcome of a psychological state, but rather the culmination of an orderly series of action-and-response sequences that displays a variety of skillful practices for doing polite resistance and other actions on Dan's part.[14]

Second, although our interactional analysis offers a picture different from the clinical one, this is not to say that clinicians are therefore mistaken or oblivious in their assessment. Rather, the way the clinicians use narrative to identify symptoms of autism in Dan's conduct is emblematic of *professional competence*: as we stated above, clinicians discover and document signs of disorder in *accountably* competent ways, which means acting in accordance with definitions in the *Diagnostic and Statistical Manual*. Additionally, they do so in ways that promote *standardization*.

Professional Competence

As a diagnostician, Jennifer's work of discovery and documentation exhibits her professional competence through *attention* to aspects of Dan's behavior that professionals consider to be relevant. Such attention simultaneously entails *disattention* to details that, for practical purposes of testing and evaluation, are considered immaterial, including features of the test's design (e.g., its constituent tasks and their ordering, coding, and scoring procedures). How clinicians administer the test also is not of explicit interest—except when an error of administration is suspected, in which case the exception serves to illustrate the rule that testing is ordinarily assumed to be unproblematic (Turowetz 2015a). The practices by which Jennifer, or any competent clinician, for that matter, displays proper "administrativeness" (Maynard and Marlaire 1992) are "specifically uninteresting" (Garfinkel 1967:9) in the sense that the tacit, embodied, taken-for-granted aspects of what she does work-wise to administer tasks and evaluate performances are so intimately ingrained in that work as to render them invisible.

Analytically, however, the "seen but unnoticed" details in the clinician's presentation of test items or activities, together with the responses they elicit, are a situated part of the activity of standardized assessment and as such deserve explication if we are fully to understand diagnosis as a socially organized activity. Much turns on this matter: if we want to understand how diagnostic actions shape the clinical and social profile of children, and how that shaping feeds into broader definitions of ability and disability, we need to know about the "praxeography" (Mol 2002) of diagnostic work: what is treated as significant and *how*, what counts as relevant and *how*, and also what is necessarily left out of the official results, as the existence of the disorder, disability, or clinical entity is brought into being. Later in this chapter (and more forcefully in chap. 8), we will direct attention to the ways that a praxeography of diagnostic work can raise the matter of autistic intelligence to more prominence.

Standardization

In the course of an autism evaluation, clinicians make use of various resources, including structured interviews with parents, informal firsthand observations of the child, third-party reports about the child (e.g., from physicians and teachers), questionnaires, checklists, and standardized assessment tools. As we have noted, for CDDC practitioners the ADOS is central to making an autism diagnosis, and, with other clinically relevant information, it is widely considered the gold standard in autism assessment. Significantly, with much research devoted to how well such instruments as the ADOS represent diagnostic criteria set out in the DSM (e.g., Evers et al. 2020), the ADOS is highly calibrated to those DSM (e.g., APA 2013) criteria. Thus, the social activities that make up the ADOS are designed to test for difficulties in two core areas: communicative social interaction and restricted or repetitive patterns of behavior. Scoring of behavior is based on how the examinee responds to the clinician's "social presses," which, following Murray (1938:115–21), are defined as external stimuli that are expected to motivate specific responses from people. The ADOS and its "presses" are meant to create "standard contexts in which interactions occur" (Lord et al. 2012:13), allowing clinicians to observe "a range of social initiations and responses" (Lord et al. 2000:205) and use their observations as indicators of behavioral patterns.

The goal of standardization is to eliminate external sources of variation in the child's performance that could confound what is being measured. Somewhat paradoxically, this means organizing the assessment environment in such a way that the environment itself can be discounted as a contributor to the child's behavior. For an exam like the ADOS, proper standardization means that the clinician and the instrument can be treated as neutral arbiters of the child's abilities and disabilities. Producing stories that focus on the child's actions while treating their own actions and the design features of the assessment tool as "empirically uninteresting" (Garfinkel 1967:7–8,263), they are tacitly affirming that standardization has been achieved and that exam results are valid. Indeed, as noted earlier, the only time clinicians topicalize their own or the exam's contributions to the child's performance is when an error of administration, and consequent failure of standardization, is suspected (Turowetz 2015a). In these cases, which are comparatively rare in our data, clinicians are responding to what could be described as a breach of *clinical common sense*. As with violations of everyday (i.e., nonclinical) common sense, their responses bring to the surface ordinarily tacit assumptions and prompt remedial efforts from coparticipants (e.g., deciding whether a result still counts as valid, etc.) By consigning the contributions of the clinician and exam to the child's performance to the background of test administration, administration of ADOS protocols may reinforce an assumption that autism is a disorder of the person that exists apart from the social environment (Mirowsky and Ross 1989). According to this view, although social relations can mediate and moderate autism's phenotypic expression (e.g., symptom frequency and intensity), its locus is not in social interaction as such. Clinically, there is no social interactional phenotype, as ultimately the disorder is thought to reside within persons, who manifest it in their behavior.

In sum, as they implement standardized assessment protocols and communicate their results to colleagues and others, clinicians by necessity (i.e., as a matter of clinical accountability) interpret children's behavior in terms of the medical model encoded in the ADOS and DSM, thereby emphasizing children's conduct and mental processes while eliding the interactional and interactive context in which such conduct occurred. A natural question is, could things be different?

Conclusion: Instantiation Stories and Intelligence

Diagnosing developmental disabilities is rarely a straightforward matter. This is especially true of psychiatric disorders without known biomarkers. We explore this issue in some depth in chapter 7. For the time being, it is enough to say that the challenges of "doing diagnosis" in reliable, standardized ways are considerable. In addition to having no known biomarkers, autism shares symptoms with a number of other disorders of childhood, including ADHD, obsessive-compulsive disorder, language disorders (e.g., apraxia of speech, specific language disorder), anxiety, motor delays, and gastrointestinal diseases. Furthermore, as we discussed in chapter 2, factors such as gender, race, and socioeconomic status have been shown to influence diagnostic outcomes. Add to all this the fact that each child—no matter what their demographic characteristics may be—is unique, and we can appreciate just how complex the diagnostic process can be. And yet despite all of this, children do emerge from diagnostic clinics with profiles that reliably fit the DSM categories. At the same time, though, the generality of such diagnoses can elide much information that captures the uniqueness of any child. What and where is this information?

We have shown how clinicians use a combination of standardized instruments, such as tests, checklists, and interview schedules, as well as third-party reports and firsthand observations, to generate diagnostic information. Then, by way of narrative, clinicians tell tendency and instantiation stories, which may feature category attributions that fit children to typical or atypical modes of development. Narratively, the diagnostic stories told by clinicians center children's behaviors while backgrounding the clinicians' own contributions, and those of their assessment tools, to the children's performance.

As clinicians build a narrative case for or against diagnosis, their stories support specific diagnostic claims and are therefore evidentiary for the particular case. We have said that story types play distinct roles in the building of an overall narrative. Instantiation stories provide specific illustrations of behavior, whereas tendency stories assimilate particular instances of behavior to generalizations about children's propensities. As clinicians build toward diagnosis, we can observe a movement away from the relative concreteness of instantiation stories and toward the generality of tendency stories and typifications, both of which are more readily fitted to generic diagnostic criteria.

This movement is one of progressive *abstraction*, in the sense that it reduces concrete features of the individual child and their relationships with interaction to more anonymous descriptions.[15]

In the deliberations over Ronnie Martin, although the clinicians reported and assessed an instance in which he followed a classroom instruction about child abuse prevention to the letter, they ended up reducing it to his propensity to imitate others (the focus of their subsequent tendency stories), ultimately typifying Ronnie as literalistic and imitative rather than creative in play—all features that fit with an autism diagnosis. Accordingly, the narrative account involved subordinating specific and particular aspects of Ronnie's behavior to the general and universal.[16]

In the case of Dan Chapman, we saw the clinicians reduce the *inter*action between Dan and Jennifer to Dan's actions alone, which were then further reduced to putative psychological processes. The concreteness and consistency of Dan's conduct as he resisted Jennifer's directives, and the situated meaning that conduct may have had for him as an autonomous person responding to another person's actions, do not come into view. In other words, the clinicians neglect autism as an interactional phenotype, promoting what we can call a *reductionist phenotype*: a *dis*ability residing entirely inside Dan, such that what was originally a joint achievement—the breakdown of the Demonstration Task—is said to emanate from a static thing (i.e., a disorder) Dan is said to have.

Overall, we find that the pattern in clinical narrative is toward increasing abstraction, with instantiation stories subordinated to tendency stories, and tendency stories subordinated to diagnostic typifications. This pattern is evident in the already-mentioned imbalance between tendency and instantiation stories, where tendency stories make up about 80 percent of all stories and instantiation stories account for the remaining 20 percent. The asymmetry is even more pronounced in the written evaluations that clinicians produce for inclusion in children's medical records.[17] Furthermore, the pattern is not restricted to the contemporary data. The cases considered in this chapter are from distinct eras in which the criteria for diagnosis, the number of professionals per case, and the average length of an evaluation were different: Ronnie Martin was evaluated in 1985, and Dan Chapman in 2014.[18] And yet the proportions of story types across time are remarkably similar. Therefore, it seems that in addition to narrative organization being a stable feature of the interaction order of the clinic, the relative distribution of tendency and instantiation stories is similarly robust (Maynard and Turowetz 2019).

This robustness has to do, at least in part, with the institutional objectives of the clinic as it operates with a medical model of disorder and diagnosis.

Since the goal is to fit particular individuals to generic diagnostic categories, tendency stories are useful for how they move in the direction of increasing abstraction, specifically of the subtractive kind. That is, they strip the particulars of the case away by summarizing them as tendencies, more precisely the tendencies enumerated in diagnostic criteria: a statement like "she has trouble with joint attention," for example, more readily fits with the criterion "deficits in non-verbal communicative behaviors" (per DSM-5) than does a story about a single occasion where the child "looked away from me when I showed her a toy." This means that while both instantiation and tendency stories provide evidence for typifications—the upshots that most directly name or index diagnostic criteria (e.g., "s/he *is* literal") and that include diagnostic conclusions as such (e.g., "s/he *has* autism")—clinicians rely mostly on generalizing about behaviors, rather than reporting on such behaviors in more discrete terms.

In the staffing (or informing) interview with families, clinicians again predominantly tell tendency stories, with very few instantiations. Parents, who are of course more knowledgeable about a child's conduct outside the clinic, also tell more tendency than instantiation stories, although the latter make up a larger proportion of their contributions to diagnostic narrative. Further, clinicians produce proportionately more stories (in the range of 75–90%) and typifying components compared with parents overall, and stories from parents are regularly in second position—that is, they follow a clinician's report, usually in an aligning way. This pattern, in which clinicians tell more stories than parents and use them in first rather than responsive positions, may be one way in which the participants orient epistemically (Heritage 2012) to clinicians' expertise and institutionalized authority to diagnose.

DEFICIT VS. COMPETENCE

First-order competencies—the many skills, abilities, and methods of sensemaking that are usually off-record in terms of gauging the second-order competence tests formally measure (Maynard and Marlaire 1992; Maynard and Turowetz 2017b)—present opportunities for clinicians, and ultimately caretakers, to inspect the child's sensemaking practices on their own terms, rather than pathologizing or ignoring them in accordance with the prerogatives of professionalized and standardized common sense, as encoded in diagnostic instruments. Indeed, a matter, per chapters 4 and 5, to be elaborated further in our concluding chapter (8), is that inspecting ostensibly "incompetent" test performances can reveal the *presence* of first-order competencies— "autistic intelligence"—where initially only absences (e.g., of ability) seemed

apparent. And such inquiry, in turn, widens ethnomethodological and related investigations, insofar as it means probing the features of common sense
itself as much as the reasoning behind expressions that threaten it. As Garfinkel (1967:31, original emphasis) once observed, "Not a method of understanding *but immensely various methods* of understanding are the sociologist's hitherto unstudied and critical phenomena."[19] When the child's private
methods of sensemaking are made publicly available and intelligible, the
strange becomes familiar and the groundwork is laid for achieving mutual
understanding.

Of the types of stories clinicians tell, instantiation stories have the great-
est potential for capturing children's methods, or at least hinting at skills that
the diagnostic process routinely misses. In practice, these stories vary con-
siderably in the amount of detail they provide. And like tendency stories,
they usually emphasize the child's actions rather than their interactions with
the clinician and assessment tool. Nonetheless, more details are captured by
stories that incorporate temporal sequencing (i.e., first x happened, then y)
than those that enfold temporally situated actions and reactions into general
tendencies (i.e., "he does a lot of x") or typified attributes (i.e., "she is y"). For
this reason, although, in their own right, instantiation stories sometimes can
obscure a child's sensemaking methods, they can also serve as points of entry
into the child's world and unique sensibilities, particularly when seen as opportunities to inquire more deeply about a focal behavior—to raise questions
and open new lines of investigation, rather than closing them down. Consider, for example, the following instantiation stories about Ronnie Martin
and Dan Chapman.

Instantiation Story about Ronnie Martin

The instantiation story about the "child abuse movie" represents a missed
opportunity to inquire into Ronnie's sensemaking practices. The clinicians
treated it as a humorous anecdote and evidence of the absence of flexible thinking on Ronnie's part, without asking what skills might be present in Ronnie's
behavior. Here, we can observe that Ronnie's sense that his father's directive to
"pick up his toys" was abusive, though evincing a literal understanding of the
movie's message, exhibits strong forms of first-order competence and autistic
intelligence. It is not only that literalism is a skill (as with Tony's orientation to
the "What do you do when" exercise recounted in chap. 5), but also that Ronnie displayed an ability to remember and follow multistep instructions, take
them seriously, apply them to a situation, and orient to an everyday moral
order regarding who is entitled to require compliance from whom within a

local course of action. These abilities represent realms of skill, competence, and autistic intelligence that could help caregivers and others (e.g., teachers) to understand Ronnie and his style of learning, teach him more effectively, and adjust the fit of his social environment to his particularities.

Instantiation Story about Dan Chapman

In his medical record, to which clinicians have access and which they are expected to read before conducting their examinations (they are permitted to bill for such time), there are strong indications that Dan could be a trouble-maker at school.

We discussed this matter in chapter 1; the following is verbatim (except for pseudonyms) from the record: "Dan's special education teacher, Terri Smith, shared a note that Dan seems to have more 'good' days than 'bad' days but his bad days at school involve verbally and/or physically aggressive behavior. His teacher noted that Dan has had three 'major meltdowns' since starting at his new school. These incidences have required seclusion and/or restraint procedures to be implemented."

Seclusion and restraint procedures are of questionable effectiveness (Reisinger 2016) and legality (Butler 2019), and other aspects of this report raise issues regarding what are known as "triggers" and how they can set off emotional dysregulation in persons with autism (Mazefsky et al. 2013). Like the reports about testing that we have discussed in this chapter, the depiction here elides both the role of other participants and any aspects of the setting or environment to which Dan's "aggressive" or other behavior may be responses. We suggest that our interactional approach sheds light on, or brings to the surface, the behavior of one person and that of other persons as well as objects in the social environment to which that behavior is intimately related.[20]

Jennifer's instantiation story about Dan and his behavior relative to the Demonstration Task is relevant here. As told, the story focuses on Dan's actions rather than his interactions with Jennifer. Even as Jennifer told it, the story of "Dan's failure" to complete the Demonstration Task represents a missed opportunity to ask what it was about the situation, including Jennifer's directives, that Dan could have been responding to. Unlike tendency stories, Jennifer's instantiation story preserves enough detail about the original interaction for clinicians and possibly his mother, Betsy, to ask different questions of it—not just about what may have been happening in Dan's mind but also in what may have been happening in his give and take with Jennifer during the assessment process. Instead of psychologizing Dan's actions, we might wonder what would have happened if the story had been treated as an opportunity to probe the assessment situation itself more deeply. In that case, it might have produced an account of the behavior more in line with our interactional analysis, which not only redistributes responsibility for the failure to both parties but shows something of an apparent contrast to Dan's school experiences. In a relatively friendly environment—as indicated in Jennifer's attempts at coaxing his compliance—Dan's resistance to her rather dogged directives[21] was politely repetitive, consistently quiet, and ultimately withdrawing rather than challenging or aggressive. This matters because it implies that minimization of more threatening or hostile directives in other social contexts, such as school, could reduce Dan's aggressions and disruptions.

Hence, it may be that the scant attention to instantiation stories—the imbalance in diagnosis whereby tendency stories outweigh them—combined with dismissive, suppressive, humorous, psychologizing, and other common ways of orienting to them when they do occur (Wiscons 2020)—suppresses information relevant to working with children such as Dan and Ronnie in terms of their embodied skills and first-order competencies. Others have argued along these lines, highlighting assets surrounding the orientation to detail in autism (Happé 1999) and ways that "formative" assessments (Erickson 2007; Heritage 2013; Heritage and Heritage 2013) based on a child's personal and idiosyncratic qualities can facilitate learning. If we deem autism to be an interactional phenotype, it means highlighting the potential of instantiation stories to direct inquiry toward interaction, rather than away from it. Then, a robust praxeography of diagnostic work may raise the matter of autistic intelligence to more prominence and motivate a different approach to evaluating and diagnosing autism. Such an approach could potentially supplement or complement the DSM's focus on deficits with an appreciation of interactional differences and the contributions of children *and* clinicians (or others, such as caregivers or teachers) *and* facets of the instrumental environment to autistic symptomatology.[22] The suggestion is not that institutionalized diagnostic practices need to be expunged entirely but instead that they may have within them unexploited possibilities for capturing the particularities of a child and thereby providing, rather than only a subtractive abstraction, a diagnostic mosaic.

Is Autism Real?

In earlier chapters, we saw that Dan Chapman presented a very mixed clinical picture, even though he ultimately qualified for an autism diagnosis. When discussing his case with the pediatrician Leah Grant, psychologist Jennifer Erickson expressed surprise that Dan "came out so high" on the ADOS, because "he did so many nice things," had a number of "pretty nice" responses, and displayed no "inappropriate gestures." When presenting the diagnosis to his mother, Betsy Chapman, Jennifer was more circumspect, saying that Dan "did show some signs that are consistent with being on the autism spectrum." Again, though, she also mentioned Dan's "nice things," "really nice strengths," being "appropriate," and doing a "nice job transitioning" as positives from her assessment.

While Dan's ADOS score was elevated enough to be unambiguous, Jennifer's surprise at the results, along with the mixed picture she presented to Leah and to Dan's mother, points to the uncertainty that can surround diagnosis and that is more extreme in some cases (Hayes et al. 2021; Hollin 2017).[1] In fact, Betsy reported during the informing interview that it had been difficult to find consistent diagnostic information for Dan and that although the doctors she consulted tried different medications, "nothing really worked" (staffing transcript:13). While this perhaps suggests indeterminacy rather than uncertainty, it indicates that from a medical point of view, the source of Dan's difficulties was far from definitive.[2] If things are so ambiguous, can autism be said to be real?

In this chapter, we explore how clinicians make sense of ambiguity, which is sometimes due to equivocal evidence. We also describe two practices for delivering diagnostic news and the ways clinicians use them to communicate diagnosis and manage parents' expectations, particularly when those expectations are at odds with the outcome. The first practice, which we call *cautious optimism*, involves announcing that a child qualifies for an autism diagnosis and following the announcement with a cautiously optimistic prognosis. The second practice, which we call *cautious pessimism*, does the inverse by provisionally ruling out a diagnosis of autism while acknowledging that the child has real problems that warrant evaluation (Halkowski 2006) and are "doctorable" (Heritage and Robinson 2006)—medically relevant and potentially treatable. The official recognition of problems and their treatability implies that no blame lies with either the parents or child as such. Both practices (cautious optimism and cautious pessimism) are common in our data and not only in borderline cases, but they are particularly visible in such cases, which is why focus on them here.

Ambiguity and Reality

Ambiguous cases of diagnosis raise a related issue. The objective reality of autism has long been a source of controversy. Does the recent upsurge in autism diagnoses reflect a change in the number of children affected by autism or the development of more sensitive methods for its detection (see chap. 2)? Is autism one or many? Is there a different autism phenotype for girls than for boys? How many "eccentric" artists, writers, and scientists from the past were actually on the spectrum before the terminology existed? The variety of stances on such matters can be gleaned from the following passages:

> Compared to other branches of medicine, psychiatric diagnosis is highly subjective. Take pneumonia, for example. The most common severe form of the disease is caused by the bacterium *Streptococcus pneumoniae*. Whether it afflicts a slum dweller in Brazil or a rice farmer in Bangladesh, it is exactly the same disease. You can see the bacterium under a microscope, you can devise a way to treat it, and the treatment will be the same no matter where you are. Now take a disorder like autism. You cannot see autism under a microscope or discover it through a lab test. The only evidence we have that someone has autism is the individual's behavior. There is little agreement, even in a single culture, about exactly what it is or how to treat it. (Grinker 2007:2)

✳

> A consensus has begun to emerge that autism (or some percentage of autism spectrum disorders) is caused by a not-yet understood confluence of genetic predisposition and environmental influence. Beyond these orthodoxies, however, the disorder remains nebulous. One reason is that the diagnostic categories themselves are constantly evolving. (Osteen 2008:9)

*

The determination of which symptoms constitute difference and which constitute impairment remains vague. (Nadesan 2005:208)

As these quotes suggest, whatever autism is, it cannot be reduced to a faulty nucleotide, missing gene, or misfolded protein that we might detect in the laboratory. Indeed, autism seems fungible—it is something of a moving target: the diagnosis has changed enough in the past few decades that it is not even clear that today's children with autism are "the same" as yesterday's.[3] To address this matter, we return to our own stance regarding autism and also reconsider autism as a social interactional phenotype.

BRACKETING THE AUTISM DIAGNOSIS

We have said that our stance toward autism is grounded in a phenomenological sensibility that suspends judgment about whether or not it is real.[4] Accordingly, in our analysis we have put the syndrome in "brackets," neither committing ourselves to its existence nor taking the stance that it does *not* "really" exist. The latter position could be compatible with seeing autism as a social construction.[5] Our orientation is different from either of these views and involves agnosticism that follows from what we said in chapter 2 about Pollner's (1974), Latour's (2004), and Mol's (2002) ways of putting the concerns of professionals and lay people at the center of analysis. It is these actors who principally wrestle with autism's reality, and they often are ambivalent about a particular child's qualifications, which may reflect how evidence itself can be ambiguous.

Because each child enters the clinic with a unique biography and set of challenges, some degree of ambiguity will be present in many cases of autism diagnosis. A common source of ambiguity is discrepant information about the child. For example, parents, teachers, and clinicians may provide different ratings of the child's social competence, creating a potential "reality disjuncture" (Pollner 1974) by producing seemingly incompatible versions of the child. Once again, this was the case with Dan Chapman, who as we saw in chapter 2 received different scores from his mother and teacher on the Child Behavior Checklist (CBCL), with the mother rating him higher (more impaired) than the teacher. He also scored just below the threshold for autism on the Social Communication Questionnaire (SCQ) filled out by his mother, whereas the clinician, on the basis of the ADOS, found that he qualified for an autism diagnosis.

One practice for resolving such discrepancies is to discount an information source as unreliable. Thus, in the case of Emmett Hanson (case 15 in our
recent data), a five-year-old boy who was diagnosed with autism, the clinical
psychologist told her speech pathologist colleague that Emmett's mother did
not seem to understand the Vineland Adaptive Behavior Scales (a measure
of adaptive functioning that parents are often asked to fill out) and "totally
overrated him." Another practice is to weight some sources more heavily than
others: in Dan's case, the clinicians seem to have treated his ADOS score as
definitive, aligning his ratings on the CBCL to the ADOS by suggesting that
the latter gave a more accurate representation of his functioning.[6] These and
related practices for making sense of discrepant information operate under
and preserve the assumption that there is only one true version of the child
across all environments: Dan cannot *really* be more socially competent in
school than at home, and Emmett *really* cannot be more socially competent
at home than in the clinic. At most, they can *appear* more competent, though
their underlying level of competence remains unchanged.[7]

In many cases, however, the ambiguities are more persistent and not as
easily resolved. A child could receive a high score on the ADOS but show
social strengths inconsistent with that score at other points in the evaluation
process. Or an ADOS score might be under the threshold for autism, but the
clinicians, suspecting that symptoms were too subtle to detect, could nonetheless advise parents to monitor the child's behavior as they age and social
situations become more complex and demanding. In these cases, clinicians
will often adopt a wait-and-see stance, giving a provisional diagnosis or a provisional non-diagnosis. Such tentative conclusions can be difficult for parents
to hear because they are lacking in not only definitive explanations for the
child's problems but also in any consequent suggestions about what can be
done. In our view, tentativeness derives in part from the way that autism is a
social interactional phenotype.

BACK TO THE SOCIAL INTERACTIONAL PHENOTYPE

We have shown that autism assessment is an interactional and interactive phenomenon. The assessment tools do not, by themselves, passively detect autism in the way a genetic test may be said to do for Down syndrome. Rather,
diagnosing autism is a complex process in which clinicians use standardized
instruments and observations to elicit, code, count, and classify social behavior. We have seen that narrative plays a central role in that process, as
clinicians use storytelling to make sense of observations and arrive at defen-
sible findings. The tacit preferences clinicians orient in telling these stories,

however, lead them to disattend—and in effect erase—their own contributions, and those of their assessment tools, to the behavior they observe. In
these stories, autistic behavior seems to emanate from the child alone, quite
independent of the social order of the clinic, which instead comes across as
a neutral arena where the child's symptoms can become manifest.[8] Accordingly, through narrative practices, the clinicians arrive at an institutionally
accountable diagnosis whose features conform to the DSM's (APA 2013) definition of autism as an enduring disorder of the person that is fundamentally
indifferent to the outside environment.

What does all this mean for the question of whether autism is real? We
already described our position as one of phenomenological agnosticism,
but a slightly different way of putting it is to say that we understand the reality of autism as being tied to the social order properties for its detection
and accountability—the ways in which it is documented through the use of
standardized assessment protocols and collectively regarded as what Latour
(2004:226–27) calls a "matter of concern." In other words, the practices for
detecting autism, including narratives that manage ambiguity and assign
weights to different information sources, are constitutive of its objectivity,
or its status as a witnessable, reportable, and consequential phenomenon for
members of a society—family, educators, therapists, and others.

Within and across phases of an evaluation, clinicians must coordinate a
range of activities—interviews with parents; pediatric medical exams; speech
and language, occupational, and psychological assessments—that bear on different aspects of diagnosis. So it is also through the work of coordination that
clinicians combine different *enactments* of autism. These variously appear, in
different testing arenas, as difficulty with expressive and receptive language
(speech and language), sensory processing issues (occupational therapy),
physical symptomology (pediatrics), cognitive differences (psychiatry), and
impaired social communication and repetitive behavior (psychology). Clinicians, by way of narrative, combine them into a unitary entity that is eventually named as autism.[9]

That autism "presents" in multiple ways even in a single clinic is apparent in cases where clinicians see different clinical objects in their respective
evaluations. For example, it may be unclear if children with language delays
are showing autism-like behavior because a specific language disorder makes
them unable to communicate and learn social skills or if the delays are in fact
manifestations of autism. In such cases, clinicians need to bring their disparate
findings together, which may require multiple narrative rounds (Turowetz
and Maynard 2017) where constraints are set on discussions, contradictory
accounts are entertained, and facts of the case are realigned in support of a

larger story line (Hayes et al. 2021). Tendency stories are especially useful in this regard, since they generalize over the kinds of specific details that appear in instantiation stories and that may even be inconsistent with DSM criteria. The same practical logic applies to all settings where autism is assembled as a social fact. In the postclinic phase of an autism career, relationships with family, peers, and institutional actors such as teachers, therapists, judges, police, case workers, insurers, and physicians further elaborate autism as a social phenomenon. The child's identity as a person with autism ultimately depends on the way these actors coordinate their practices so as to achieve the disorder's singularity amid its multiplicity (i.e., its multiple realizations across distinct environments).

ACHIEVING DIAGNOSTIC COHERENCE

A particularly striking illustration of the *achieved* character of autism's unity occurs when different organizations use distinct criteria and thereby produce discrepant versions of the person. For example, in some US states, it is possible to have an educational diagnosis of autism but not a medical one. This is because school administrators, although bound by the Individuals with Disabilities Education Act (IDEA) to determine who qualifies for special education, are not required to use DSM criteria. Instead, an evaluation committee consisting of parents, teachers, and school psychologists makes the decision, as outlined in the Code of Federal Regulations (Center for Autism Research 2020). If the school decides the child has autism for educational purposes, they may be entitled to an individualized education plan (IEP) and associated resources in school, even if they do not have a medical diagnosis that would qualify them for state services and reimbursements from insurers. Conversely, a child may have a medical diagnosis, but if school personnel determine that their condition is not severe enough to impair classroom performance, there is no educational diagnosis or commensurate programming.[10]

Thus, during the latter part of the informing interview for Dan Chapman, Leah Grant says to his mother, Betsy, "When we give a new diagnosis for a kid who's already in school, we recommend going back to the school, taking the information from our visit. . . . We'd be setting up a case conference, and kind of reevaluating what the services are that the school's giving, and . . . that he's qualified for. . . . Because Autism Spectrum Disorder is also a diagnostic classification for the school" (staffing transcript:13).

As we have said, our research is limited to the in-clinic phase of things, and we do not know what happened at Dan's school. However, we can see in the developmental pediatrician's remarks that there is ambiguity as to what will happen at the school in terms of diagnosis and provision of services. In some cases, parents may have to fight the school for diagnosis and services, even though the clinic documents an autism diagnosis.

When there are "medical" and "educational" diagnoses, and if they are in conflict, which version of the child is the "real" one? How can a child, because of different standards, have autism at one time and not at another, or in one place and not another? Our answer is that contradictory diagnostic outcomes are *all real* insofar as actors in an accredited setting constitute them as objective "matters of concern" (Latour 2004) within their respective orders of practice. Whether and how the distinct versions of the child cohere is sometimes, but not always, a problem for agents (e.g., parents, clinicians, educators), and in such cases the analyst's task is to attend to the procedures through which such coherence is achieved. In other words, from our ethnomethodological perspective, the analyst's concern is to explain how coherence (or lack thereof) is made into a problem by members of a given setting (be it the clinic or school) and with which practices they resolve that problem.

In what follows, we examine three cases in which clinicians and families treat the appropriateness of an autism diagnosis for a child as a problem. In these cases, there are interactional sequences whereby participants orient to the relevance and consequences of the diagnosis. Clinicians work to manage the ambiguity surrounding symptoms and diagnosis, parents respond in discrete ways, and the parties all cooperatively assemble autism as either a present or a potential feature of the child. In the cases we scrutinize—one in which the child is given an autism diagnosis and two in which autism is ruled out—participants orient to the question of whether autism is *real for this child* as a local matter of concern.[11]

Cautious Optimism

In chapter 5, we met Sara Brennan (case 34), who was three years old when she arrived at the CDDC. Although Sara's medical records stated that she lagged behind her peers in language development and social skills and was prone to inflexible behavior and tantrums, in the clinic she was lively and socially engaging. However, Sara inexplicably faltered on the Demonstration Task when she produced a sneeze instead of showing and telling how to brush one's teeth. In fact, Sara displayed inconsistencies throughout her evaluation, prompting Dr. Ruth McCain, the psychologist who evaluated her, to express ambivalence about the diagnosis during a case conference with Dr. Aaron Schultz, the speech pathologist who observed Ruth's administration of the ADOS:

TRANSCRIPT 7.1A: CASE 34: PRESTF2:1

```
 1  Ruth:   Well:: um: actually I was surprised at how well she ↑did on
 2          [a lot of things to be honest and so [(.) um: I was gonna
 3  Aar:    [Yeah (Nodding))                     [#(      )#
 4  Ruth:   =actually score it before I even .h 'cos I don't- I'm not I don't
 5          think it's clear. I mean she has some:: um: definite atypicalities?
 6          [to her and um and (then) she's repetitive and she's kind of rigid.
 7  Aar:    [Yup. ((Nodding))
 8  Ruth:   Um: but she has she's: has really nice requests, she has really
 9          nice gestures [.hh (.) um that she's using (.) appropriately=
10  Aar:                  [Yup.
11  Ruth:   =to get her (.) thoughts (that) needs to communicate across?
12  Aar:    Mm hmm.
```

Ruth's expression of surprise (lines 1–2) turns out to be a narrative preface, which she elaborates by saying that she needs to tally Sara's score "before" (line 4) making a decision, since the diagnosis is not "clear" (lines 4–5). In doing so, Ruth may be suggesting an implicit contrast between cases where she knows the outcome before even calculating a score—cases where the child's performance is not "surprising"[12]—and this one. Ruth then produces an "I mean" utterance that projects a defense of her assessment (cf. Maynard 2013), which she accomplishes with typifying upshots (e.g., "she has," "she is") about Sara's "atypicalities," repetitiveness, and rigidity (lines 5–6), followed by a contrastive (*but*-prefaced) list of the child's developmentally typical tendencies: "nice requests," "gestures . . . that she's using appropriately" (lines 8–9, 11).

Such ambivalence is expressed throughout Ruth and Aaron's review of Sara's ADOS performance. Aaron tells an instantiation story that illustrates the complexities involved in making sense of Sara's behavior. He describes how at one point she was "pretending to be the mommy" in an imaginary picnic, which he assesses as "a nice role-play thing." However, he goes on to qualify that assessment, saying, "But then I kinda didn't know what to make of it because it seemed, ah, her way of making things be about her." Ruth aligns to and elaborates on Aaron's story, saying, "Yeah. Yeah like she was getting rid of me in the play." This is a tendency story, as it suggests that the exclusionary behavior happened on multiple occasions.

The way that Ruth and Aaron understand what Sara was doing during the "picnic" matters. If they decide she was engaged in successful role play, it would mean she was displaying a skill that is known to be problematic for autistic children. If, however, the clinicians see her actions as exhibits of rigidity, or inept and egocentric play, they can be considered manifestations of autism. The borderline between these interpretations is permeable, but once it becomes firmly drawn, it has crucial implications for diagnosis and a child's ensuing moral career (Goffman 1961) as typically or atypically developing.

Ruth and Aaron proceed to comment on Sara's problematic gesturing, lack of eye contact, rigidity, and repetitiveness in play, with Ruth concluding that those "are her main weaknesses." Slightly later, she asks Aaron if he saw "any initiation of joint attention" on Sara's part. She starts a story about Sara's performance on a task involving a remote-controlled toy bunny, saying that Sara "did a nice job," but aborts this utterance to note that she (Ruth) made a mistake "the first time I did it" (summoned Sara) because the bunny was under a blanket.[13] However, Aaron, positioning himself as a story-consociate (Lerner 1992)—a knowledgeable contributor to the diagnostic narrative—introduces mention of the "third time" Ruth made a bid for Sara's attention. He observes that Ruth "really had to get [her] full body" into getting Sara to respond. In so doing, he builds a preface in contradistinction to Ruth's projected story about a "nice job" into one about Sara's failure at joint attention—another symptom of autism, and one that the bunny task is designed to measure.

Ruth responds with a second story that reflexively elaborates Aaron's first story. In reference to a task where Ruth and Sara played a game in which Ruth blew up a balloon, released it, and encouraged Sara to bring it back to her for another round (they went through several), Ruth produces a typification regarding "eye contact" (below, extract 7.1b, line 1), followed by a tendency story (lines 2–3, "She was looking") that suggests lack of eye contact. Ruth then produces an instantiation story in which she describes and reenacts (lines 6–7) how Sara blew on her finger to tacitly request that Ruth blow up the balloon but nonetheless only "looked at" Ruth momentarily and was otherwise focused on the balloon (lines 5, 7–9; see fig. 7.1).

This story seems designed for Aaron to hear it as evidence of Sara orienting to objects instead of people, which is considered a sign of autism.

TRANSCRIPT 7.1B: CASE 34: PRESTF2:4

```
 1  Ruth:   =She doesn't have a clear:: even with her eye contact isn't
 2          clearly: eye contact (or) with the balloon? She was looking at the
 3          balloon she wasn't looking at me.
 4  Aar:    Okay.
 5  Ruth:   Um: (no/the) when she [did ↑THIS: she did look at me=
 6  Ruth:                         [((Puts finger to mouth))
 7  Ruth:   =when she went ((blows on finger)) like that? She looked at me but
 8          it was very: >fast< and she'd go right to the balloon and she was
 9          really focused on my mouth and the balloon?=
10  Aar:    =(That's): I saw that a lot . . .
```

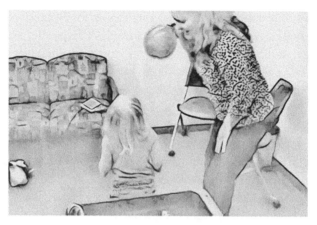

FIGURE 7.1

Ruth's story also describes Sara as not making eye contact with Ruth—"she was really focused on my mouth" (lines 8–9)—another characteristic commonly associated with autism. At line 10, Aaron aligns ("I saw that a lot"), and projects a further story in which he describes instances of fleeting eye contact. However, the ambivalence about Sara's symptoms continues, as when slightly later Aaron goes on to say, "Well there was the one time when she had the book open, and she said, 'uh oh,' then pointed to it and looked right at you, and looked back to the book." Ruth acknowledges this report with an "okay." Shortly thereafter, Aaron says, "I gotta run and get ready for number two" (another patient).

Now it was time for Ruth to consult with Leah Grant, the developmental pediatrician who had been the first clinician to see Sara and her family that day. Ruth had not yet had a chance to score the ADOS, so the discussion centered on informal observations made in the context of administering the exam. Ruth paged through her ADOS test booklet, consulting her notes. As she narrates her observations to Leah, Ruth evinces diagnostic ambivalence through her use of *contrastive* elements (cf. Goldknopf 2002:74–77). She does this in a patterned way where she describes and positively assesses a behavior, then produces a contrast marker (*but*, or *not*) followed by a further assessment that names a behavior associated with autism. These further assessments both diminish the earlier positive assessment and implicate an autism diagnosis (Case 34PRESTF:1,1,3):

"I can just tell you quick that she had some nice strengths still, but she was pretty rigid in her play." [preface]

"So with the balloon play especially, she did a really nice requesting with gestures, but it wasn't really with eye contact, and she would look right at the balloon instead of at me" [tendency].

"The way that we code with this, she has a lot of the skills that you would see; they're just not great." [typifying]

In sequential terms, these contrastive devices position the final, downgrading phrase as strongly "implicative" for further discourse (Schegloff and Sacks 1973:296), which enables interactional progressivity toward the autism diagnosis. However, a coherent narrative in Sara's case only comes together after Ruth has a chance to score the ADOS and when Leah and Ruth meet with the family— mother, father, Sara, and her younger sister—during the informing interview.

THE DIAGNOSTIC MOMENT FOR SARA

Sara's case was complicated. While she showed symptoms of autism, including rigidity, inflexibility, and problems with communication, she also had many strengths, as the clinicians repeatedly observed. When Ruth scored the ADOS, however, she found that Sara qualified for the ASD diagnosis. Anticipating the delivery of their findings, the clinicians observed that the parents were in a fragile place. Leah commented that she sensed some hostility from Sara's mother toward her father, who had mostly sat in silence as the mother answered Leah's questions. And Leah proposed how raising a challenging child may have been taking a toll on the marriage. Accordingly, when delivering the diagnosis to the parents, they proceeded carefully, offering empathy and understanding as Sara's mother, Stephanie, reacted to the news. Although at first showing strong emotion, subsequently Stephanie was cautiously optimistic, in line with the way the clinicians were framing the news.

As Ruth and Leah talk, Sara and her younger sister are playing with toys nearby in the same room. Leah opens the conversation by briefly summarizing the family's journey to the clinic, which she acknowledges has been difficult. She then offers the floor to Ruth, who goes on to describe the testing she did with Sara and present the diagnosis. Using a *so*-preface to project an upshot to the testing (line 1),[14] Ruth reports that Sara "<u>did</u> meet the cutoff" for autism (lines 2–3).[15]

TRANSCRIPT 7.1C: CASE 34: STF:3

```
1  Ruth:   So ↑having said all (of) that (.) she di:d (.) she did meet
2          the ↓cutoff fo:r an autism spectrum disorder (.) in terms of
3          .h what I saw in the: uh (.) in the assessment today.
```

```
 4          (0.2)
 5  Steph:  So what does that mean. ((Mother furrows brow; Father nods))
 6          (0.2)
 7  Ruth:   It ↑means ↓tha:t we ca:n go ahead and give her a diagnosis
 8          (.) of aut[ism.
 9  Steph:            [((Looks down; puts hands over face and cries))
10          (.)
11  Ruth:   I kn- I know that's really a difficult thing to hear.
12          (.)
13  Steph:  It just ((muffled; crying voice)) in a way it's a relief but
14          at the same time it's not. .h ((removes hands from face))
15  Ruth:   Yeah
```

At line 5, Stephanie asks for clarification (on post-announcement meaning assessments, cf. Maynard 2006), and Ruth explains, "It means that we can go ahead and give her a diagnosis of autism" (lines 7–8). Stephanie starts to sob, but after Ruth expresses empathy at line 11, she displays an ambivalent stance toward the diagnosis (lines 13–14), including "relief" (line 13), that may reflect the feelings of many parents upon hearing their child has autism.

Leah now enters the discussion (not on transcript), describing the diagnosis as "really hard" and "not as clear cut" as in other cases she sees. She repeats that Sara "does meet the cutoff" on the ADOS, adding that the diagnosis also fits with Sara's "history and the things that you [the parents] told me," but then offers an optimistic prognosis, saying that "because she's so young and because she has so many strengths . . . what we're gonna do is . . . we're gonna give her the diagnosis of autism today and we're gonna call it a provisional diagnosis."

Leah also recommends that "we reassess" before Sara starts kindergarten, and continues (Case 34 STF:4): "It may be that in a couple of years it's still pretty clear that that diagnosis is a good fit for her. There are a very small number of kids and we don't even understand exactly why this is . . . who don't seem to fit the criteria a couple years down the road . . . we think and we hope it may have something to do with really putting all the right supports in place for them." Leah is constructing a narrative about a "possible future" (Gibson 2011), in which Sara may turn out to be like a category of children who, after a few years, no longer "fit the criteria." At the end, she shifts into the subjunctive mood, saying that "we" (a reference to herself and fellow professionals) "think . . . and hope" that interventions and supports are the reason children improve. The upshot is that with the right treatment, Sara *may* eventually function as a neurotypical child does.

Leah then goes on to say that "even if" the diagnosis sticks, Sara is still a "very bright little girl" with many strengths. Sara's mother contributes to this bright-side projection, recounting her own experience with a man who comes into her workplace every day, goes through the same routine, and leaves. She says that while her coworkers think he is strange, she recognizes that he is autistic. Finally, she offers her own optimistic upshot: this man's parents have done well with him, so although there will be challenges, there is hope for Sara (implying a positive role for her husband and herself in Sara's development).

Stephanie's contribution provides a further illustration of how parents can participate in the structural organization of diagnosis through forms of narrative recipiency. Parents' stories shape what the diagnosis means for each specific child, often helping to align generic diagnostic criteria to the particularities of a single individual, though in some instances they will overtly challenge clinicians.[16] For their part, clinicians regularly couple announcements of autism with hypothetical stories about the future, putting a positive slant on ostensibly bad news and projecting the experience of a relatively benign social world (Maynard 2003:chap. 6) for the child and family despite the diagnosis.

Cautious Pessimism

If confirming a diagnosis of autism can end on a cautiously optimistic note, the apparently "good" news that a child does not have autism can go in the opposite direction. Such news may engender what we call *cautious pessimism*. In fact, parents sometimes are quite distraught by the news that their child does not have autism. This is because a not-autism finding leaves "symptom residue" (Maynard and Frankel 2006) in its wake, meaning that the child's troubles and challenges remain unexplained. At the same time, such a finding may raise the possibility that the difficulties are due to poor parenting or that the parents are being irresponsible by worrying too much about their child's mental health (e.g., they could be over-monitoring the child's behavior; cf. Halkowski 2006).

Aware of possible parental sensitivities when ruling out autism, clinicians avoid giving a no-problem diagnosis in any comprehensive way. Instead, they affirm that the child *does* have problems but that autism is not the best way to describe them. In this way, they reassure the parents that the child's problems fall within the purview of medicine—that they are clinically relevant (cf. Heritage and Robinson 2006) and that it may be possible to obtain services to treat them, even if they do not meet the criteria for an autism spectrum disorder. Our first example of cautious pessimism, involving Lily Wren, is brief, as it mainly illustrates how a parent can resist a delivery of diagnostic news presented as "good" because it rules out autism. Our second example and analysis of cautious pessimism is longer. It involves Max Bailey (whose performance on the Demonstration Task is seen in chap. 5) and illustrates the matter of ambiguity in a more complex manner.

LILY WREN: GETTING SERVICES

A year before her 2013 visit to CDDC, Lily Wren, a seven-year-and-nine-month-old girl, had been diagnosed with intellectual disability and attention deficit disorder. Three months previous to the current visit, a CDDC developmental pediatrician, Dr. Patricia Owens, had seen Lily, noted a variety of problems, and recommended a new psychological assessment because of the mother's concerns about the possibility of autism. The mother, Anna Wren, was concerned about Lily's impulsive behavior, difficulty comprehending directions, episodes of staring, repetitive talk, and other difficulties. She was most especially interested in the possibility of autism.

For this visit at CDDC, Aaron Schultz, the clinic's speech pathologist (who also saw Sara Brennan), examined Lily and determined that her language skills were at about a four-year-old level, or three years behind her chronological age. Furthermore, during a pre-staffing conference, both Aaron and Dr. Ellen Miller, the psychologist who had administered the Vineland Adaptive Behavior Skills and Child Behavior Checklist instruments along with the ADOS, agreed that autism was not indicated. A medical resident was observing. Subsequently, the two clinicians, Ellen and Aaron, and the resident met with Anna, Anna's partner, George, and Lily's father, William (who, with amicable arrangements, was also a caretaker for Lily), for the informing interview.

Near the very beginning, Ellen (lines 1–2 below) rules out an autism diagnosis, which she frames as "good news." During this delivery, but not marked on the transcript, she gazes briefly at Aaron, who nods several times in response. Thus, it is something of a collaborative presentation. However, notice that after completing her utterance at line 2, which is a point where "turn transition" (Sacks, Schegloff, and Jefferson 1974) is relevant, Ellen draws an inbreath (".hh") and hesitates with "um::." This is an initial indication that Anna is refraining from taking a turn at talk, and subsequently, there is a silence (line 3), indicating full-blown withholding from talk on Anna's part, which shows resistance to the "good news" characterization. Ellen continues with "on the one hand" (line 4), which projects a contrast between what is "kind of nice to hear" when someone "does have something like that" (lines 4–5). As her turn goes on, Ellen begins a "because then" clause (end of line 6,

line 8), but Anna comes in with a candidate completion (Lerner 1996) of Ellen's utterance (line 9), "we want some kind of a diagnosis," while in overlap
(line 10), Ellen loudly says, "AN ANSWER." With "I know, I know" (line 12),
Ellen also claims understanding of what Anna asserts that she wants.

TRANSCRIPT 7.2: CASE 17: STF:1:19

```
 1  Ellen:  So .hh ↑good ↓new:s is that she doesn't (.) have an autism
 2           spectrum disorder. .hh um:
 3           (0.7)
 4  Ellen:  On- on the one hand it- (.) you know it can be (0.5) kind of
 5           nice to hear that someone (0.2) does have something like that
 6           >when you're in a situation< [like you're in, because=
 7  Anna:                                 [Yeah
 8  Ellen:  =then [it's like-
 9  Anna:         [We want some kind of a diag[nosis.    ]=
10  Ellen:                                     [AN ANSWER.]=
11  Anna:   =[(      )]
12  Ell:    =[I know. ] I [know.
13  Dad:                  [Yeah [(   )
14  Anna:                 [You- you do have a (      )
15  Lily:                 [My tummy hurts [really bad.
16  Ellen:                                [Right. Right. I mean it's
17           really is mixed feelings.=Um .hhh but (0.2) the- the good news
18           is that you know autism spectrum disorders like they're life
19           lo:n:g, and and- we don't have (0.7) really: (.) there's a lot
20           of things that we don't know about how to help people with
21           them.=.hhh um:
22           (1.2)
23  Ellen:  So: she- she:: (0.9) she does have (.) other: diagnoses going on
24           I think that we can give her that will help her get services.
25           Which: is really what you want.
```

After some overlapping talk, including Lily's complaint about her stomach
(line 15), Ellen pursues the matter of no autism as "good news," suggesting
that this is because "autism spectrum disorders" are "life lo:n:g" and that there
is a lack of knowledge about how to deal with the condition (lines 18–20).
This addition elaborates the "good news" framing by providing a reason why
the parents should be happy their child does not have autism. Still, at line 22,
Anna refrains from uptake, and Ellen now offers a cautiously pessimistic take
on Lily's situation: although she does not have autism, there are "other diagnoses going on" that will help the family procure treatment for their child
(lines 23–24). In this way, Ellen reassures the parents that there is a medical
explanation for Lily's problems—that they are doctorable and will make her
eligible for services.

MAX BAILEY: WAIT AND SEE

Max Bailey (case 18) is another one of the children whose performance on the Demonstration Task was discussed in chapter 5. Max was five years old in 2013, when he was evaluated at the CDDC upon referral from his pediatrician. Referral documents in his medical record give an initial sense of ambiguity regarding Max's difficulties. These are verbatim reports, with only the names altered:

> Max's mother reported that Max does make social approaches to others. He will often approach others asking a question to which he already knows the answer; his parents interpret this as an effort to start an interaction with others. Having reciprocal conversation is difficult for Max. He becomes excited around other children and is interested in them, but he does not seem to know how to interact with peers. His mother said that Max appears to ignore peers who approach him. He is very happy to play near peers and does not seem aware at all that he is completely unengaged with them. He will respond to adults and will seek adults out. He is very good at doing pretend play.

> ✳

> Max also misses verbal social information. He often requires directions to be given multiple times before they register with him. This requires a lot of extra time and effort from his teachers. He relies on routines. Once they are established, he will notice any changes to the routine and ask about the change, although he is not distressed by a change in his routine.

> ✳

> Max also has unusual interests. He has had an interest in makes and models of vehicles, and he would ask adults what make and model their car was, without regard for the appropriateness of asking for this information in a given social situation. He now has a strong interest in Legos and especially in the instructions for Legos. He sleeps with an instruction booklet, and he often asks about the order of steps to building a structure. While Max has these interests, he can be diverted from them. If told once or twice that it is not time to talk about one of these topics, he can move away to something else. These interests have never interfered with his ability to do other things, according to his mother.

There hardly could be more equivocation about characteristics of autism. Max is interested in other children but does not know how to approach them except through questions to which he knows the answers. He often ignores others who approach him, apparently "unaware" of his disengagement, but he does respond to adults, and he engages in "pretend play." He requires multiple directions to understand what he is to do and relies on routines, but is not distressed when there are changes to the routines. Max has unusual interests in cars and does not realize he is inappropriate in expressing these interests, but is not rigid in their pursuit. Given these characteristics, the final evaluation may be surprising.

At CDDC, Max was initially seen by an occupational therapist, a developmental pediatrician, and a speech pathologist. The speech and language evaluation confirmed, per the medical record, "moderately to severely delayed language skills compared to peers his age, with language skills between a 3- to 4-year-old level." On a subsequent visit, psychologist Dr. Ellen Miller, who also saw Lily Wren, evaluated Max. She administered the ADOS along with tests of cognitive ability and adaptive behaviors. Although finding some symptoms of autism, Ellen concluded, after scoring the ADOS and reviewing the other assessments, that Max did not meet the threshold for autism. On ADOS-2, Max scored at 5, which was, as she put it in her written report, "below the cutoff of 8 considered suggestive of an ASD." Still, she also noted that, although he "showed a number of strengths in terms of social communication," he exhibited limited (a) use of eye gaze, (b) reciprocal communication, (c) rapport, and (d) flexibility in speech. Given that the other clinicians saw Max on a different day and were not available when Ellen conducted her evaluations, there was no pre-staffing conference. Once Ellen had completed her interviews and tests, she went directly to the informing interview phase of the visit.

THE DIAGNOSTIC MOMENT FOR MAX

In delivering her results to Max's mother, Marge Bailey,[17] Ellen hedges the news. She is careful to acknowledge the legitimacy of the parents' (and others') concerns, claiming that the referral to CDDC was warranted. At lines 1–2 and 4 below, Ellen issues a pre-announcement, briefly summarizing the testing she did with Max. She then produces a *so*-prefaced announcement of the news (lines 4–5). Her claim to not give a "final diagnosis" suggests a qualification, and after Marge produces a minimal news receipt (line 6), Ellen begins to elaborate, "co-implicating" her perspective (cf. Maynard 1992) by referencing what "you [Marge] said" (line 7). Ellen breaks off her turn when Max initiates a short exchange with his mother (line 8), but then, upon resumption, she assesses Max as "so mild" (line 9) and appears to initiate an *if* clause at the end of that utterance. At this point, Marge provides a candidate completion of the clause and adds an agreement token ("If he does yeah," line 10), which Ellen collaboratively completes (line 11; cf. Lerner 1996), stressing the conditional nature of the "mild" disorder by putting vocal emphasis on "if." Marge responds with strong agreement ("That's right," line 12).

TRANSCRIPT 7.3A: CASE 18: STF:3

```
 1   Ellen:   O:kay so um so (like you know I've been doing) cognitive
 2            [testing with hi:m [an:d um testing for an autism spectrum=
 3   Marge:   [Sure              [Yeah
 4   Ellen:   =disorder.=So .hh the- (no//now) I'm not giving a final
 5            diagnosis of an autism spectrum disorder, .hh=
 6   Marge:   =Mm hmm=
 7   Ellen:   =Um: (0.4) I think he's a little like- like you said he's:-
 8   . . .    ((7 transcript lines dealing with question from Max omitted))
 9   Ellen:   He's (sort/so)- he's so mi:l:d if- if=
10   Marge:   =If he does [yeah=
11   Ellen:               [If he does have [one.
12   Marge:                                [That's (right).
13            (.)
14   Ellen:   .hh He ↑doesn't meet the criteria on the- on the ADOS? (which
15            is) (.) an autism [diagnostic observation schedule. .hh um:
16   Marge:                     [Mm hmm.
17            (0.6)
18   Ellen:   Eh- he got a f- a fi:ve, and the cutoff is eight. (So he didn't
19            meet    )
20   . . .    ((5 transcript lines dealing with Max and toys omitted))
21   Ellen:   But he's the kinda kid who: um (0.7) m:ight like in- in la:ter
22            like in middle school, (and some)- everybody has a hard time in
23            middle school right?
24            (.)
25   Ellen:   um: but if- if you start to see- (0.3) well if you see concerns
26            at any time [but in particular like loo:king .hh for um social=
27   Marge:               [Okay
28   Ellen:   =challenges [around that age and=
29   Marge:               [Mm hmm
30   Marge:   =In middle school. Okay.
```

Following a micropause (line 13), Ellen elaborates (lines 14–15), *citing* (Maynard 2004) or *explicating* (Peräkylä 1998) Max's ADOS score (lines 18–19) as evidence. Then, after a brief exchange with Max (line 20), who has unloaded a bucket of toys onto the floor, Ellen produces a category attribution, assimilating Max to a larger group of children ("he's the kinda kid," line 21) who might experience challenges in middle school (lines 22–23) and advising Marge to monitor Max's development for "social challenges" in particular (lines 26, 28). Thus, through a prognostic narrative about a possible future (Gibson 2011) for Max, Ellen acknowledges that autism may yet be the appropriate diagnosis for him.

Immediately after excerpt 7.3a, Ellen states that symptoms can become more visible even as early as fourth grade, as social relationships become more complex and demanding (not shown). Marge asks if autism can be diagnosed that late, and Ellen says yes, adding that her specialty is diagnosing and treating adolescents and adults with autism. She then reaffirms the possibility of "later" diagnosis (below, line 1) and goes on to assess the referral as a "good" one (lines 3,6)—in other words, relevant to have consulted CDDC about—citing the "intense" quality of Max's social interactions as reasonable grounds (lines 8, 12–13).

TRANSCRIPT 7.3B: CASE 18: STF:3

```
 1   Ellen:   Um so (0.3) so yeah so I mean people can be diagnosed later
 2            (0.3) and- and a thing is- is that there are some-
 3            [(0.4) some (0.5) ↑things that [(I)- and- and this is a=
 4            [((Max talking in overlap))
 5   Marge:                                  [Yes.
 6   Ellen:   =good referral.
 7            (.)
 8   Ellen:   You know. [And there's some good reasons to think that he (.)=
 9   Marge:             [Ye:s.
10   Marge:   =Yeah.
11            (.)
12   Ellen:   could have a- ay uh- a social quality (and/to) his interactions
13            (0.2) [are ↓really intense.
14   Max:           [((indecipherable talking))
15            ((Ellen and Marge have a brief exchange with Max about a toy))
16   Ellen:   Um (0.3) so- (0.4) so: (.) um: (.) so yeah I mean he's g- he's
17            got these >couple things< but the social quality of his
18            interactions=
19   Marge:   =Yeah=
20   Ellen:   =really is nice once you have his attention.
```

Following an upshot (lines 16–18) that typifies the "couple of things" (i.e., symptoms) Max has, Ellen (line 20) adds the qualification that the social quality of his interactions "really is nice once you have his attention." As the discussion continues (not shown), Ellen also raises the possibility of an ADHD diagnosis but hedges on this as well, saying that given Max's young age, "it could just be an inattention kind of thing" and that she "would hate to put this lifelong label on him." They also briefly discuss services (also not shown), with Marge reporting that Max has never received services from his school district and Ellen advising her to seek private support, stating: "I don't think he [Max] necessarily has autism spectrum disorder but he's got some differences."

In short, Ellen affirms the legitimacy of the parents' concerns. Further, although Max does not meet criteria for autism, the overall assessment is far from a no-problem one. Instead, as Ellen hedges, she holds open the possibility that Max may have autism, while also proposing the possibility of an alternate diagnosis, ADHD. Thus, the ostensibly "good" news that Max does not have autism is tempered by assertions that there are problems that could worsen over time, such that vigilant monitoring is advised.

Conclusion: The Ambiguity of Diagnosis

We have suggested that autism becomes a diagnostic entity through interaction and the talk-based procedures by which clinicians resolve its often ambiguous and uncertain qualities. Autism as a diagnosis is not an ostensive, definitive object. Nor is it a social construction, though as a diagnosis, it is achieved and made accountable through practices of narrative and talk in interaction. Yet, by itself, narrative does not resolve the ambiguity and uncertainty surrounding diagnosis. If the news is "bad," such that clinicians do diagnose autism, they may suggest an optimistic exit from the topic by stressing the potential for improvement with early and intensive intervention. Conversely, if the news is ostensibly "good" because a child does not have autism, clinicians attenuate any "symptom residue" (Maynard and Frankel 2006) with reassurances to parents that the child's problems do exist and that they may be treatable.[18]

In the three borderline cases analyzed in this chapter, the clinicians constitute autism as an ontological entity that can be difficult to detect but that is in principle objectively real and recognizable. The uncertainty belongs to the work of detection and contingent features of each case, rather than to the diagnostic object itself. Accordingly, Leah states that although Sara *probably* has autism, her symptoms could improve in the future to the point where she no longer meets diagnostic criteria. However, immediately after raising this possibility, Leah was quick to dispel the idea that Sara can "grow out of autism"—if it does turn out that Sara no longer meets criteria, it would be because she did not have autism to begin with: "Y'know I never- I always tell people, I never say people *grow out* of autism ((makes 'air quotes' gesture)). But I think that sometimes the features at a young age, you know sometimes it's just . . . it's not a hundred percent clear" (Case 34_STF, lines 162–63).

The implication seems to be that the ADOS might have produced a false positive or, in diagnostic nomenclature, was lacking in specificity for this borderline case. The error is not the fault of the test or the diagnostic criteria but is due to Sara's early age; if she were "school age," Leah explains, there would be no ambiguity: "Y'know when we make the diagnosis in a school age child, there's no question that that diagnosis is gonna continue to fit over time . . . even though how the child looks over time may- may grow and change, and they may develop new skills" (Case 34_STF, lines 170–74).

Leah's line of reasoning preserves a *clinical* understanding that autism is something a person can *either* have *or* not have and that once someone has autism, they can never not have it, even if they improve to the point where their symptoms are less detectable, as with author Kamran Nazeer (2006), whose autism was not at all evident by the time he became an adult. In this way, Leah and colleagues manage the boundaries of the diagnosis, creating an age-graded space where a margin of error can make results inconclusive. Inside that margin, autism's boundaries become more porous, making complex cases harder to classify.

In two other cases, both involving Ellen Miller as psychologist, and each ruling out autism, the parents are assured that there are "other diagnoses" and that "services" are available (Lily). In Max's case, the conclusion is that if he does have autism, it is too subtle to affirm at present but may become more visible as he ages and as his social circumstances change.

Clinicians practice cautious optimism or pessimism, in varying degrees, in all of the cases in our data, but in the face of heightened uncertainty and ambiguity, these practices can have the added effect of securing parents' alignment to a likewise uncertain prognosis, as exemplified in clinicians' stories about possible futures. In all, our analysis suggests that the question forming the title for this chapter needs to be revised. The question is not *whether* autism is real but in *what ways* it can be said to be real. Whether or not a child qualifies for the diagnosis, and "what autism is" more generally, can be said to live in the ways that clinicians, parents, and others work with children, on the ground and using the tools and instruments at hand, to engage, elicit, respond to, and make sense of behavior that then is diagnostically treated as conforming or not conforming to the official, DSM-based definition of autism at a given time and place.

8

Interaction and the Particular Autistic Person

In 1963, the National Autistic Society (NAS), a charitable foundation in Britain, adopted a puzzle piece as its logo. On the piece was a picture of a weeping child (see fig. 8.1). Created by Gerald Gasson, an early board member and parent of an autistic child, the logo symbolized the puzzlement he and other parents experienced as they attempted to understand their children and guide them through largely uncharted territory. With its tearful child, the image also suggested autistic individuals somehow "suffered" from the condition (Muzikar 2019). As might be expected, this image of autism became very controversial, and the NAS has since switched logos.

Carissa Paccerelli, who identifies as an "autism advocate," has drawn a chalk-art image to protest the treatment of autistic people as puzzles rather than persons (see fig. 8.2). According to her website, Paccerelli "has been drawing and painting since age three." Now an award-winning artist in her twenties, she was diagnosed as being on the autism spectrum at age six. In a sense, our book is meant to raise a protest similar to Paccerelli's, at least in its challenge to the reductionism that autism diagnosis involves when it highlights generic features of a child and neglects the particularities and forms of intelligence—the personhood—the child evinces.

Yet puzzle imagery has been persistent in public discussions about autism. As Grinker and Mandell (2015:643) remark, "The puzzle piece as a symbol for autism awareness, advocacy, and services is ubiquitous." Despite the objections of autistic persons (Gernsbacher et al. 2018:119), the organization Autism Speaks uses a single blue puzzle piece as its logo, the Autism Society of America has a ribbon with different colored puzzle pieces as its trademark, and many books on autism, along with internet sites, depict puzzle pieces on their covers or pages, often using the word *puzzle* in their titles.

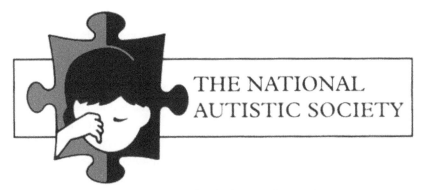

FIGURE 8.1. Gerald Gasson logo for the National Autistic Society

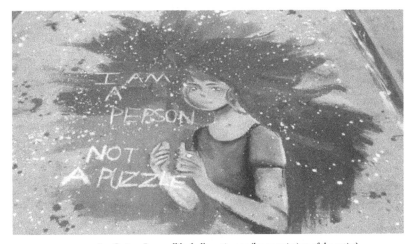

FIGURE 8.2. Carissa Paccerelli's chalk-art image (by permission of the artist)

This pervasiveness also exists in scientific organizations and literature (Gernsbacher et al. 2018:118).

In sociology, a book by Eyal and colleagues (2010) titled *The Autism Matrix*, from which we have drawn copiously in our own research, has a cover design featuring dozens of puzzle pieces configured into the sort of matrix alluded to by its title. That matrix, however, encompasses much more than individuals with autism—for example, the first chapter is called "The Puzzle of Variation in Autism Rates." Accordingly, the way in which the term is used matters. As far as diagnosis is concerned, our view is that so long as there are developmental concerns about a child, "presenting symptoms" in the clinic do, and will continue to, constitute a puzzle to be solved. This is not unique to autism but is true of all diagnoses, organic and psychiatric alike. As Foucault

(1973) documents, Western medicine has been making a puzzle of patients, with the express aim of identifying "disordered" pieces, since Enlightenment-era practitioners replaced premodern holistic conceptions of patienthood with modern mechanistic ones.

Still, a problem with the analogy is the assumption that when one encounters a candidate for autism diagnosis, there are identical pieces to be found and they can be fit into uniform labels derived from the DSM. The pieces are assumed to be damaged pieces of the genome, alterations to neurochemistry and biology—some structural or functional component of the brain—faulty aspects of cognition, or any combination of elements thought to lie *behind* the child's behavior. What matters is that these elements are considered universal and in some sense *more essential* than the behavior they are taken to explain: the pieces are seen as generative of the behavioral picture, which gets reduced to an epiphenomenon of the genetics, cognition, or neurobiology believed to underlie it. As a result, the way a child's actions-in-interaction are themselves socially organized phenomena—interactional phenotypes—is missed, as are forms of competence that the child may deploy while dealing with other participants and instrumental aspects of the setting. Overall, assuming the existence of pieces whose proper assembly explains the diagnosis of an autistic child misses the individuality—the "personhood"—of the child, as it is constituted in space and time as the child engages with other participants and the manipulative affordances of the social environment.

The tension in modern diagnosis between particular persons and the generic categories applied to them permeates the interaction order of the clinic. But given this interaction order and the sociohistorical relations that gave rise to it, we might nonetheless ask how practitioners can balance individuality and generality. One step in that direction would be to link the practices of puzzle solving to the picture that emerges, such that the picture's synoptic quality has unique aspects to it formed from those practices.[1] For example, in the case of a favorite over-the-counter puzzle—let's say Denali (formerly Mount McKinley)—much as the end product could look the "same" each time it is put together, it still could be differentiated according to the time, place, and interactional facets of its assembly. The Denali that is constructed when vacationing in a mountain cabin is different from the Denali that is made on the dining room table during a holiday. Who was there, what order pieces were found in, who found them, and how they were found would all be distinctive. The final puzzle is a unique confluence, not an inert reification—although the pieces do place restrictions on what can be depicted (e.g., they can only depict Denali and not, say, a skyscraper).[2] In short, it matters who puts the puzzle together, and where and how they do so together (or do not).

Our inquiry has shown that, although it is possible to generate an abstract, generic, or synoptic picture through testing and diagnosis, it is also possible to learn about the detailed practices at the level of everyday interactions contributing to these pictures in distinctive ways. If we shift attention away from puzzle pieces as neurobiological or neuropsychological to the realm of actions and interactions and their emplacement in settings where diagnosis is made to happen, then the pieces have new dimensions. Rather being representations of preexistent, background conditions or states, they can foreground aspects of actions and interactions that exhibit sensitivity to the particular facets of the person being evaluated. Even as clinicians may need to assimilate children to abstract diagnostic categories that paint a synoptic picture, perhaps we can, following Garfinkel (e.g., 1996:6), ask "what more" there is to children's and clinicians' actions and their emplacement in diagnostic settings. Independently of their official structural, or second-order performances, "what else" is it that children do in relationship with copresent others (clinicians, parents, caretakers) and devices or instruments that are often left out of the official records that document an autism spectrum disorder? Can the what-more and what-else be incorporated into clinical assessments to form descriptions that go beyond synopsis to capture personhood and embodied action? In short, how may diagnosis become more sensitive to *who* is being diagnosed and *how* they do things rather than to *what* they have?

At the same time as we are raising questions about autism diagnosis, we mean to stretch the boundaries of our own ethnomethodological, conversation analytic, and interaction order enterprise. The orders of practice that we have described and analyzed include both commonsense and "un-commonsense" competencies, the latter including self-attentive exhibits of autistic intelligence. To the degree that common sense can adapt to that intelligence, the seeming fixity of the taken-for-granted is more fluid than Garfinkel's (1967:chap. 2) "breaching demonstrations" suggest. This point is actually consistent with his own research, which we discuss later in the chapter, but here it can be noted that, besides highlighting intransigent exhibits of common sense, Garfinkel (1967:31) also states, "Not *a* method of understanding but *immensely various* methods of understanding are the sociologist's hitherto unstudied and critical phenomena." Consistent with this, when we recognize and appreciate autistic intelligence for its "haves," per Mukhopadhyay (2003), we see that it involves strengths as well as challenges and that it forms a panoply that situates the person as a specific individual with particular characteristics and skills or "methods of understanding." Knowing about those characteristics and skills provides an avenue for reaching and building on what the child already knows and does, and can be informative for configuring, or

reconfiguring, the social environments in which that child exists as an interactional being.

This concluding chapter, then, brings together the analyses in previous chapters, presenting a review of key findings and a framework for understanding autism not as solely in terms of the brains and bodies of those on the spectrum but
as an interactional and interactive phenomenon existing in spaces populated
by commonsense actors with their artifacts (be they assessment instruments,
toys and objects at home, or curricular programs at school), on the one hand,
and the children who come to be seen as being on the autism spectrum, on
the other. We align with others who understand autism in terms of difference,
not deficit, and raise the possibility of a diagnostic process that highlights the
particularities of the child, rather than only the generic attributes that qualify
them for the diagnosis.

Along these lines, we observe that the puzzlement associated with autism
is not a one-way street: those on the spectrum are often as baffled by neurotypical or commonsense behavior as neurotypical or commonsense actors
are by autistic behavior. As Temple Grandin memorably put it, navigating
the neurotypical world can make someone on the spectrum feel like "an anthropologist on Mars" (O. Sacks 1993:112; O. Sacks 1995). In shifting the focus
from deficit to difference and to what people are doing together to create
mutual unintelligibility (which we recognize is a kind of oxymoron), we raise
the possibility not only of making common sense accessible to those with
autism—the goal of myriad autism therapies—*but of making autism accessible
and intelligible to those immersed in a commonsense world.*

A Commonsense Approach to Autism

In chapter 3, we had a close look at the beginning of Dan Chapman's evaluation with Jenifer Erickson. In preparation for the ADOS, she offered Dan the
choice of having his mother stay in the room or leave. Dan utterly avoided
answering the offer, and Jennifer and Betsy eventually decided the matter
themselves. Neither Dan's behavior nor Jennifer's later narrative about it were
diagnostic per se. However, they show all the elements that we have been
pursuing in our approach to autism diagnosis. As such, the behavior and the
subsequent narrative lend to a review of those elements, including common
sense, autistic intelligence, storytelling, and the particularization of autism.
How is it possible to make the world of autism familiar, or has Grinker (2007)
has put it, something "unstrange" that can be "remapped?"

Whether inside or outside the clinic, the everyday world is pervaded
by the presence of common sense in interaction. Dan is enveloped in an

environment of tacit understandings and practices from the very outset of his visit to CDDC and during the assessment process itself. Recall that by *common sense* we refer to all that participants take for granted about how to "do things" intelligibly and meaningfully in the social world. When at the outset of her evaluation Jennifer says, "Dan, it's up to you, do you want your mom in the room for this?" she is making an offer and projecting the relevance of an immediate yes or no type of reply. Like the overwhelming bulk of social actions performed in everyday life, Jennifer's utterance does not have a name (i.e., Jennifer does not say, "Dan, I'm making you *an offer*") or other markers of the action it embodies (cf. Levinson 1983:263–68) attached to it. However, for one who does not readily access commonsense understandings, the confusion can be palpable, as it seemed to be for Dan.

The social force of common sense is underlain by expectations that, following Garfinkel (1963; 1967), we have called "trust conditions." Competent members of a society (1) presuppose the relevance of their own tacit knowledge about social actions, (2) assume that others possess this knowledge as well, and (3) assume that as they assume others will adhere to this knowledge, so too will others make this assumption about them. When anomalous behavior violates those assumptions or conditions of trust, it is highly disruptive and can evoke manifestations of emotion that are otherwise held at bay. In Garfinkel's (1963; 1967) experimental disruptions, targets could become angry very quickly. With more naturalistic disruptions, such as those induced when an autistic individual seems to transgress common sense, parents and others in the immediate environment can become frustrated (Frankel 1982:36), depressed, or angry (Benson and Karlof 2009).[3] More benignly, others may treat transgressive matters with laughter and humor, even though in public there is the matter of feeling shamed (Park 1967:107). The strategy of humorous treatment may be akin to an artistic imagination, allowing, per Shklovsky (1990[1929]), for unlocking or interrupting habitual orientations to appreciate the possibilities for fresh understandings that inhere in transgressive acts.[4] In any case, it is the violation of trust conditions that is at issue: the child's nonadherence to deeply rooted, tacit understandings that suffuse everyday life and experience for commonsense actors.

COMMON SENSE IN THE CLINIC

Common sense pervades the interaction order of the clinic as much as it does everyday life. For a clear example, in chapter 4 we discussed the Brigance subtest called "Knows What to Do in Different Situations," which asks the child to answer questions such as, "What do you do when you're hungry?" To receive full points, the child is required not only to produce a sensible reply (e.g., "you eat") but also to grasp the more tacit assumptions that ground the social activity of testing. Among other things, this means understanding that question-answer sequences are to be treated separately, rather than merging them in the way we saw Tony Smith do in chapter 5.

Another example is the use of "presses" on the ADOS (see chap. 6). The ADOS manual states that in evaluating a child's behavior, the examiner is to use "a hierarchy of structured and unstructured social presses," such as playing with a balloon to see if a child will ask to have it blown up or stating that one has pets at home to see if the child will ask about them. Stated plainly, the idea is to "elicit spontaneous behaviors in standardized contexts" (Lord et al. 2000:205). The ADOS is meant to assess the child's "participation in social exchanges" (Lord, DiLavore, and Gotham 2012:13), exchanges that are, at bottom, nothing other than ones that involve the use of common sense.

To follow the logic of the ADOS design—and the diagnostic criteria it operationalizes—is to say that those who are diagnosed with autism are those who *fail at commonsense competence*, whether it involves putting a picture "where it goes" because it matches another graphic item, answering questions about feelings, characterizing items in terms of contrasts (e.g., tall vs. short, empty vs. full), assembling a puzzle according to what it is said to picture, demonstrating how to brush one's teeth, showing proper "eye contact," initiating joint attention, and so forth. Indeed, the sheer pervasiveness of the commonsense perspective, both in everyday contexts and in the clinic, means that it is usually beyond overt reflection, much less interrogation.

The fact that common sense usually does not raise questions has to do with the matter of *trust* that we have described. The stakes of noncompliance with common sense are high. When participants mutually take the tacit realm for granted, it is reassurance that they inhabit a shared social world with an objective or real existence. Socks go on feet; feeling angry is like rumbling in your stomach; the opposite of short is tall; disparate pieces of a puzzle with partial graphic representations can be assembled to form a coherent picture; showing how to brush your teeth simply involves describing and performing the acts of putting toothpaste on a brush, wetting it under a faucet, and rubbing the brush across the teeth; co-playing with objects means initiating and responding to another participant through bodily orientation and gaze direction; and so on. Any breakdown in the collaborative practices through which these activities are assembled means that the activities themselves, and the way they endow the social world with its sensuous and sensible character, are impossible. And so too, therefore, is our perception of having a real world.

Common Sense and the Interactional Phenotype

Common sense is a public feature of interaction, rather than a private property of cognition or mind. This is doubly so in that it depends on participants being co-oriented to its implementation whenever they fashion social actions *and* responses. Yet this sociological point has gone unrecognized in the vast literature on the neurobiology of autism and other disorders. So long as it is ignored, the search for autism's causes and correlates can at best provide only a partial understanding of the disorder. Neurobiology already faces steep challenges in identifying genomic sites of disorder, reliable brain anomalies, and the mechanisms or pathways that connect them to actual behavior. Beyond those challenges, efforts to grasp neurobiological effects in relation to what people can accomplish in terms of home, school, and community participation will fall short of identifying what autism means phenomenologically. That is, it will fail to grasp persons as they are in their actual, real-time interactions with others in concrete settings of daily or clinical life.[5]

Our point is not that neurobiological investigations are in any sense misguided, or that disability has no genetic or genomic basis, but that human experience, in all of its complexity, needs to be at the center of the story.[6] Fitzgerald (2017:162), reflecting on what a brain scientist has said to him, captures the matter: "At stake, here, is a loop from some kind of phenotypic abnormality (for example, red hair) to society and the environment (different treatment of people with red hair), to anatomy and the body (brain changes on the basis of this treatment), and back out to behavior (a whole host of clinical symptoms that are produced by those brain changes)." To put it succinctly, just as disease and disability at the cellular, genetic, and neurological levels are extremely complex, so are phenotypic "conditions" themselves difficult to define and describe with precision. This is what the concept of the phenotypic bottleneck (Freese 2008) entails: a recognition that the effects of neurobiology are neither singular behaviors nor traits but complex forms of conduct coproduced with other humans and emplaced material forms (Gieryn 2000)—what Latour (1987) calls actants: instruments, toys, and other objects.

If behavior is indelibly behavior-in-interaction, it is not enough to consider both "genetics" and "environment" in understanding the autism phenotype. This is why we refer to the *interactional* phenotype for autism and propose a new understanding of autistic intelligence, one that goes beyond how Kanner and Asperger used it to refer to savant-type talents. To get a better handle on social interactional phenotypes, investigative resources—both "pure" and "applied"—would need to be allocated more evenly across social, linguistic, occupational therapeutic, and behavioral sciences, not just "natural" ones such as genetics and neurobiology.

AN ETHNOMETHODOLOGICAL AND
CONVERSATION ANALYTIC APPROACH

As sociologists, our way of getting at the interactional phenotype is to investigate how it is assembled at a particular site, the clinic, which operates against the background of historically specific, more or less unified medical discourses about autism and its effects. There is no better example of this unity than the criteria for autism listed in the *Diagnostic and Statistical Manual* of the American Psychiatric Association (APA 2013) and the World Health Organization's *International Classification of Diseases* (WHO 2018), which, despite some differences (Doernberg and Hollander 2016), have increasingly converged in recent years. To the degree that the ADOS, ADI-R, and other assessment tools are correlated with the DSM and the ICD, they constitute *protocols* for making diagnostic decisions. By prescribing what needs to occur in domains of application, a protocol, in the words of Lynch and colleagues (2008:88–89), "is an ideal-typical set of instructions formulated independently of any particular attempt to do what it says." Because of its ideal-typical character, implementing a protocol may prevent practitioners from attending to important nuances inhabiting its domains of application (Maynard 2019:20; Maynard and Turowetz 2020).

The nuances of the testing environment are many. They encompass such administrative practices as asking questions, issuing directives, and otherwise initiating interactional sequences (Talkington and Maynard 2021). Nuances include design features of an instrument itself, and the scripts that examiners are expected to follow. The details of actual implementation can affect a child's understanding of what is being asked of them and how they fashion their responses, which means that those responses can provide valuable information about the child as an individual, rather than solely as a member of a diagnostic category. Accordingly, we need ways of penetrating beyond the categories that populate medical discourse to grasp the interactional practices that bring those categories to life and the tacit, often invisible competencies on which they depend. Such grasp requires an interactional gaze.

As sociologists whose approach is rooted in ethnomethodology and conversation analysis, and Goffman's (1959a; 1983) studies of "moral careers" and the interaction order, we take off from what Hacking (2002:100) describes as the too-often-overlooked "ordinary dynamics of human interaction." Because these dynamics reside in the silences, hesitations, overlapping utterances, bodily motions, and other pervasive characteristics of everyday life, we make use of recordings and specialized transcripts to capture them in their details. Conversation analysis in particular offers a set of analytic strategies for examining how participants perform, recognize, and respond to social actions on a turn-by-turn basis. As such, it can be readily attuned to what Lord and colleagues (2020:2) describe as the "heterogeneity both within and between individuals with autism, and outcomes across the lifespan." The heterogeneous and the particular are what get exhibited in and as autistic intelligence and are precisely what get turned up through close analysis of interaction.

Autistic Intelligence

Autistic intelligence is something we all have. Drawing on the Greek word, it is an acumen that, if not entirely private, is at least self-attentive in the sense that its expression draws on meanings bound to the speaker's own world that are not shared by coparticipants (cf. Heritage 1998). In chapter 4 (note 4), we further specified autistic intelligence as stimulus-bound, additive, locally oriented, and literal. In that sense, autistic meanings may be *un*common and make interaction and joint effort difficult if not impossible. As an example, we mentioned comedian George Carlin's riff on the common English phrase "Have a nice day," which is ordinarily used as a salutation at the close of a social encounter, but which can be treated as a command or imperative if taken literally. As a way of doing comedy, this sort of punning is intentional. If comedy is not the intent, a literal response such as "Why should I" (have a nice day), or "Let somebody else have one" not only would seem abrasive but could engender prolonged attempts to repair understandings.

AUTISM AS SELF-ATTENTIVENESS

When a comedian engages in purposeful punning, its use is autistically intelligent in a strategic way. If successful, it generates laughter. However, when such intelligence is exhibited by a "neurotypical" individual for nonstrategic reasons—that is, by accident—then it can be corrected. Consider an example from the podcast *This American Life* where the host, Ira Glass, is interviewing a scientist, the executive director of the Earth Sciences Teacher Association, about whether climate change should be taught in schools. After the first part of her presentation, in which she discusses evidence that the earth is warming up, the following exchange occurs:

GLASS: Okay, so that's the first part of your presentation. What's the second
     part? I understand it has to do with something called ice cores?
JOHNSON: Yeah, so there's these really cool ice cores—cool, I didn't mean as
     a pun, actually—they have drilled these things now for decades.

When Johnson does a "self-initiated" (Schegloff, Jefferson, and Sacks 1977) *re-pair* on her infelicitous use of "cool," we listeners can understand that she meant
something like "interesting" or "intriguing" or "amazing," as she goes on to ex-
plain how these ice cores, dug out of the ground, can provide an annual record
of the earth's temperature going back hundreds of thousands of years.[7]

What may distinguish the autistic from the nonautistic is not self-
attentiveness or ego-focused orientations to a private world per se, but rather the
fixedness with which this occurs. That is, as Shore (2003:50) has put it (see chap. 4,
note 2), "most people experience autistic traits at one time or another," but it is
when "these traits are strong and numerous enough to significantly impact daily
functioning" that autism becomes a relevant diagnosis. However, it is not as if such
auto-involvement is entirely voluntary: the heightened sensitivities to sound,
touch, sight (lighting, for example), and other senses that people with autism are
known to experience mean that self-attentiveness is hardly a choice.[8] If the person neither self-corrects nor responds to efforts by others to restore mutuality,
it may seem as though they are committing an intentional and personal affront
(Duchan 1998). But the fact remains that this seeming indifference to others
is not personal (i.e., intentionally aimed at others) so much as a means of self-
maintenance that is often practiced in full awareness of how others perceive it.[9]

Nonetheless, as we have observed, commonsense actors may respond with
anger, or sometimes laughter, to the autistic person's refusal or inability to
participate in the ordinary, taken-for-granted realms of everyday life. These
strong displays of affect signal the deep, embodied investment these actors
have in common sense and their resistance to actions that make it strange.
But because the tendency to fixate on a private world is not easily remedied in
autism, commonsense actors would be well served to work *with* those on the
spectrum to make the strangeness more familiar and less alien. We will have
more to say about this matter shortly, but an initial way to make strangeness
more familiar is to appreciate the *un*common intelligence it expresses.

THE SUBTERRANEAN PERVASIVENESS OF
AUTISTIC INTELLIGENCE

When a child gives a correct answer to a prompt (such as matching a picture in hand to one in a booklet) or shows other behavior that exhibits social

awareness, it involves both first-order or fundamental, and second-order or structural competence. First-order competence includes such skills as understanding and complying with instructions, showing co-orientation, and introducing or producing sequentially relevant responses. Second-order competence, on the other hand, includes the ability to exhibit decentered knowledge that is abstracted from lived experience. In the sense that it incorporates tacit understandings that go beyond literalism, it is structural rather than fundamental. While first-order competence facilitates the display of second-order competence, it usually operates beneath the surface of ordinary perception—but in a more concrete sense than the inexplicitness of common sense.[10] Asking or answering a question, reaching for an object, and shaking one's head in response to a directive are all examples of first-order competence. Furthermore, when such competence does surface, particularly in instances where tacit assumptions are violated, it is frequently treated as evidence of the violator's incompetence, rather than as an opportunity to explore their sensemaking methods (or the tacit bases of mundane common sense, for that matter). Autistic intelligence may surface during children's failures to display second-order competence but frequently gets ignored or interpreted as deficits and deficiencies. Displays of associative thinking, for example, are seen as evidence of disability, as strange rather than as legitimate, if different, contributions to a dialogue.

Understanding that a question has been asked and giving an answer, or using gaze to engage with an object—even in the absence of co-orientation by other participants—are practices that may be purposeful. Their apparent randomness conceals an order implicit, for example, in the child's preoccupation with the local world where they are planted, or their active appraisal of affordances provided by the social environment. Spinning like a fan to preserve a sense of one's own bodily integrity, requesting a small toy presented by a clinician in between her directives to match pictures, assembling question-answer sequences into a narrative, filling the answer slots that follow questions with names of objects provided by a visual/tactile space, arranging puzzle pieces according to their sensuous or tactile contours, resisting entreaties to choose from options for a next task, declining to demonstrate a mundane daily task or taking it in a nonnormative direction, and being involved with a balloon to the neglect of a coparticipant may all exhibit first-order competence, even if the display of second-order competence being requested does not emerge and may even be impeded by the deployment of fundamental competence.

Autistic intelligence is not an incidental part of clinical testing or everyday life. As the example in chapter 3 involving Jennifer's offer to Dan illustrates, a child who seems out of sync and withdrawn from a commonsense environment may in fact be making sophisticated moves in response to an awkward situation. Moreover, the child may show autistic intelligence not just in one sphere or task but in starkly different assessment environments. As we saw in chapters 4 and 5, different children may perform the same task in ways that exhibit divergent forms of autistic intelligence. Autism biography and autobiography document many other unique forms of competence at home, at work, and in professional environments, whether it is an ability to "think in pictures" (Grandin 1995), handle the complexities of ordinary conversation through puppetry (cf. Andre in Nazeer 2006; Williams 1992:51–53), perform in and appreciate a variety of musical genres (Bakan 2018), engage in sophisticated forms of logical thinking (cf. Jessie Park in Park 2001:chap. 5), draw on kinesthetic sensibilities in place of, or in addition to, visual and auditory ways of sensemaking (Donna Williams in Biklen 2002:19; cf. Higashida 2013), or learn the ways of human communication and emotional experience by observing and engaging with gorillas (Prince-Hughes 2004:131–53).[11]

Because autistic intelligence so often exists at a subterranean level in interaction, appreciating it requires special forms of attentiveness. As autism narrative reveals, individuals with autism and their caretakers may be aware of such intelligence, and in the clinic, it sometimes appears in instantiation stories. That autistic intelligence is commonly missed does not mean parents and clinicians are not fully capable of attending to it: think of Sue Lehr (chap. 1) responding to her screaming son's typed message by "tilting" him, or the Suskinds' discovery that they can enter Owen's world through Disney talk, or the mother in Morocco who understands her nonverbal son's seemingly random laughter as responsive to a question asked by his speech therapist and the joint laughter that occurs once she explains what is going on, or the psychologist at CDDC who, after reporting to the parents of a boy that she would like to see him do "a little bit more of imaginary play," produces instantiation stories about how "he did feed the baby [doll] spontaneously . . . and he bathed the baby . . . [and] had the baby blow out the candles [during an ADOS 'pretend birthday party']" (Wiscons 2020).

While examples such as these show parents and clinicians making observations about mere moments and details of interaction, these moments and details evince competencies on which it is possible to build for any number of purposes, including reducing or redirecting challenging behavior and expanding skills into other realms of social activity. Although specific examples of autistic intelligence do come up in the course of instantiation stories, at present, they are subordinated to narratives about the child's global tendencies, especially those that fit with generic diagnostic criteria. Perhaps more can be done to explore these instances of autistically competent behavior to advance the very goals for which diagnosis reaches: among other things, providing structure, adducing expertise, imposing order, separating what is valid from what is not, integrating community values, and restoring relationships between individuals and the groups to which they belong (Jutel 2009).[12]

The Narrative Organization of Diagnosis

We have highlighted autistic intelligence, but of course the diagnostic process is one that necessitates looking for disease and disability. In examining the implementation of assessment instruments, we have contributed to the "sociology of testing" (Brown, 1990, 1995; Pinch 1993), taking seriously "the technoscientific nature" of clinical practices (Casper and Berg 1995:398–99) to grasp analytically the deployment of psychometric evaluation technology in the autism clinic. Standardization creates equivalences across children and contexts, which are necessary for assimilating disparate individuals to uniform categories (Bowker and Star 1999; Porter 1995). Although a great deal of "tinkering, repairing, subverting, or circumventing prescriptions of the standard are necessary to make standards work" (Timmermans and Epstein 2010:81), instruments such as the Autism Diagnostic Observation Schedule provide a blueprint or script for establishing an interactional environment where children's abilities may be elicited and a framework for evaluating them.

Studies in the sociology of diagnosis (Brown 1995:39) emphasize the social and political contexts in which "conflicted diagnoses" exhibit manifestations of power and control. Previous conversation analytic research about diagnosis has focused on primary care medicine (Heath 1992; Heritage and McArthur 2019; Peräkylä 1998); cancer (Lutfey and Maynard 1998); genetics and genomics (Stivers and Timmermans 2016; Stivers and Timmermans 2017); and developmental disabilities (Gill and Maynard 1995; Maynard 1989), but all concentrate on the delivery and reception of diagnosis, rather than *the orderly interactional processes by which clinicians arrive at a diagnosis in the first place*. Research in these two domains of inquiry—social and political structures of diagnosis and its delivery by health care practitioners—has usefully documented the macro-institutional milieus of diagnosis, and the local particulars of its presentation.

Our own investigation, located between the larger institutional environment and the situated delivery of diagnostic news, has examined the large and uncharted domain of *doing diagnosis*—how clinicians perform assessments, formulate findings, decide what those findings mean, and determine how to categorize patients (chap. 6). Unlike other research that relies upon post facto accounts or online (i.e., "thinking aloud") commentary by clinicians as they reason about stylized vignettes and that focuses on cognitive processes located "in the mind" of the clinician (e.g., Garb 1998), our study centers the interactions through which clinical data are assembled and interpreted. This approach has the advantage of being able to identify collective sensemaking practices that, because of their own tacit or taken-for-granted character, are not transparent to researchers or practitioners and that only become accessible when diagnostic work is analyzed naturalistically and in real time.

We have shown how clinicians adapt ordinary storytelling competencies to the institutional objectives of the clinic as they determine the "facts of the case," fit them to DSM criteria, and deliver their findings to families. Further, we have shown that these stories are organized in terms of a narrative structure consisting of four components: a preface, tendency or instantiation stories about a child's behavior, typifying upshots that make categorical claims about the child, and story recipiency, which is performed by clinicians, family members, and others during and upon completion of the sequence. Recipients may also contribute further stories to the overall narrative, which gradually materializes in favor of or against a given diagnosis. In ethnomethodological terms, narrative consists of methods for achieving diagnoses that are endogenous to the interaction order of the clinic. As such, narrative practices are not merely a supplement to diagnostic protocols but an indispensable part of how those protocols are applied, interpreted, and made to work in practice.

THE GENERIC REACH OF NARRATIVE ANALYSIS

That diagnosis involves narrative is not an entirely new idea, but previous research in medical sociology has treated the process as one in which patients have their own "lay" stories, which they bring to the medical encounter and which may compete with or become absorbed into a more authoritative clinical story, be it about heart disease, cancer, or more benign ailments (cf. Charon 2006; Frank, 1995; Freidson 1970:chap. 12, chap. 13; Mishler 1984). It is certainly true that careful listening to a patient's story on the clinician's part can mean better understanding and care. "While not all illnesses can be diagnosed," Jutel (2009:287) writes, "their narratives are the starting point for diagnosis." Nonetheless, as our data show, stories are not simply pitted one against another or abstracted from the patient's "lifeworld" and re-narrated in the "voice of medicine" (Mishler 1984); rather, they are cooperatively assembled by speakers and recipients over a sequence of turns for myriad local purposes: agreeing, disagreeing, evidencing, elaborating, challenging, repairing, inviting shared laughter, and so forth.

For autism diagnosis in particular, not much documentation exists regarding the stories that families or individuals bring to the clinical encounter, possibly because the process is weighted toward the DSM, what it requires in terms of testing and classification, and how lay stories can become "transformed into medical accounts upon their telling" (Jutel 2009:287). In autism clinics, as our data show, professionals will ask parents about the child and get informal feedback, in addition to soliciting their stories as they help to construct the overall diagnostic narrative. However, more formally, parents fill out structured questionnaires and answer questions from the Autism Diagnostic Interview, and the professionals have their own protocols to follow.

Clinical reliance on reductive assessments and other protocols may be why elsewhere there is an outpouring of "autism narrative" (Hacking 2009) in the form of biography, autobiography, and novelistic storytelling, as well as cinematic and other multimedia portrayals. These may bypass clinical versions of autism to offer social critique through a kind of celebration of disruptiveness that asks about the meaning of autism's "flawed existence" (Mitchell and Snyder 2001:49, 54–55). As Osteen (2008:17) has put it, "a tension between narrative order and narrative disruption—whether figured as relentless repetition or as outbreaks of chaos—runs through virtually all family autism stories." This aligns with our perspective on autism as a breach or violation of common sense.

More generally, we can observe that all disease and disability involve violation, whether organic, social, or some relation between the two. Even when clear biomarkers are involved, the process of converting evidence into diagnostic categories remains a complex matter, such that our analysis may also apply to nonpsychiatric conditions with well-established etiologies. Consider the words of physician Alvan Feinstein (1973:212): "Diagnostic reasoning in modern medicine is a process of converting observed evidence into the names of diseases." This reasoning is thought to be different for organic/physical conditions than for mental/psychiatric ones, and in ways that parallel the difference between the natural and human sciences (Foucault 1987). However, in organic medicine, it is well recognized that the use of laboratory science, anatomic pathology, and medical imaging is not as straightforward as is often assumed and that the processes of testing and interpreting results are both subject to error. Diagnosis in organic medicine, even with sophisticated and reliable ways to detect physiological markers, remains a complex endeavor in which test findings must be integrated with patient history, symptoms, physical exams, and so forth (Balogh, Miller, and Ball 2015:41).[13]

The complex, contingent, time-based process that Balogh, Mill, and Ball (2015) describe in their US Academy of Medicine report is also characteristic of autism diagnosis, even though (or possibly *because*) the latter lacks biomarkers or other "hard" indicators. If, in general, "diagnoses are the classification tools of medicine" (Jutel 2009:278), or as Abbott (1988:40) says, "diagnosis takes information into the professional knowledge system and treatment brings instructions back out from it," then our study regarding narrative structure as an interactional phenomenon may be applicable to many other diagnostic endeavors besides autism (and we shall get to the "treatment" part shortly).[14]

Certainly, in some contexts, as Glenn and Koschmann (2005) show, diagnosis may be different from narrative, as in problem-based learning (PBL) tutorials where students are given photographs or videos of simulated patients and told to use the information to produce, test, and evaluate diagnostic *hypotheses*, to which other participants then respond (cf. Koschmann, Glenn, and Conlee 2000). These hypotheses may range from words or phrases naming a medical condition to more elaborate and "uncertainty"-marked propositions that can be confirmed or disconfirmed, accepted or rejected, through subsequent discussion. Given the authors' examples of PBL, storytelling may or may not figure in the process, though overall it seems mostly driven by the back and forth of hypothesis and response. So while we are far from claiming that the narrative structure of diagnosis is universal, or that it is the only dynamic involved, it may bear consideration in documenting the hands-on nature of determining other diagnoses besides autism (cf. Hayes et al. 2020:14).

INSTANTIATION STORIES AND THEIR TRANSMISSIONS

Within the narrative structure we have identified is a tension among the naturally occurring stories in our data. Tendency stories reduce situated events to global behavior patterns, whereas instantiation stories describe, and potentially preserve, the details of such events through more gestalt-like abstractions (Maynard and Turowetz 2019). We have shown how tendency stories operate through quantification: "he did all at age level," "he shows many of the signs of autism," "she does a lot of repetition," "he did a lotta this [grimacing]," "it was always about X," "when he has to take those skills and apply it, that's where he falls down," and "he tends to perseverate." These stories, as we noted in chapter 6, account for about 80 percent of all that clinicians produce, in part because they readily lend to upshots (e.g., "he *has x*," "she *is y*") that are readily fitted to diagnostic criteria (Maynard and Turowetz 2017a).

Instantiation stories, by contrast, describe single episodes of behavior. Even when providing evidence for upshots, they preserve something of the time and place of the event, along with its interactional and interactive components (other participants, instruments, objects) and details related to a child's performance. This means that such stories at least have the potential to help us access the child's embedded sensemaking practices, or what we are calling their uncommon sense and autistic intelligence. In other words, rather than describing *a child* with autism, such stories describe *this child* with autism and their unique ways of acting in relation to other people in the social world. *They transmit something of who the child is as an intelligent being.*

The imbalance between tendency and instantiation stories means that the diagnostic picture for a child comes to resemble the generic descriptions in the DSM. Furthermore, when clinicians or others do produce an instantiation story, it is often a humorous anecdote, as in the report about Ronnie Martin misunderstanding the video about child abuse (chap. 6). Or the story psychologizes a behavior, as when the clinicians gloss Tony Smith's rejection of help as "emerging pride and independence" (chap. 5) or Dan's withdrawal from the ADOS as "feeling put on the spot" (chap. 6) and his indecision about his mother being in the room as "being uncomfortable" (chap. 3). In our view such treatments are only partial and represent a missed opportunity. A different, perhaps complementary approach is to inspect these instances for what they can reveal about the interactional (coparticipatory) and interactive (material) environments where the behavior occurred, and the child's strategies in relation to those environments.

If, as we have argued, autism is deeply related to the organization of interaction and the configuration of social settings, then instantiation stories can also reach beyond diagnosis to inform recommendations for how to work with a child in the home, at school, and in other settings where they may experience challenges. The competencies that surface in these stories can be harnessed not only to help the child adjust to their environment but to adjust the particulars of that environment to the child. Thus, in Dan Chapman's case, we might speculate (as we did in chap. 5 and 6) that if he could skillfully manage the awkward demands placed on him in an unfamiliar clinical setting, then surely the problems he experiences in other contexts do not reside entirely with him. They also implicate features of the environment—including the way others may give him directives and respond to him—as contributors to his antisocial behavior.[15] Here as elsewhere, the burden of adjustment should reside not only with children like Dan but also with their coparticipants and the settings in which they are members.

Making the Strange Familiar: Accessing Other Worlds

Although our approach to autism assessment and the interaction order of the clinic is rooted in ethnomethodology, we are aware that the ethnomethodological study of common sense can give the impression that it is rigid, unyielding, and generative of strong reactionary emotions. This is the message readers might take from Garfinkel's (1967) reports about his breaching experiments, for example. In chapter 1, we described how quickly the unwitting "subjects" of these experiments reacted when their tacit everyday expectations were disrupted and how they often made angry imputations about the experimenter's psychological motives. From such demonstrations, it is easy to infer that common sense is unyielding, static, and inert.

However, in writing about autism generally, the anthropologist Grinker (2007:13), whose approach we discussed in chapter 1 and who is the father of a daughter on the spectrum, has stated: "Our goal is to make the strange familiar. Indeed, with every day that passes, as autism advocates, parents, and researchers teach us about the complexity of human behavior, autism seems less exotic and more 'unstrange,' a word invented by the poet e.e. cummings in an untitled poem rebuking societies in the thrall of conformity."[16]

Because instantiation stories can to some degree capture real, situated experiences, they present opportunities for clinicians and family members to focus away from the breach of common sense, temper the emotional response it frequently triggers, and engage the reasoning of the person doing the breaching. In this respect, they can be similar to autism biography and autobiography. For example, when Sue Lehr (via Solomon 2012) describes her experience in the mall with her son Ben, she provides enough detail to give the reader access to both her response to Ben's challenging conduct and the in situ autistic intelligence that conduct exhibited. Lucy Blackman (1999), Haoki Higashida (2013), Dawn Prince-Hughes (2004), Temple Grandin (2006), John Robison (2007), Tito Mukhopadhyay (2003), Donna Williams (1992), and many others retrospectively take us inside the forms of intelligence they manifest in social environments, allowing us to become familiar with what seems like strange and disruptive behavior to those around them. In a way that Garfinkel's (1967) classic analysis of artificial disruptions or breaches to ordinary common sense usually does not, close-hand accounts go beyond the commonsense arena to give us access to the reasoning practices of an actual breaching actor.[17]

The strategy for making the strange familiar is somehow to gain access to the worlds of those who commit breaches—the strangers themselves. In an apt parable, attributed to a Boston psychiatrist by the name of Pierre Johannet and retold by a supervising therapist, Nancy Reiser, at the Putnam's Children Center in Roxbury, Massachusetts, Shore (2003) asks us to imagine trying to reach "a young prince locked inside a huge castle."[18] We have to cross a moat filled with alligators, find a way into the castle, get past armed guards, locate a secret stairway to the highest tower, and find a key to unlock the heavy door. Once inside, we find the child looking out a window, and he does not greet us.

If we walk over to him, the strategy is for us to look out the window and eventually speak quietly about what we see. Eventually, if we "have been careful and respectful enough, and noticed the 'right' things . . . the child may turn to acknowledge that he is no longer alone." And ultimately, after spending a long time in the tower, it can happen that the child notices the door, leads us to it, opens it, takes our hand, and guides us past the obstacles to the outside world, exploring it with us, and, finally, says, "Farewell, I'm ready to explore with others and by myself."

The metaphor captures what it takes to gain access to another person's world when that person is on the spectrum.[19] Like fairy tales sometimes do, it can romanticize what is often an arduous journey in which the seeker becomes a follower. However, it is a journey that many parents and caretakers have undertaken successfully, even with the most challenging and challenged of children. Consider Chris, the son of Bill and Jae Davis (Solomon 2012:285):

> Chris didn't sleep. He flapped his hands. He injured himself. He smeared himself with feces and flung it at his parents. He bit himself. He gouged at his eyes. He stared at the ceiling fan for hours on end. Jae had intuited that Chris would need infinite patience, and a progressive approach to things he found difficult, including intimacy itself. She and Bill broke everything into small tasks. "It was like, 'Can I just touch you?' 'Oh, thank you so much. You're great,'" Bill said. "He wouldn't walk to the end of the block. So I would take him half a block and say, 'What a great walk!'"
>
> Chris had difficulty understanding cause and effect. He liked the motion of the car and screamed every time it stopped for a red light. Jae made red and green cards, and whenever the car approached a red light, she would show him the red one, and when it was time to go, she would show him the green. Once he understood the correlation, the screaming stopped.

Parents and others often show themselves to be exceptionally capable of entering the world of their child and acting on the child's uncommon sense to build collaborative endeavors.

ALTERATIONS IN COMMONSENSE REASONING

If ethnomethodology seems to depict common sense, and the social organization it embodies, as fixed and rigid, ethnomethodological studies also offer clues that commonsense reasoning is not necessarily that way. To see this, we need to consult earlier writings about the demonstrations reported in *Studies in Ethnomethodology* (Garfinkel 1967). In what is known as the "trust" paper, published four years earlier, Garfinkel (1963:222–23) reports on an instance that failed to produce the usual indignation and moral imputations. The experimenter, whom we will call Andrea, replied to a question from her husband, Mark, about whether she remembered to drop off shirts at the laundry, by saying, "What shirts did you mean, and what did you mean by having them 'dropped' off?" Initially, Mark was puzzled and indignant, but when Andrea persisted with her stance, eventually Mark "reflected on what I said, then changed the entire perspective as though we were playing a game, that it was all a joke." He did this by decomposing—artfully, we might say—her questions into their elementary parts and turning them back on her. And Andrea goes on, "He seemed to enjoy the joke." As Heritage (1984b:82) observes about this episode, "The potentially anomic features of the interaction with the associated elements of moral outrage, which began to surface in the early parts of the interaction, were thereby attenuated and ultimately cut short."

Mark's skillful rejoinders to Andrea are cousins to Sue Lehr's handling of her son Ben's "meltdown" at the bottom of a mall escalator. To revisit this episode analytically, we can observe how Sue disciplines herself through close attention to her son's trajectory, rather than, for example, yelling at him or asking the security guard for help. Having prepared for the situation by bringing a keyboard device, and even while entertaining rather panicky ideas about how things might look to bystanders, she allows time for Ben to type, "hit me." By continuing to pay attention in a concrete way to his behavior, she permits a next step in which Ben, exhibiting his autistic intelligence, types, "like a record player." As Mark did, Sue makes space for reflection, decomposes the episode into elementary parts, and deals with them in a way that preserves their integrity. She is fully inside Ben's castle, and to follow the parable, "careful and respectful" in a way that results in full-bore acknowledgment.

The example of Andrea and Mark connects with Garfinkel's (1963:201–6) report about another of his famous breaching experiments, which involved an experimenter starting the game of tic-tac-toe with another person. Following that person's placement of an X in a square on the game's grid, the experimenter would erase it and put it in another square. Regularly, subjects reacted by attempting to normalize such a discrepancy. If they did so while orienting to the basic rules of tic-tac-toe, they experienced a state of senselessness (Garfinkel 1963:206). However, *if* they interpreted the experimenter's move as initiating a new game, subjects "showed little disturbance." Accordingly, when those whose common sense was rendered strange could react with humor—by sensing a joke on the part of the violator, or by "switching" games—their sense of disturbance was vastly attenuated. They successfully crossed the bridge into another world than the taken-for-granted one, and thereby made the strange become familiar.

In accord with this pattern is research on parental acceptance of autism's difference, which shows that while high acceptance is *not* related to objective measures of severity, it *is* related to low subjective levels of stress. This is because, as Gernsbacher (2015:9) states, parents who score high on acceptance of disability "are adept at reframing their situation"—in our terms, questioning what is taken for granted and making the strange familiar by adopting a stance that is different because it is intimately related to the world of the autistic person rather than the commonsense one.

Diagnosis, Treatment, and the Prosthetic Environment

The area of treatment for autism is large and diverse, and it is not a topic we can address fully. Indeed, the very notion of "treatment" is contentious, insofar as it implicates a deficit picture of autism. Our own research has not concerned treatment recommendations as such, though we do think it carries implications for the design of "prosthetic environments" that can better accommodate children and adults on the spectrum and that could include relationships with therapists and other professionals. According to Holmes (1990:341), "A prosthetic environment enables a person to continue to be challenged and productive . . . clearly defined and regimented in order that the child or adult with autism feels secure and less anxious, and in turn, better able to focus on learning and productivity." Such an environment is geared to the individual and is less structurally defined or regimented than the official therapies for autism.

These official therapies include, most prominently, Applied Behavior Analysis (ABA), but also Treatment and Education of Autistic and Related Communications Handicapped Children (TEACCH), Perceptual-Motor Therapy (PIT), Sensory Integration Therapy (SIT), and the Floor Time or Relationship-Based (DIR) model,[20] among others (see the table in Eyal et al. 2010:252).[21] These therapeutic modalities fit three categories: they can be "bottom up," working from elementary behavior and communications to more complex conduct; "top down," representing for the child what he or she intends but cannot communicate; or aimed to effect the brain directly, as in PIT or SIT. In practice, Eyal and colleagues (2010:254) suggest, the differences are not very stark, as each approach has a mixture of the three categories of therapy while emphasizing one over the others.

Critics have argued that these and other therapies devalue difference by forcing autistic individuals to conform to neurotypical social and behavioral norms. These criticisms, many of which come from the neurodiversity movement (Ortega 2009) but some of which come from other sources (Bumiller 2008:976; Hacking 2007:311), point to the dehumanizing effects of therapy.

While these arguments are entirely valid, others have observed that the therapeutic picture as a whole is in fact more complicated.

As Eyal and colleagues (2010:264) write: "Autism therapies are technologies of the autistic self, and they reconfigure the goal of treatment. They come equipped with a whole host of prosthetic devices—PECS[22] books, personal communication computers, wristbands, and more. They are meant to be tunable to the child's individual strengths and weaknesses, and calculated to extend outward and blend into the environment."

Autism therapies offer the possibility of making the strange familiar *if* they allow for understanding the world of autism and for reconfiguring the interactional and interactive environments in which autistic individuals reside. Again drawing on Eyal and colleagues (2010:264): "The idea of the 'prosthetic environment' is, in some sense, paradoxical. It aims at achieving maximum independence, autonomy, agency, and sociability—all the trappings of the modern subject—yet these are often achieved—better, approximated—through hybrid arrangements involving therapists and parents who prompt the child or translate his utterances and behaviors, computers that project typed or touched words, or environments geared to the child's sensory sensitivities or distractive proclivities."

To return to our theme and the parable of the castle, the challenge is in accessing the world of the autistic person and knowing the ways that behavioral and social interactional details matter. At the same time, the challenge runs in the reverse direction. Neurotypicals must make commonsense reasoning accessible to persons with autism. To make sense together and achieve mutual intelligibility, participants in interaction must engage in a process of reciprocal accommodation. And this can only happen if therapy is seen as a two-way street that is more collaborative than remedial, so that therapist and client learn from one another with the goal of mutual understanding, rather than somehow fixing a broken or deficient person.

A Potential Role for Instantiation Stories in Fashioning Recommendations

Although clinicians are not readily able to draw on instantiation stories for making recommendations—in part because of the time and resource constraints described in chapter 6—we have argued that they nonetheless have the potential to provide greater access to the child's world than do tendency stories. In chapter 6, we used the cases of Dan Chapman and Ronnie Martin to illustrate the sorts of off-record competences that instantiation stories can document. We recognize that such stories, in themselves, are accounts or reports that still gloss much detail. However, more so than other kinds of stories, they capture interactional practices that can be explicated to bring features of *both* common sense and autistic intelligence into greater relief. For one further illustration, we will consider another episode from the case of Tony Smith, whom we met in chapter 5.

Recall the variety of autistic intelligence that Tony exhibited on different clinical tests. One of those was the "cow puzzle" subtest on the Psychoeducational Profile: Laura Sims placed a stack of tiles in front of Tony, said, "You try this puzzle for me," and asked, "Can you make a picture of a cow?" Roughly speaking, Tony was uncooperative or noncompliant, and Laura finally gave up, saying "Okay, hey, you know what? We've got another puzzle here to make . . . let's put the cow away. We're all done with the cow." Tony replied, "We all done with the cow," and the two of them proceeded to pick up the puzzle pieces and change activities.

This was not the end of the matter, however. As we also saw in chapter 5, Laura and the other clinicians treated the cow puzzle event with a story. During the informing interview, they shared the event with Tony's parents and teachers, putting a gloss on it that we called *anecdotal optimism*. Laura described how Tony *tended* to react to offers of help, saying, "A while ago, he wanted help with everything. And now, when you want to offer help, he's sort of rejecting." Molly, the psychiatrist, concurred: "And it goes along with the emergence of his showing pride in being able to do things." Laura and Molly psychologize Tony's actions, attributing them to an internal developmental process and leaving it at that.

However, if we inspect the original interaction closely, we can see how both Tony's ultimate noncompliance and occasional displays of compliance are joint achievements by himself and Laura acting in concert. At places in the interaction where Laura relinquishes the expectation that Tony should comply with her directives, including those that offer help (lines 1, 3, 5 below; fig. 8.3a), and instead aligns to Tony's counter-directive not to help (line 6) and watches his activity (lines 9–11; fig. 8.3b), then subsequent to *her* directives (lines 12, 14; fig. 8.3c), he complies (lines 13, 15; fig. 8.3d).

TRANSCRIPT 8.3: CASE M:1

```
1   Laura:   Want me to show you?
2            (1.5)
3   Laura:   Loo:k I'll make a COW for you.
4            (0.9)
5   Laura:   I'll help you, put that one here.
6   Tony:    Eh- [No don't help me::!
7   Laura:       [You-
8   Laura:   You wanna try it yourself?
9            (6.0)
```

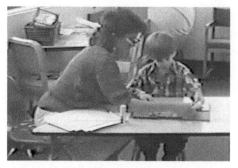

FIGURE 8.3A. I'll help you, put that one here (line 5).

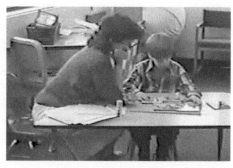

FIGURE 8.3B. You wanna try it yourself (line 8).

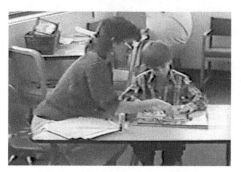

FIGURE 8.3C. Turn this one arou::nd (line 12).

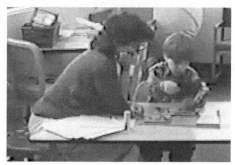

FIGURE 8.3D. ((Tony turns the piece)) (line 13).

```
10   Laura:   Oka:::y?
11            (5.2)
12   Laura:   Turn this one arou::nd. °Turn this one arou:nd.°
13            (2.8) ((Tony turns the piece))
14   Laura:   One muh- all:: the way around.
15            (2.0) ((Tony turns further))
16   Laura:   Oka::y?
```

To summarize: Tony had oriented to the puzzle in a very tactile way and demanded that Laura watch him. After Laura complies with his counter-directives (fig. 8.3b), Tony follows her directives to turn the puzzle pieces around, acceding to her prioritization of the puzzle's two-dimensional properties and claims about how it should look. In terms of its sequential placement, Tony's compliance is in line with research showing that *follow-in* directives—those that trail a child's focus of attention—obtain more compliance than *initiating* directives, possibly enhancing speech comprehension and production in the process (Brigham et al. 2010; Haebig, McDuffie, and Weismer 2013; Mirenda and Donnellan 1986; Siller and Sigman 2002).

At the autism-only school where Tan and Eyal (2015) conducted ethnographic research, instructors found "that by following the child they discover what interests him or her, using it as a hook to engage the child in a joint activity, thereby practicing with the child how to form relationships with others around them." And so, while it is not necessarily wrong to say that Tony is "rejecting" offers of help and "showing pride," that is not the entire story. By paying close attention to Tony's sequentially relevant initiatives, it is possible to access his world and learn how to work with his behavior, in this case by following rather than attempting to lead him.[23] This means aligning to his own directives and recognizing the competences they embody, even if those competences are not called for or measured by the test. In this way, it becomes possible to move Tony in different and teachable directions while also widening our own sense of what intelligent behavior looks like.

In chapter 5, we reviewed the saying "If you know one person with autism, you know one person with autism," which has become something of a cliché. Nonetheless, the phrase does capture the enormous heterogeneity among those who are diagnosed with autism.[24] Given that heterogeneity, when we think about how to design prosthetic environments that will maximize the autistic individual's participation in social life, it is extremely important to capture the particulars of that person's challenges *and* their skills. Equally, it is important to locate those challenges in mutual failures of sensemaking, rather than by pathologizing the person with autism for their failure to comport with neurotypical or commonsense expectations. After all, it is just as true to say that the neurotypical person is not comporting with autistic expectations. But to the extent that the autistic person's expectations are private and therefore uncommon, we need to find ways to make them public and accessible to commonsense reasoning (without necessarily assimilating them to that reasoning).

With regard to the critically important diagnostic process, our analysis suggests that we can be detailed about the kinds of diagnostic assessment and narrative practices that could better facilitate access to the child's world, making it possible to learn about and appreciate the forms of intelligence it comprises—even as we remain mindful of the problems diagnosis poses and of diagnostic manuals' orientation toward deficit. Documenting autistic intelligence and first-order competence is crucial for designing environments, including their technological aspects, that autistic individuals can successfully share.[25]

The design of the individual child's environment, in other words, can be built so that its interactional and interactive features enhance that child's discernable first-order, fundamental competence and autistic intelligence while minimizing, if not eliminating entirely, aspects of the environment that make the child's differences disabling—in other words, *those aspects that turn difference into deficit and disability.* Indeed, if we think of such design in terms of accommodation, then as Gernsbacher (2015) states the matter, we also can anticipate that many people will end up reaping the advantages of these accommodations beyond their direct beneficiaries, whether in the manner of curb cuts, whose original purpose was to facilitate the use of wheelchairs but which also wound up accommodating shopping carts, bicycles, and the use of canes or other implements for walking; elimination of labels in clothing, to which many people are sensitive; or allowing extended time for test taking, which alleviates pressure unnecessary to the assessment of skill in any number of domains.[26] In our terms, altering and adapting common sense—making the strange familiar—enhances the corporate lives of adapters as much as those for whom adaptations are made.[27]

In sum, shifting from the currently dominant conception of autism as disorder to an alternative conception of autism as difference will involve recognizing autism as a phenotype located in interactional and interactive environments, rather than in the head or body of the person alone. It will also mean bringing the elements of autism we have examined—common sense, interaction, autistic intelligence, narrative sensemaking—into the foreground and fashioning diagnoses that do not pathologize neurodiversity but identify and work with the challenges it can create in a world based on common sense. Although there will always be a certain tension between the generalizing thrust of diagnosis and the particularization necessary to appreciate autism as difference, our findings suggest possibilities. The diagnostic process could achieve a better balance between the generic and the particular by attending to the coproduced features of autism in interaction, for example by reducing the tendency-instantiation story ratio, producing instantiation stories that foreground what child and clinician are doing *together*—instead of the child's actions only—and treating a broader variety of events as worthy of telling in the first place. Ultimately, the shift would direct attention, not "upward," from situated practices and sensemaking toward a generic diagnosis, but "downward" toward the practices that make diagnosis possible in the first place.

Acknowledgments

Doug Maynard

My son Theodore was diagnosed in fifth grade with what was then called high-functioning autism or Asperger's syndrome. Because of the challenges that he had presented, virtually since early childhood, and which became exacerbated in the schooling context, we had asked an expert psychologist to examine him. When she completed her extensive evaluation, we were surprised by the diagnosis, but it began to help us make sense of the difficulties we were experiencing both at home and at school with our son.

However, our family experiences with Theo are not described or referenced in this book, partly out of respect for his privacy, partly because this is a coauthored text that would have made my reflections out of sync in our joint narrative flow, and, finally, because our collaborative aim is to capture the world of testing and diagnosis in terms that are intrinsic to the data we collected. That said, my experiences as a father matter in many ways for the understandings I bring to this research. However much I have learned about autism through investigating, reading, and hearing or reviewing the work of experts in the field, Theo has been by far my biggest teacher. There is an unsurpassable integrity that he, like others on the spectrum, exhibits. That integrity is utterly dependable, it can draw you to live in the moment, and when we (my wife and I) really watch, listen, or engage with him in ways that match his integrity, it is always a gift. And as he has grown older, and as we have learned more, so the challenges have receded, and the seeds of his original joyful presence, for some time seemingly in the background, have utterly increased and come to the fore. They have blossomed.

My academic interest in autism predates the birth and diagnosis of our son, however. As a postdoctoral fellow in the Department of Psychiatry at the University of Wisconsin in the early 1980s, I was given a collection of audio recordings by Bonnie Svarstad and Helene Lipton, the analysis of which they had already completed. These were informing interviews from a clinic for developmental disabilities, and they awakened my interest in that field. They had cases of autism that were, in the 1970s, considered to be a form of child-hood psychosis. With this seed data, I was able to obtain a grant (#17803) from the National Institutes of Health to collect more such data by way of video recordings in a different clinic. That data (from 1985–86) also included cases in which children were given an autism diagnosis or the related (1980s) diagnosis of atypical pervasive developmental disorder.

My sociological orientation in the field of ethnomethodology is a natural home for understanding about disability, and particularly autism, because these conditions reveal so much about what we take for granted in ordinary social life. So both of these data sets piqued my interest to analyze autism by ethnomethodological study and by the related field of conversation analysis. In many ways, and apart from the role of my family experience related to au-tism, this book for me is a culmination of these substantive, theoretical, and methodological interests. I am grateful to the teachers in my field, including Harold Garfinkel, Gail Jefferson, and Emanuel Schegloff, for both the inter-personal learning experiences and the intellectual heft from their writings that infuse much of our analysis. Don Zimmerman, Tom Wilson, and Melvin Pollner were more immediate teachers during my graduate school experience at the University of California, Santa Barbara, and while attending classes that Pollner taught at the University of California, Los Angeles. I also owe an enormous debt to the worldwide set of scholars in these fields from my own and later generations. Not least are the many undergraduates in my classes, who have listened, read materials, and heard me talk about these interests for many years. Over time, even before I embarked on this book project, my graduate students became roped into the various autism interests and other ethnomethodological or conversation analytic projects that I was develop-ing, and I remain very thankful for all the enthusiasm and independence of thinking they brought, which greatly enhanced my own intellectual endeav-ors. Jason Turowetz was once my graduate student, and, over the years, I have enjoyed his becoming a full-fledged and awesome collaborator and coauthor on this book.

We (Jason Turowetz and I) have had many chances to present our work at professional meetings, where, again, the feedback has often been invaluable. I particularly want to thank colleagues at the Academy of Finland–funded Finnish Centre of Excellence in Intersubjectivity in Interaction in Helsinki, Finland, where I was hosted over the five years of the Centre's duration from 2012–17. Regularly, I was able to discuss and present embryonic aspects of our research and get excellent feedback from Anssi Peräkylä, Marja-Leena Sorjonen, and their students, postdoctoral fellows, and colleagues, including Jörg Bergmann from the University of Bielefeld in Germany. At the University of Wisconsin–Madison, my home institution, I have had the support of colleagues from the Department of Sociology and intellectual and material backing from the Center for the Demography of Health and Aging, and the Waisman Center. The University of Wisconsin Graduate School provided much-needed seed money for pilot projects that enabled successful grant applications to the National Institutes of Health and the National Science Foundation. As well, I remain very grateful to the Holtz Center for Science and Technology Studies at the University of Wisconsin, which provided both material and intellectual support over the duration of this project.

Besides Theo, the other members of my family have been my constants. Our daughter Jessica, a practitioner of traditional Chinese medicine and an acupuncturist, has the right balance of intellectual rigor, clinical understanding, Eastern and Western medicinal knowledge, and other qualities that make us proud parents. I can only hope that this book lives up to her high standards. And, from day one, she has been a loving older sister to Theo; the care they show for one another—along with Jessica's partner Kirk Moorhead—is also an inspiration.

In the acknowledgments to *Studies in Ethnomethodology*, Harold Garfinkel, whose precision of expression can be, as he used to say, "just right," wrote this about Arlene Garfinkel, whom my spouse and I also had the pleasure to know: "My lovely wife knows this book with me" (p. xi). Well, Joan Maynard knows *this* book with *me*. Together we raised our children while I was reading and writing in the field of autism studies (and wider domains of sociology, ethnomethodology, and conversation analysis); together we learned about what it is like to raise a child who is on the spectrum; together—because of her unending interest and support, including a steady supply of resources that I may not have otherwise come across—we have brought my part of this manuscript to completion. This book is dedicated to all my close family, but I also want to acknowledge my brother Tom, who, over the years, fed me a steady stream of journalist accounts regarding autism, and my brother Ron, a medical anthropologist, who read an early version of the entire manuscript and gave us some critically helpful feedback. Over time, Tom and Ron (and their own families) have been valuable supporters of Theo and Jessica as well.

Jason Turowetz

This book has been several years in the making, and it represents my and Doug's effort to do some justice to the complexity of autism as it is experienced by children on the spectrum and by those who assess and diagnose it. The many hours I have spent reading, recording, interviewing, viewing and re-viewing tapes, transcribing, and discussing my thoughts with friends and colleagues have provided me with a deep appreciation for what we call the "uncommon sense" exhibited by autistic children, as well as a sense of hu-mility that comes from realizing just how little I know about it, even after all this time. It was a privilege to observe and learn from these children, whose unique ways of understanding the world we have attempted to convey, how-ever imperfectly, in this book's pages.

I would like to thank the Social Sciences and Humanities Research Coun-cil of Canada (SSHRC) for supporting my first four years as a graduate stu-dent at the University of Wisconsin–Madison, where I learned about ethno-methodology and conversation analysis and developed the skills that I took into the field while conducting the research for this book. Thanks also to the Robert F. and Jean E. Holtz Center for Science and Technology Studies at University of Wisconsin–Madison for funding conference travel; the Robert Wood Johnson Foundation Health & Society Scholars Program at the Uni-versity of Wisconsin–Madison for supporting my fieldwork and writing with the Population Health Dissertation Grant; and the Morse Fellows Society for the Study of Developmental Psychopathology at the University of Wisconsin–Madison's Waisman Center, which in addition to providing financial support also connected me with an interdisciplinary group of scholars working at the cutting edge of autism research.

On a more personal note, thanks to the family and friends who have pro-vided companionship and encouragement throughout the research and writ-ing process. My parents and siblings have been a constant source of support and understanding at every stage of my career. I would not be writing these words without them. I have benefited greatly over the years from conversa-tions with Gina Longo, Waverly Duck, Rahul Mahajan, David Schelly, Matt Hollander, Clemens Eisenmann, Anne Rawls, Jeff Denis, and others who have offered feedback and advice at various stages of the project, as well as friend-ship and support. Finally, thank you to my wonderful wife, Sabrina, and our daughter, Violette, for their endless love, encouragement, and inspiration.

Doug Maynard and Jason Turowetz

First and foremost, we want to jointly thank the clinicians and staff at CDDC for allowing us to observe them in the course of their work and for generously participating in discussions and interviews, even as they juggled demanding schedules. They graciously allowed us not only to observe but also to shadow, ask questions, look over their shoulders, and otherwise intrude as we learned about their work. We also wish to thank the several dozen families and children who participated in our research, many of whom selflessly expressed the hope, when we asked for permission to record their evaluations, that others would benefit from their participation. We were total strangers, given access to one of the most important and vulnerable moments of their lives. This book simply would not have been possible without their cooperation. For other families who potentially may benefit from our research, we hope it lives up to the expectations of those who generously participated in our study.

We are also most grateful for sources of funding that sustained this project over a number of years. A grant from the National Science Foundation (No. 1257065) made it possible for us (Maynard and Turowetz), along with Research Assistants T. A. McDonald, Trini Stickle, and Adam Talkington, and Dr. Waverly Duck, who was on research leave from the University of Pittsburgh, to collect data at the site we call Central Developmental Disabilities Clinic (CDDC). Back on campus, the Waisman Center at the University of Wisconsin–Madison, and its University Center for Excellence in Developmental Disabilities grant (NICHD No. P30 HD03352), allowed us lab space for processing our data and the arduous task of transcription. Marsha Mailick, the director of the Waisman Center, was particularly helpful in making this arrangement for us. When he was still at the University of Wisconsin–Madison and the director of the Research Corps at the Waisman Center, Leonard Abbeduto, now the director of the University of California Davis MIND Institute, was an early supporter of our research. Our investigations were also supported by a grant to the Center for Demography of Health and Aging (P30 AG017266) at the University of Wisconsin–Madison.

Finally, we are grateful for the exceptionally helpful written and oral feedback on previous drafts or in-progress work from colleagues. In some cases, it was long discussions about our data. In other cases, it was feedback on particular chapters. And in a few cases, it was reading the entire manuscript. So, one way or the other, our heartfelt thanks go to Somer Bishop, Galina Bolden, Steve Clayman, Joe Conti, Dagoberto Cortez, Leann DaWalt, Waverly Duck, Clemens Eisenmann, Jeremy Freese, Joan Fujimura, Virginia Gill, Mike Halpin, Matthew Hollander, John Heritage, Annemarie Jutel, John Martin, Jenny Mandelbaum, Lindsay McCary, Jason Nolen, Alberto Palloni, Anssi Peräkylä, John Rae, Jeff Robinson, and Tanya Stivers. Nora Cate Schaeffer provided links, journalistic accounts, and other resources for our endeavors. This book was originally contracted with the University of Chicago Press when the late Doug Mitchell was the social science editor, and we regret that he is not here to see the final product. Elizabeth Branch Dyson has ably taken the editorial position and helped to shepherd this book through final reviews, making extremely supportive as well as beneficial suggestions for revision along the way. Reviewers of our book for the Press also made valuable comments, and we hope they will see changes in the manuscript that we have made in response. Lucas Wiscons, besides working with our project data for his own research, has been an invaluable source of insight and, more practically, the one who got this manuscript into shape, following detailed protocols for submission to the University of Chicago Press. We are particularly in his debt for that.

Notes

Chapter One

1. All names connected with our data in this and subsequent chapters, including personal and geographic references, are pseudonyms.

2. A pseudonym.

3. This is one of three data sets (recordings of clinical interactions) that we have. See the description of our collections in the section on the Interaction Order of the Clinic at the end of the chapter.

4. Survey research provides some insight into the preclinic, in-clinic, and postclinic phases of the autism career but mostly focuses on levels of satisfaction with the overall diagnostic process, including levels of support after diagnosis. See, for example, research drawing on the experiences of those who receive the diagnosis (Jones et al. 2014); for research on the parents' point of view, see Howlin and Moore (1997).

5. In this book, we vacillate between formal (Dr. Grant) and informal references (Leah) to the professionals. This reflects the practices we encountered in the clinic, where staff mostly used first names with one another. Parents, when they had occasion to address a clinician, also vacillated between formal and informal usages.

6. References to the Diagnostic and Statistical Manuals will be denoted by "APA," the acronym for the American Psychiatric Association.

7. We say more about our training experience in chap. 5.

8. A number of sociological and anthropological investigators (Cicourel 1974; Corsaro 1979; Ochs 1979) have studied children's taken-for-granted knowledge, using other terms to describe commonsense understanding and index what Briggs (1986:75) calls the "conventionalized expectations" and "metacommunicative" features of everyday and interview-based talk.

9. The matter of tacitness and implicitness can be complex. Roughly, an explicit version of an action would contain some kind of marker, as in "I promise I will meet you on Friday at 2 p.m.," where the beginning phrase ("I promise") formulates the kind of action being produced. This can be compared with "See you on Friday at 2," which can be considered a commitment of the "promising" type, but the promise is tacit and implicit rather than overt and explicit. For discussion, see Levinson (1983:263–76), and Sidnell and Enfield (2014:426–28).

10. Our approach is captured succinctly in a study (Saenz, Black, and Pelegrini 1999:123) about imputations of social competence in children diagnosed with Specific Language Impairment

(SLI): "These data would suggest that incompetence is not the sole possession of the individual and that children should not be evaluated as having 'social problems' that are intrinsic to their nature. Rather, portraits of competence and incompetence should be regarded as complex constructions, which can differ with the situation."

Accordingly, our analytic approach to autism goes beyond the child to the social environment in which their actions occur and are then interpreted as symptoms of disorder, and it has implications for other evaluations and diagnostic processes beyond autism. See the collection of studies (Kovarsky, Duchan, and Maxwell 1999) in which the Saenz and colleagues (1999) paper appears.

11. A recent paper (Vivanti 2020) raises the question, "What is the most appropriate way to talk about individuals with a diagnosis of Autism? Should we stop saying 'person with autism,' and use 'autistic person' instead?" With some qualifications, and on the basis of considerations from other research and writings about the issue, including from the neurodiversity movement, the answer this editorial provides is in favor of "autistic person." In this book, we are following this practice except when other locutions may be relevant, given the context. For other discussions favoring the practice of referring to an "autistic person," see Gernsbacher (2017) and Baron-Cohen (2017).

12. The British autism researcher—and mother of an autistic daughter—Lorna Wing (1973:111) may be the first to have referred to how parents can have access to "the special language of their own autistic child." See the discussion in Hart (2014:291–92), who remarks, "This language is not only verbal; it includes seemingly cacophonous gestures, vocalizations and ritualistic behavioral patterns."

13. For a contrary view and findings suggesting the opposite—i.e., that echolalia is not what its name implies and is interactionally meaningful in a variety of ways—see Kawashima and Maynard (2019), Prizant and Duchan (1981), Sterponi and Shankey (2014), Stribling, Rae, and Dickerson (2007), Tarplee and Barrow (1999), and Wootton (1999).

14. As Suskind (2014:134) observes, "what had been happening naturally and forcefully, day by day, year to year, inside our home: the judgments . . . widely accepted suppositions about those with so-called 'intellectual disabilities'—were being dislodged, often against our will, and replaced with a much deeper understanding."

15. Briefly, by *first-order competence* we mean the basic or fundamental competences required to participate in social life (e.g., recognizing a question as a question and being able to produce an answer in response). We distinguish this from second-order, structural competence, which builds on first-order competence and involves participating in more elaborate, sustained social activities, which include the use and implementation of tacit knowledge.

16. We had the impression that, in addition to expecting the diagnosis, Betsy had been hoping for it, though she did not say so in so many words. As we discuss later in the book (especially in chap. 7), it was not uncommon for parents to want a diagnosis like autism, which could explain their child's troubles and make them eligible for much-needed services. Even among these parents, though, news of autism was not welcomed as uniformly good; reactions were frequently ambivalent, and clinicians and parents worked jointly to realize the news (or rather aspects of the news) as "good" or "bad."

17. We suspect that, if the cases in our 1972 and 1985 collections could be re-examined using today's diagnostic criteria, they would each have higher proportions of autism diagnoses.

Chapter Two

1. Our overview draws from various sources. See for example the research of Barker and Galardi (2015); Evans (2013); Eyal (2013); Eyal, Hart, Onculer et al. (2010); Frith (2003); Grinker

(2007); Nadesan (2005); Sheffer (2018); Silverman (2012); and Wolff (2004). Journalistic accounts include Donvan and Zucker (2016); Feinstein (2010); and Silberman (2015).

2. We are indebted to Schegloff's (2007b) use of the term "talk-in-interaction."

3. Autism is what Hacking (1999:103) has called an "interactive" kind of disorder, meaning that it is the kind of classification that may affect not only those to whom it is applied but also "the larger matrix of institutions and practices surrounding this classification." Fully answering our hypothetical and counterfactual question would necessitate a larger historical and sociological inquiry of the sort that Hacking (1999) himself engaged in with regard to madness and child abuse, for example. See also Hacking (1998) on transient mental illness.

4. Wing (1991:115) notes that Asperger's term was "autistic psychopathy," which was misleading because it implied abnormality of personality. She declared "Asperger's Syndrome" as the "preferred" term so that autism was not equated with sociopathic behavior.

5. For a detailed overview of the history and controversies surrounding the DSM-5, we draw on a variety of sources (Paris and Phillips 2013; Sweet and Decoteau 2017; Whooley and Horwitz 2013).

6. The international picture is more complicated. For a long time, standardized assessments and classifications were not available internationally, and studies across countries and nationalities are expensive to conduct (Grinker, Yeargin-Allsopp, and Boyle 2011:116). A host of obstacles stand in the way: the reliability of school and other reports; the question of whether diagnosis matters when services are not available; opposition to research on conditions that are not perceived as life-threatening, given more pressing (i.e., life-threatening) diseases; and concerns about social stigma (Grinker, Yeargin-Allsopp, and Boyle 2011:118). For more recent and in-depth chapters on cultural factors affecting the diagnosis of autism, see Fein and Rios (2018). In particular, for France see Chamak and Bonniau (2013), for Brazil see Rios and Andrada (2015), and for Costa Rica, see Schelly, Jiménez, and Solis (2015). And, for a critical autism studies approach, which draws on the notion of "epistemic communities" to explore culturally varying knowledges about autism, see O'Dell and colleagues (2016).

7. See chap. 3 and Hacking (2009).

8. Eyal et al. (2010) and Eyal (2013) draw on "actor-network theory" (e.g., Callon 1999; Latour 1987; Latour 1999; Law 2009) in the science, technology, and society (STS) literature.

9. However, the social movements originating in parental advocacy for autism are not uniform in their orientations, particularly when members of a specific racial and national group have migrated to separate countries with differing cultures of receptivity to the group and the health status of members. See for example Decoteau's (2017) study of Somalis in Minneapolis and Toronto, their different epistemic communities, and distinct ways of mobilizing for children who become diagnosed with ASD.

10. Having an extended timeline is well-documented in research on laboratories and investigators whose efforts are devoted to finding genetic bases for alcoholism through research on rats. As Nelson (2018:78) reports, "Researchers managed what they perceived to be overly confident and socially irresponsible knowledge claims by expanding the field's temporal horizons back out again, pushing clinical scenarios into the far distant future and introducing potential complications that made it seem unlikely that clinical applications would be coming any time soon." See also Fortun's (2001:145) succinct and well-supported comment, deriving from his extensive ethnographic investigations (Fortun 2005; Fortun 2008) of deCODE Genetics Inc. and its efforts in Iceland to establish a universal database of medical records that would facilitate the human genome project: "The many stories about genomics that appear increasingly on

television, in newspapers and magazines, and on the Internet reinforce the standard story that this is an industry based on genetic information. But to the extent that we can say it is 'based' on anything, the genomics industry is based on the *promise* of genetic information . . . what genetic information *may become* in the anticipated, contingent future."

In short, as Fortun (2001:144) puts it, "The science and business of genomics is fundamentally anticipatory."

11. Regarding RDoC, see, for example, the National Institute of Mental Health (2019) website. A further consequence of the neuromolecular gaze is that the environment is underemphasized if not entirely excluded in the search for causality (Nadesan 2005:148, 160; Silverman 2012:142; Singh 2016:98). Related to this, the resources devoted to genomic research from both public and private sources has been enormous. For example, when it became possible to scan whole genomes with great magnification and detect chromosomal deviations by identifying spontaneously generated (rather than inherited) copy number variations (i.e., de novo CNVs), the National Institutes of Health disbursed $15 million in 2013 alone for CNV autism research projects. Private research foundations also contributed, and in that year, 291 studies focused on CNVs and autism appeared (Singh 2016:98). Overall, between federal and private agencies devoted to autism, hundreds of millions of dollars are allocated to autism research each year, with a heavy emphasis on genetic understandings (Singh 2016:63–64). In 2013, the NIH itself spent $186 million on autism research, with the federal government and its leaders orienting to "cure," which translates to a disease framework (Pitney 2015:41–43) and prioritizes genetic research.

12. See Dreaver and colleagues (2020:1658) and their advocacy of a "bio-psycho-social" approach to understanding ASD, and of addressing problems of employment specifically. For more general statements regarding what Engel (1980) famously called the "biopsychosocial" model in medicine, see Frankel, Quill, and McDaniel's (2003) edited volume on this topic, and see Aharoni and colleagues (2019:465) on a "biopsychosocial framework" that incorporates "dynamic, bidirectional interactions between the brain and social environments."

13. Also see Nelson's (2018) study of experimental approaches to, and practices for, finding the genetics of rat behavior (the goal of which is to extrapolate to humans). Investigated close up, these approaches and practices, involving the epistemologies and ontologies related to lab work, do not fit the stereotype of reductionism often attributed to them.

14. On the history of the microarray technology development and efforts to find genetic markers for human traits and diseases, and in the process to ascribe group-based differences at the level of DNA sequencing, see Rajagopalan and Fujimura (2018). On how such history has resulted in a social construction of race, see Fujimura and colleagues (2014).

15. For an example with regard to autism, see Weiss and Arking (2009).

16. Relying on data from the Genome Wide Association Studies (GWAS), the practice has been to "measure hundreds of thousands or more alleles like scattershot across the genome . . . scientists could throw thousands of strands of spaghetti against the wall and see which stuck—that is, conduct a hypothesis-free investigation and see what 'pops out' in the data" (Conley and Fletcher 2017:44). However, rare variants, which characterize many mutations, will not emerge. They are invisible to GWAS.

17. However, in the United States, these communities, and their access to genetic testing, reflect patterns of stratification in the wider society (Clarke et al. 2003:170; Navon 2019:207).

18. The documentary is called "Autism under the Lens" and is part of the Home Box Office series entitled *VICE*. The writer is Reid Cherlin, the correspondent is Gianna Toboni, the producer is Seth Dalton, the editor is Greg Wright, and the directory of photography for the

segment is Daniel Hollis. Mr. Robison's statement is at about twenty-three minutes and thirty-five seconds into the video.

19. However, see the discussion in Abbeduto, McDuffie, and Thurman's (2014) research suggesting the importance of differences in symptoms, behaviors, and developmental trajectories between those with comorbid FXS and those diagnosed with ASD but not FXS. For in-depth analysis of the autism–fragile X relationship and the genetics thereof, see Navon (2019:chap. 3).

20. Mol (e.g., 2002:35) distinguishes "clinical atherosclerosis" from "pathological atherosclerosis," the former having to do with a patient's symptomology and the latter involving that which is "visible under the microscope." Similarly, following Navon (2011) and Navon and Eyal (2016), we could distinguish between clinical autism and pathological autism—what a child may present and what the lab may turn up independently of such presentation. Finally, when there is the possibility of a genetic mutation, such as is caused by a microdeletion on the genome, there are both advantages and disadvantages in its discovery. For discussion, see Navon (2019:chap. 6, chap. 7).

21. The relation between genetic substrates and phenotypes is considered to be mediated by endophenotypes, such as neurotransmitters (Nadesan 2005:155–56; Schnittker 2017:213–19). As Gottesman and Gould (2003:636) put it, endophenotypes "represent simpler clues to genetic underpinnings than the disease syndrome itself . . . psychiatric diagnoses can be decomposed or deconstructed, which can result in more straightforward—and successful—genetic analysis."

22. Compatible with the notion of phenotypic bottleneck is what Fitzgerald (2017:11, original emphasis) has to say about "tracing autism"—"a structure of looping interactions between biological marks and social world, somehow distinct *from* one another but also irretrievably entangled *in* one another." Fitzgerald (2017:11) draws an example from a psychiatrist who posits a person with language problems such that people in the social environment "react differently to them, so this very small and innate molecular difference would radically alter that person's social surroundings," with further "looping" back into the biology of the brain.

23. It is not as if the neurobiological correlates of social interaction can be conceived as static entities either. As Haraway (1997:142) observes: "The processes 'inside' bodies—such as the cascades of action that constitute an organism or that constitute the play of genes and other entities that go to make up a cell—are interactions, not frozen things. For humans, a word like gene specifies a multifaceted set of interactions among people and nonhumans in historically contingent, practical, knowledge-making work. A gene is not a thing, much less a 'master molecule' or a self-contained code. Instead, the term gene signifies a node of durable action where many actors, human and nonhuman, meet."

24. Science and technology scholars have developed a lucid critique of the notion of personalized medicine (PM) that stems from the Human Genome Project's proposal that medicine and health care should be tailored closely to individual characteristics by differentiating disease entities according to a person's unique biology. Although applicable to common complex diseases, efforts to apply genomic medicine to mental health, including ASD, raise many concerns allied to those we have already articulated (Rüppel and Voigt 2019). Prainsack (2017:chap. 7) develops the idea that people are relational beings and that the unit of analysis for understanding mental health should be "interactions between people." Complementary to biological and neurological information, dynamic social information about the person could make for true personalized medicine. That is, we need "sociomarkers" in addition to "biomarkers." In practical terms, it needs to be noted that, although it could be said that in this book we are going after "sociomark-ers," our concerns are starkly different from personalized medicine in autism, where the goal is

to identify genetic causes of autism at the molecular level in order to fashion specific treatments for individual patients (cf. Navon 2019:161–63). When we discuss the particularizing of diagnosis, our goal is to capture the organization of relationships in which autism in its gestalt or mosaic qualities (Hacking 2009; Maynard and Turowetz 2019) is manifest because of individualized forms of intelligence being expressed on the surface of interaction.

25. We should add that the professionals we studied were nothing if not careful, cautious, and concerned to do right by the children and families with whom they work. Clinicians know full well that there is no biological marker for autism; that it is a behavioral syndrome that affects some children more severely than others; that its definition has changed over time; that competing interpretations easily emerge from their observations; and that there exist both aggrandizing and stigmatizing attitudes toward autism in the wider society. Thus, they are far from naive or uninformed participants who perform diagnosis mechanically. It is our aim to capture the deeply socially organized details of how they manage to coordinate their actions with those of children, families, and others to conduct evaluations and decide whether or not a child—whom they have not sought out but who has come before them—qualifies for an autism spectrum disorder. In a phrase, the goal is to examine clinicians' sensemaking practices and their consequences.

Chapter Three

1. Depending on a child's developmental level, clinicians administering the ADOS have options for including parents in the examining room. When administering ADOS Module T (for toddlers), Module 1 (for children thirty-one months and older who do not consistently use phrase speech), and Module 2 (for children of any age who use phrase speech but are not verbally fluent), clinicians are directed to include parents during testing, as some "presses" or attempts to engage the child may involve their participation. For Modules 3 (for verbally fluent children and young adolescents) and 4 (for verbally fluent older adolescents and adults), the manual for administering the ADOS (Lord et al. 2012:20) states, "a parent/caregiver should not be in the room during the administration unless there is an unusual circumstance that calls for his/her presence (e.g., if the child is very young)."

2. And Goffman (1963:70) further defines the "away" as "taking the form of what is variously called reverie, brown study, woolgathering, daydreaming, or autistic thinking."

3. For discussion regarding "acquiescent" responses in the context of disability testing, see Rapley (2004:chap. 3).

4. We are taking a stance inspired by phenomenology, through which it is possible to "bracket" or hold in abeyance a commitment as to whether Dan is "autistic" or "typical." This stance, otherwise referred to as a transcendental reduction or epoche (Husserl 1970), allows for the suspension of such judgments to describe wider aspects of human and social experience.

5. A detailed review of the speech act theorists, as well as sociolinguistic, discourse analytic, pragmatic, and applied linguistic scholarship, can be found in Maynard and Turowetz (2013a).

6. The relation of the interaction order and its elements to larger forms of social organization is a complex matter (Boden and Zimmerman 1991; Drew and Heritage 1992). For recent treatment of the issues in regard to race, see the collection of papers in Rawls, Whitehead, and Duck (2020); regarding gender, see Speer and Stokoe (2011); and for a general review, see Heritage and Maynard (in press).

7. These data, collected for other studies (Lipton and Svarstad 1977; Svarstad and Lipton 1977) and given to us by the coauthors, are used in only a limited way in this book. However, see

Maynard (1989), and for more extensive description of the entire collection of data, see Maynard and Turowetz (2019).

8. For a more extensive set of considerations regarding data collection, see Mondada (2013). For considerations about CA strictures applied to language use and autism from a linguistic anthropology perspective, see Sterponi, de Kirby, and Shankey (2015).

9. The term *autism narrative* is also not to be confused with the diagnostic narratives we will discuss in chap. 6 and 7.

10. Adapted from Jefferson (1974), "Error Correction as an Interactional Resource." See also: Atkinson and Heritage (1984:ix-vi), and Hepburn and Bolden (2013:57–76). Nonvocal, embodied aspects of interaction are transcribed in complementary ways (Heath and Luff 2012:283-307).

Chapter Four

1. Thirty years, ago, Brown (1990:389[143]) noted how "increasing faith" in the DSM "is central to the new biopsychiatry."

2. For a thoroughgoing contemporary investigation of gaze patterns in interactions involving autistic children, see Korkiagangas (2018).

3. When we use the term *autistic intelligence*, we are not suggesting that there is only one form of such intelligence. It should be understood, rather, as a collective noun that encompasses many varieties of self-attentive intelligence. As such, any given case of autistic intelligence represents but one instance of such intelligence among many.

4. Beyond self-attentiveness, Maynard (2005) has identified four features of autistic intelligence that distinguish it from common sense. Comparing the answers given by neurotypical and autistic individuals to "What Do You Do When" questions (e.g., "what do you do when *x* happens?"), he describes autistic intelligence as (1) additive and stimulus-bound, (2) local, (3) literal, and (4) constructive. It is *additive* and *stimulus-bound* in its tendency to focus on parts rather than wholes, which can include, for example, focusing on the actions (e.g., questions and answers) that constitute a social activity (e.g., testing) instead of orienting to the activity itself; *local* in its orientation to specific as opposed to global features of objects—for example, equating all dogs with one specific dog; *literal* in its orientation to fixed meanings and rules; and constructive in Sacks's (1989[1964]: 223) sense of "taking . . . pieces and adding them up in some way." Common sense, by comparison, orients to *gestalt-wholes* over parts, is *global* and abstract rather than local and concrete, *idiomatic* in its apprehension of the nonliteral meanings of words and actions, and *composite*, in contrast to *constructive* (Sacks 1989[1964]) in its orientation to meanings that incorporate commonly held but tacit elaborations on the particularities of conduct. It is also other-attentive in a way that autistic intelligence is not, a point we expand upon in this chapter and in chap. 8. These distinctions should not be taken to imply that people with autism cannot reason in commonsense ways, or that nonautistic people never exhibit autistic intelligence. Rather, they are meant to identify a method (or collection of methods) of sensemaking characteristic of those identified as autistic—methods in which such individuals are more likely than others to engage and become immersed. Autistic intelligence does not reside "inside" of autistic people any more than common sense resides in or is unique to non-autistic people.

5. Regarding the "poetics" of everyday talk, see the conversation analytic literature, including papers by Jefferson (1996) and Schegloff (2003b; 2003c) and lectures by Sacks (1992a; 1992b).

6. Hacking (2009:1472–73) uses both of these (Mukhopadhyay's and Grandin's) comments to offer a brief critique of the "theory of mind" hypothesis and to suggest that those who have

more severe autism than Mukhopadhyay or Grandin and "who communicate very little" may "also understand, in a quite specific way, far more than is evident to the outsider."

7. For a thorough-going treatment of the phenomenon of recruitment in interaction—how participants deploy linguistic and embodied practices to seek assistance for everyday tasks—see Kendrick and Drew (2016).

8. In his critique of the "metric society"—and parallel to Donaldson (1978)—Mau (2019) observes how quantification (which diagnostic testing entails) is an act of translation that involves "disembedding" and stripping away "local knowledge and the context of social practices in order to obtain more abstract information that can be recombined and amalgamated with information from other sources."

9. In various places in his published lectures, Sacks (e.g., 1992a:Part II, Fall 1965, Lecture 5) discusses "tying rules," or mechanisms for how segments of conversation can be connected verbally and in other ways with one another.

10. In chap. 5, we will examine another child's performance on this subtest and see how, in some of his answers, he may notice patterns in detail that are invisible to the commonsense eye, even though his answers lack in structural competence.

11. For how parents, in a team-wise fashion, may manage "self-stimming" (i.e., sensory stimulating) behavior, see Maynard, McDonald, and Stickle (2016).

12. This toy is a wheel-like object. When used with its wooden structure, it is manipulative and visual. The child places the wheel at the top of the structure and watches it roll down the four layers of track that guide it to the bottom of the structure. Usually, the child will repeat the exercise several times. After the several unsuccessful efforts to have Marcus do the Picture Similarities task (which we analyze later in the section), Peg brings out the wooden structure and hands the toy wheel to him. He then enthusiastically engages with it.

13. Unfortunately, due to the logistics of getting our camera set up for recording this part of the Marcus visit, we were unable to record the very beginning of this testing interview. Our video of the encounter begins with line 1 in transcript 4.2.

14. As Sidnell (2007:392) observes, "look-prefaced" utterances can launch a course of action and may "pre-empt some course of action which might otherwise have occurred in its place."

15. Several details can be noticed here. First, in line with patterns that Rossi (2014) identifies in the use and nonuse of language in requesting, Marcus initially requests the toy, which is in visual range for both participants, nonvocally with an open hand gesture. When that fails, he produces the apparent "to me" verbalizations at lines 21 and 22. Still, his gaze is directed at the toy and only momentarily at the clinician, which may be consistent with younger children's use of reaching gestures to request (Rossano and Liebal 2014:360).

16. On the basis of the overall evaluation process, Peg later informs Marcus's mother that her son qualifies for the ASD diagnosis. See Turowetz and Maynard (2016).

17. An exception is at lines 18–19, when Marcus reaches for the toy, and Peg, after another directive to "show me," very quickly nods and says "yes" in an acknowledgment of Marcus's reaching gesture.

18. This is a one-way mirror, behind which is an observation room. Those in the examination room see the mirror, while those in the observation room observe them through the glass. A video camera is recording the interaction through the glass.

19. See Fein (2020:104–15) and the discussion of self-conscious agency that an individual on the spectrum may exert in particular contexts.

20. With regard to classroom teacher-student interactions, see Corsaro, Molinari, and Rosier (2002), who show how ambiguous classroom instructions can be and find that even when teachers carefully articulate instructional rubrics, children may still be confused about what they are being asked to do. Such patterns present the issue of whether children are being tested on abilities to disambiguate presentations of stimulus items, in addition to whatever substantive domain (such as the meaning of emotion words) a question enacts, or whether it is the substantive domain simpliciter that is under review.

21. Many people with autism have difficulty lying or saying anything that is not completely true. Andre's clever workaround was to put the untruth in the mouth of a puppet, thereby absolving himself of responsibility for what was said.

Chapter Five

1. This example is explored in more detail in Maynard and Marlaire (1992) and Maynard and Turowetz (2017b), where we also discuss inadvertent signals from (a) the design of the instrument and (b) the clinician's behavioral cues that could be contributing to Lyn's incorrect answering. In this chapter, such features of testing are discussed below in examples involving Tony Smith.

2. More technically, the diagnosis involved five multiaxial components, the first three of which constituted the official diagnostic assessment. Clinicians diagnosed infantile autism on axis I and "unspecific" mental retardation on axis II, while also raising the possibility of an axis III diagnosis of seizure disorder and suggesting the need for further evaluation of Tony's symptoms (Turowetz and Maynard 2017).

3. For an investigation that is relevant to the sorts of *and-* linkages in this episode, but specifically concerned with the ways that *and*-prefaced questions can be linked to preceding question-answer pairs, see Heritage and Sorjonen (1994).

4. For a fuller and more technical analysis of this episode and the overall subtest of which it is a part, see Maynard (2005).

5. The story that Donaldson relates is from the first volume of Laurie Lee's (1959) three-volume autobiography.

6. Nelson (2018:10, 12) refers to the "'extrafactual' work of the laboratory—work done to validate models or understand laboratory environments that is not specifically aimed at producing experimental data, but supports and shapes this process." Clinical assessment shares such "extrafactual" features, including how these features may invisibly figure into what becomes documented as the child's own performance.

7. For a more thorough analysis of this episode, see Maynard and Turowetz (in press). Also, we return to the episode in chap. 8.

8. In the phraseology of the clinic, this knowledge could be used to develop more targeted and effective "treatment recommendations." We hesitate to use this term, however, since as neurodiversity advocates have pointed out, it can formulate autism as something that needs to be fixed or "cured" (Ortega 2009; Shields and Beversdorf 2020). Our own orientation is toward the possibility of mutual adjustments between the common sense of neurotypical actors and the uncommon sense of neurodiverse actors, a point we anticipated in chap. 1 with the notion of learning the "language of autism" and on which we elaborate in chap. 8 when we discuss the matter of prosthetic environments.

9. More specifically: "This activity assesses the participant's ability to communicate about a familiar series of actions using gesture or mime with accompanying language, and to report on a routine event" (Lord et al. 2012:113).

10. For a more detailed analysis of this episode, see Maynard and Turowetz (in press).

11. This is an instance of how clinicians sometimes improvise to deal with overfull schedules. As we observe in chap. 1, clinicians must continually find ways to balance efficiency and thoroughness, especially in the face of resource constraints and an increasing demand for autism evaluations.

12. On the phenomenon of "scaffolding" for tasks and activities involving autistic children, see Stribling and Rae (2010) and Ramey and Rae (2015).

13. There is a part c ("Failure to develop and maintain peer relationships appropriate to developmental level"), but the Demonstration Task is not relevant for this.

14. For more extended consideration of this matter pertaining to Dan and to incidents involving autistic individuals' interactions with police, see Maynard (2019) and Maynard and Turowetz (2020).

15. An expert clinician who reviewed our manuscript observes that it is incorrect to introduce the Demonstration Task as "silly," as it could destandardize the assessment. In reliability trainings, instructors stress that such introductions are to be avoided.

16. To anticipate our discussion in chap. 6, the abstraction in instantiation stories has to do with how the conduct of the child and relevant others is isolated from the larger environment, but in a way that can provide for a more rounded and particularistic appreciation of their individuality than is common in diagnostic practice. We propose that within the context of the clinic, closer attention to autistic intelligence and its relationship to what we're calling second-order competence can involve that sort of holistic abstraction (cf. Cassirer 1953[1923]; Köhler 1947; Martin 2011; Maynard and Turowetz 2019), which Hacking's (2009) work on autism narrative highlights. That sort of attention, in turn, could foster recognition and appreciation of the uncommon sense that shows up regularly in the context of *both* the child's successes *and* their failures to display the kind of second-order competence that diagnostic instruments are designed to assess.

Chapter Six

1. For the conversation analytic approach that informs our approach to narrative, in addition to Sacks (1984) and his lectures (Sacks 1992a; 1992b), see Jefferson (1978) and Mandelbaum (2003; 2013).

2. Other researchers have also documented the use of narrative in clinical settings. For example, in their study of doctors who diagnose genetic disorders in prenatal and infant babies, Timmermans and Buchbinder (2013:chap. 4) describe a practice they call "narrating objectivity," whereby physicians and parents collaborate in creating a story line about children's development. Similarly, Buckholdt and Gubrium (1979) analyze how professionals working with elderly nursing home residents and emotionally disturbed children, respectively, deliberate about clients in "staffing" meetings that are organized along the same lines as the pre-staffing conferences we observed at CDDC. Although Buckholdt and Gubrium do not use the terms *storytelling* or *narrative*, the transcripts they reproduce feature several instances of practitioners employing the story types we identify in this chapter, and often for the same purpose: diagnosis and treatment. More generally, several scholars have highlighted the role of narrative in clinical talk, but

with less focus on interaction per se than on story design and content (e.g., Hunter 1991). By contrast, our focus is primarily on the sequential and interactional organization of narrative—its achieved orderliness by two or more parties in interaction—rather than its discursive features alone or what it reveals about the "thinking styles" of physicians or patients (Turowetz and Maynard 2017).

3. We say that they *can* preserve particularities because in actual practice they are often quite terse and undetailed. Even then, however, they still preserve more of the concreteness of the original interaction than their tendency counterparts.

4. To put Ronnie's evaluation in perspective, we can compare it to the more recent ones we observed during our fieldwork. In the 1980s, an assessment at CDDC could last two to three days. In some cases six or seven specialists saw a child, and informing interviews frequently included not only the clinicians, the child, and the family but also schoolteachers and school officials. Today things are different. Changes to the way US health care is financed and organized have put pressure on clinics like CDDC to conduct evaluations more quickly than in the past—in hours, as opposed to days—and with fewer resources. Thus, most of the cases we observed from 2011–15 involved only two to three specialists, who might not all be able to see the child on the same day. Pre-staffing conferences today are less lengthy, sometimes lasting as little as five minutes, with clinicians stopping by colleagues' offices one or more times over the course of a day to share results and quickly decide on a diagnosis. Similarly, contemporary staffing interviews last thirty to forty-five minutes, whereas in the 1980s they regularly took an hour or more and could last upward of three hours.

5. See the discussion in Hayes and colleagues (2020:9–12) regarding how clinicians may cite reports of "non-present patients, their parents, partners or other informant[s]."

6. Clinicians in the Ronnie Martin case largely agreed with one another on the diagnosis and its various facets. However, stories can also be used to indicate disagreement. In other publications (Turowetz and Maynard 2017), we have explored how clinicians developed a diagnostic narrative about eight-year-old Tony Smith, whose performances on various tests we also discussed here in chap. 4. While testing Tony, several clinicians began to suspect that he suffered from a seizure disorder, as there were times when he seemed to "phase out" and appeared disoriented once his focus returned. In the pre-staffing, with psychiatrist Molly Gardner (also the psychiatrist in Ronnie Martin's case) leading the way, the clinicians agreed that Tony had autism. However, in response to Molly's claim that she saw "no evidence of seizuring," two clinicians produced a series of counter-stories that thematized Tony's "staring episodes." A third clinician eventually joined in, the three of them arguing that Tony might be suffering from a comorbid seizure disorder. This mattered, because a seizure disorder could have affected his performance on cognitive testing, which in turn would inform any estimates of how high functioning he was. Eventually, a compromise was reached after Molly proposed a drug trial to see if Tony's symptoms improved on medication. If so, this would be evidence in favor of the seizure hypothesis, whereas no effect would mean discounting that hypothesis. Although we do not know the outcome of the drug trial, what matters for our purposes is that and how the clinicians deployed competing stories in the diagnostic process, thereby constituting Tony's symptoms as ambiguous and in need of further investigation.

7. As the reader may note, our analysis has affinities with scholarship that uses membership categorization analysis (MCA), particularly studies of how categories are predicated of persons (e.g., Hester and Eglin 1997; O'Neill and LeCouteur 2014; Roca-Cuberes 2008). Where our approach differs is in its emphasis on the sequential aspects of category attribution: whereas

"MCA . . . places more emphasis on interactants' interpretive procedures than sequential structure" (Roca-Cuberes 2008:549), our approach prioritizes sequencing, such that interactants' interpretations are ascribed on the basis of their sequential location. In this respect, our approach is closer to conversation analytic work on category use (Schegloff 2007a; Schegloff 2007c; Speer and Stokoe 2011; Whitehead 2009).

8. What Bill does here is related to a practice for delivering diagnosis that Gill and Maynard (1995) have called an "incomplete syllogism," whereby the clinician lists premises from which recipients are tacitly encouraged to draw a diagnostic conclusion.

9. This phrase is taken from Jutel (2014). See also Heritage and McArthur (2019). We use it to refer to the moment when a diagnosis is determined, an event that can be thought of as the culmination of a larger diagnostic narrative.

10. Technically, the diagnosis should be atypical pervasive developmental disorder (APDD).

11. On the complicated relationship between APDD and autism as diagnostic terms when DSM III (APA 1980) was in place, see Grinker (2007:30–31).

12. The correct term (APA 1980) would be "atypical pervasive developmental disorder."

13. Bill's emphasis on services is similar to a practice that Gill and Maynard (1995: 25–29) call "subordinating the label," where the label itself is subordinated to the services it will allow the child to receive. It serves as another reason for parents to accept the diagnosis, and thus further pushes back against resistance as the visit is coming to a close.

14. As with Ronnie Martin, we return to the matter of Dan's competence (i.e., his skillful practices and autistic intelligence) in the conclusion to this chapter.

15. As we (Maynard and Turowetz 2019) have discussed elsewhere, investigators including Cassirer (1953[1923]:6); Foucault (1973:8–9, 91); Mirowsky and Ross (1989:12); and Abbott (1988:102–3) have written about this kind of abstraction. A different kind of abstraction, per such scholars as Abbott (1988:102–3); Hacking (1999; 2009); Martin (2011:29); and Rickert (1986), involves the preservation of particularity by way of holistic or gestalt-type formulations.

16. As we will see in the next chapter, a similar abstractive pattern is also evident in ambivalent discussions about Sara Brennan (whom we met in chap. 5 as one of the children doing the Demonstration Task). Those discussions involve movement from acknowledging Sara's strengths to an instantiation story about a pretend picnic that excluded Ruth, the psychologist, from entering in, to citing tendencies toward control (directing others but not taking directions), and finally to typifying her as "rigid" and "repetitive" in her play.

17. While we do not deal with medical records in this book, we have analyzed them elsewhere (Turowetz and Maynard 2019). To briefly summarize our findings, we can note that medical records, like conversations about diagnosis, exhibit narrative organization, being made up primarily of tendency stories and typifying upshots. However, these stories are even more terse in written form than in spoken form, and they further elide the contributions of social context to the child's performance in the clinic. In addition to manifesting the institutionalized expectations of the clinic, textual practices comport with the requirements of other institutional actors engaged in people-processing. Schools, hospitals, clinics, insurers, therapists, courts, and related institutions require actionable diagnoses based on the medical model—fidelity to which is a condition of their perceived legitimacy—which the records produced by clinicians provide. For a discussion of the relationship between medical records and forensic records produced by police, see Maynard (2019) and Maynard and Turowetz (2020). We once again mention that the postclinic career of children whom the CDDC evaluates is a topic that we cannot address (because of the limitations of our project and data) and that deserves attention in its own right.

18. While we do not fully use the 1972 dataset in this book (but see Maynard [2019]), it is noteworthy that the narrative patterns for diagnosis we observed in 2014 and 1985 at CDDC are also evident in the 1972 collection.

19. For a thoroughgoing study of skills and forms of reasoning in "domains of mundane expertise," such as playing games of checkers, assembling jigsaw puzzles, making origami models, and conducting psychological experiments, see Livingston's (2008) aptly entitled *Ethnographies of Reason.*

20. Mrs. Chapman reported to Leah Grant, the developmental pediatrician, several instances in which Dan was treated threateningly at school. One morning when she took Dan to school, he would not exit the car when they arrived. Mrs. Chapman telephoned the school officer for help, but he took the extreme measure of coming to the car, grabbing Dan, and throwing him over his shoulder. We do not know if these instances were the ones that resulted in Dan's own reportedly "aggressive" behavior, but there is a strong possibility that there is *transpositioning* in the official reports, whereby aggressive moves by police or other authority figures, to which Dan responds in "second position," become depicted as "first position," stimulating *actions* on Dan's part that warrant and legitimize *reactions* on the part of officers. See Maynard (2019) and Maynard and Turowetz (2020).

21. The detailed formatting of these directives in terms of "entitlement," modality, and other features, are analyzed in Maynard and Turowetz (in Press). See also Curl and Drew (2008) and Craven and Potter (2010).

22. In other words, we are arguing that the uncommon sense of persons diagnosed with autism cannot be fully recognized or appreciated so long as autism is defined as an individual phenotype under approaches such as that embodied in the DSM (APA 2013) that individualize and pathologize it. Indeed, such approaches make it difficult to see inappropriate or unexpected behavior as anything other than a personal failing due to a deficit. On the other hand, if autism were understood as an interactional phenotype, one that belongs not strictly to the individual but also to the society, it might be possible to depathologize the diagnosis by encouraging and allowing commonsense actors to grasp the sensibility behind autistic behavior. We will have more to say about these matters in chap. 8.

Chapter Seven

1. See Hollin (2017) on "autistic heterogeneity" and epistemological and ontological kinds of uncertainty. Aside from uncertainty, another problem is that of contradiction, where clinicians have discrepant assessments of whether autism is present in a particular person. Hayes et al. (2021) identify a three-phase pattern of interaction through which clinicians work to resolve such discrepancies.

2. Of course, this matter is well-known among professionals who are experts in autism diagnosis. Noting the enormous variability in language acquisition and use, and in other communication skills (attention, gaze, joint engagement), temperament, and cultural background in all young children, Bishop and colleagues (2008:26) state, "The fact that there is a wide range of social and communication skills among typically developing young children presents a challenge to those trying to identify 'markers' of ASD in children of this age."

3. Again, see chap. 2. As Navon (2019:136) observes, diagnostic categories change for many reasons, such that defining, interpreting, or classifying the phenotype of a genetic mutation depends on clinical practices as much as it does on the mutation that is taken as its

biochemical cause, a matter that implicates "spirals of looping that shape medical and psychiatric classification."

4. See, for example, chap. 3, note 3.

5. For discussions—both sympathetic and critical—of autism or other developmental disabilities as a social construction, see for example Nadesan (2005), Osteen (2008), and Rapley (2004).

6. The search for definitive genetic factors, which we discuss in chap. 2, would not necessarily solve the problem of ambiguity even were it successful. As Stivers and Timmermans (2016:202) report in their study regarding next-generation genomic testing, and exome sequencing specifically, "genomic testing does not always produce causal variants but often reveals ambiguous findings that have the potential to exacerbate rather than ease the patient's diagnostic uncertainty." The authors examine the kinds of interpretive practices in which geneticists as well as parents engage to render meaning from underlying uncertainty.

7. Similarly, it is assumed that autism is something the child either has or does not have: they cannot have it in one setting and not have it in another. At most, they can *appear* more or less autistic. We expand on this point in the next section and in the conclusion to the chapter.

8. See chap. 4–6, as well as Turowetz (2015a). Also, consider the point that Siegel (2018:31), a developmental psychologist and founder/executive director of the Autism Center of Northern California with long-standing experience in autism diagnosis and treatment, makes about the process:

> The way a given child happens to react during the hour or so of an ADOS interview can be strongly influenced by whether an examiner has rapport with the child and whether the child decides he or she likes or dislikes the examiner, does or does not want to be cooperative, and so on. Turning pages, writing things down, talking too fast, not getting the child's attention before beginning a new activity, and not waiting long enough for a response may leave a child looking "worse" than the child may have seemed with a different examiner, in a different setting, or on a different day.

For recent evidence that Siegel may be right—that there may be important alterations in the bodily responses of a given child to different clinicians administering the same item in controlled room conditions—see Torres and colleagues (2020).

9. Here we draw on Mol's research on atherosclerosis (2002; cf. Timmermans and Haas 2008) and her argument that doctors, pathologists, patients, therapists, and others produce atherosclerosis as different kinds of objects (e.g., as leg pain in the doctor's office, as plaques in the pathology lab, as limited mobility in physical therapy) that they then assemble into a singular disease entity at specific times and for specific purposes.

10. Under IDEA, students with autism are not automatically entitled to special services. Instead, "eligibility for special education services is based . . . on an educational determination of disability, which involves meeting not just the criteria for a specific disability (such as autism), but also finding that a student is in need of special services" (Center for Autism Research 2020).

11. The three cases we examine involve children who are relatively "high functioning." However, indeterminacy and ambiguity may be features of diagnosis when there is more severe impairment as well. For one thing, there may be windows of development whereby some children show patterns associated with autism but grow out of them (Bishop et al. 2008:29), which is why early attempts at diagnosis can be problematic. Also, there are other developmental disorders—intellectual, expressive and receptive language, anxiety, and attention deficit/hyperactivity—and genetic disorders, such as fragile X syndrome, that "share many features with ASD" (Bishop

et al. 2008:30). Diagnostically, no matter the level of severity, a balancing act goes on between *sensitivity*, accurately "ruling in" individuals with autism, and *specificity*, or ruling out those who do not have the condition (Bishop et al. 2008:34; Schnittker 2017:42–45).

12. Other research (Hayes et al. 2020:7) has documented how clinicians may express that "they could feel or sense when a person they were assessing was autistic." Additionally, neuroscientists who study autism may share a "feeling" about diagnosis in the "affective space" they occupy (Fitzgerald 2014:245; 2017:chap. 2).

13. As we explain in chap. 6, clinicians only topicalize their own actions when an error of administration occurs or is suspected (Turowetz 2015a). Otherwise, their own detailed practices for pursuing clinical objectives do not come under scrutiny.

14. See Maynard and Turowetz (2017a:264–69) for a fuller account of the informing interview.

15. See Raymond (2016) on the use of "do-constructions" in conversation to suggest an understanding that contrasts with prior assertions or stances. Here, "she di:d (.) she did meet the cutoff," particularly the stress on the second "did," marks a contrast with the previous positive assessments and "strengths" that Ruth had listed. See also Stivers (2002:328n16), specifically on how such *do*-constructions can mark contrastive positions regarding diagnosis in medical care.

16. This happens in the case of Tanner Johnson, whose answers to ADOS questions about emotions we examined in chap. 4 (cf. Turowetz and Maynard 2017:373–75). When the psychologist, having said that Tanner qualifies for the autism diagnosis, goes on to suggest that he engages in certain behavior because of his need for sensory stimulation (common among autistic children), his mother interjects with more prosaic explanations, such as getting "excited." She also produces a "challenging question" (Bolden and Robinson 2011; Robinson and Bolden 2010) about the sensory stimulation, "Is that weird?" More technically, this is a reverse-polarity question that tacitly projects a no answer without stating it (Koshik 2005:76–77). The reader will also recall Mrs. Martin's less overt challenge to the clinicians' claims about Ronnie in chap. 6. In these cases, the parents participate in narrative sequences by taking issue with the upshots clinicians are drawing from their tendency or instantiation stories.

17. Only Max's mother was present for the visit at CDDC. At the end of the visit, they refer to meeting his dad for lunch, so he may have been at work during the interviews.

18. As Stivers and Timmermans (2017) put it, clinicians and parents may cooperatively realize the news as "bivalent"—as having a mixture of good and bad elements—and provide for affiliation on the basis of that mixture.

Chapter Eight

1. As Grinker and Mandell (2015:644) write, "Although each piece of a jigsaw puzzle is unique, the desire to work on a puzzle presupposes both that the pieces will interlock and that we know what the puzzle as a whole will look like (like the cover of the jigsaw puzzle box). But for ASD, the whole always differs."

2. We should add that for clinicians, there is the added complication that the pieces themselves are not ready-made, but must be produced out of the data (observations, exam results, etc.) before they can be assembled into a coherent diagnostic picture. This involves treating behaviors as expressions of *literalism*, *rigidity*, *sensory seeking*, and so forth, and then configuring these pieces into a picture of an *autistic child*. That picture then becomes a resource that fellow professionals and laypeople use to make sense of the child's behavior, enabling them to see "the same" pieces that were documented in the clinic across a variety of social settings.

3. That is, unless they have learned to *suspend* common sense: "When Granny Eva fell downstairs and hurt her hand quite badly, she called out, 'George, can you help me?' George trilled, 'No, I can't,' as he ran gaily past" (Moore, 2004:275). Granny, Moore observes, "asked a question; he supplied an answer," and "he doesn't mind what she thinks of his response." Moore goes on: "It's not exactly that he doesn't care, it's that he hasn't got the capacity to consider the issue." Moore (2004), who is George's mother, has learned to suspend common sense, which enables her to surpass the kind of reaction that Park (1967:108) recalls initially having to the behavior of her autistic daughter Jessie, where she "would become irritated, then infuriated at behavior which looked in every way like willful disobedience." Of course, Park also eventually learned to suspend common sense, establishing the mutually intelligible world with her daughter that she would go on to describe so insightfully.

4. Per chap. 1, see also Kumagai and Wear (2014) and Pinchevski (2005).

5. As Fitzgerald (2017:137) has put it, "We can say that perhaps more than any other diagnosis, the social has always been what is actually in question in autism—that it has historically been thought of as a disorder, more than anything else, of social interaction."

6. As Lord and colleagues (2020:5) explain, "Although the study of autism risk genes in model systems has revealed a great deal about general biology, how these findings relate to the pathophysiology of autism is less clear. In general, autism risk genes tend to have a role in multiple functions in many brain regions that unfold in a spatiotemporally defined manner across development. Consequently, although manipulation of a single risk gene in a model system may lead to interesting phenotypes, including social-behavioural phenotypes in evolutionarily distant organisms, it does not necessarily illuminate its contribution to human social disability."

7. As a further example, consider a phone conversation between two friends, Emma and Nancy, where Nancy produces what's meant as a supportive offer in a self-attentive, and therefore inapposite, way. At the beginning of the phone call, Emma informs Nancy that she has a sore toe and will have difficulty walking. Despite this knowledge, Nancy goes ahead and invites Emma to go shopping with her because she, the inviter, needs a new dress for work and wants the company. However, noticing Emma's resistance to the *self*-attentive invitation, Nancy offers to pick her up—to drive her to the store. She also uses a device that can further repair her invitation: the "I-mean prefaced utterance" (Maynard 2016). The caller goes on to say, "I mean can I get you something. . . . I mean you don't have to walk around because all I'm gonna do is just go up [to] their patio dresses." In this way, Nancy shifts to an other-attentive stance that recognizes, and attempts to repair, the problem with her prior action.

8. As Moore (2004:89), the mother of two boys on the spectrum, has said:

> I believe that more attention needs to be paid to the physical symptoms. The constraints these place on the life of an autist can be a great barrier to social integration and learning. Imagine how you would feel about going to school or to work if strip lighting caused you violent discomfort, or the smell of a certain cleaning fluid made you want to vomit. Then add the problem that you are unlikely to be able to communicate these difficulties to anyone with the power to help you. How daunting and impenetrable the neurotypical world must seem! No wonder so many autists retreat into their own.

See also the lucid autobiographical account of autistic sensuousness and sensibility, *The Reason I Jump: The Inner Voice of a Thirteen-Year-Old Boy with Autism* (Higashida 2013).

9. "Autism is not a polite disorder," Rubin (2005:86) observes, "nor does it care what others perceive as being wrong or right." Recall from chap. 4 Mukhopadhyay's (2003:23) contradiction

of his clinicians' proposal that he did not know what was "going on around him." See also Fein (2015:104, original emphasis) on teenage Kevin's assertion that he avoided showering when he was young because it was too monotonous:

> People think like: oh this person doesn't understand that it's important to shower if you have Asperger's. But no: it's a personal decision . . . they might fully understand and be like, well, if you're going to judge me based on whether I'm showering, I don't want to be friends with you.

Such awareness and strategic action belies "theory of mind" conceptions of autism, which posit that people on the spectrum lack the ability to infer what others are thinking (cf. Hacking 2009:1470).

10. In characterizing first-order competence as subterranean, we mean that it underlies much that we do at a more surface level. However, although commonly ignored or missed, such competence is there for the looking and overt formulating, as when "have a nice day" is treated literally as a command or imperative of sorts. Common sense, we have said, is tacit (rather than subterranean) and involves complex understandings that are not easily seen or articulated. That "have a nice" day can be a salutation requires the invocation of a complex of unstated forms of sensemaking that are difficult to articulate. For another example: When Edna calls her sister on a land-line telephone and says, "Your line's been busy," the utterance as a "fishing" device (Pomerantz 1980), asking for an explanation without overtly requesting it, and also as an implicit form of complaining, involves layers of "community" or commonsense understandings for which, à la Garfinkel (1967), there is no easy or complete summary; such easiness or completeness is "impossible."

11. As Fein (2015:238) succinctly puts the matter: "Responding to autism requires us not to reduce it to individual or societal dimensions but to conceptualize it in all its fullness, as it is lived and construed and manifested across its variety of enactments."

12. A section on "How to Interpret the DAS-II" in a manual that is co-authored by the developer of the Differential Abilities Scale (Elliott 1990) states, "Observations of testing behaviors may help in interpreting the results of Picture Similarities," and poses the following questions (Dumont et al. 2009:203):

> Does the child demonstrate impulsive behaviors, such as responding too rapidly without carefully checking their response or not carefully examining the pictures to determine the subtle differences between them? Does the child have difficulty placing the pictures accurately on the target page, possibly indicating a fine-motor problem? Does language help or hinder the child's responses? Is there any indication that the child does not know what many of the pictures represent? Does the child appear to have problems understanding the directions, or does the child appear to use verbalization to help solve the items? Does the child require many items to be explained on the specific items that require teaching after failure?

The goal of interpreting a child's performance on the subtest is laudable. However, it can be noted that these questions all presume or perpetuate a deficit picture regarding a child's performance. References are to difficulties, problems, and absences of various kinds. An orientation to autistic intelligence instead asks about presences, skills, and competencies upon which development potentially can be based. See chap. 4 and the Marcus Davidson example.

13. Moreover, even when biogenetic markers for a disease have been identified, they can make the diagnostic process more complex by fragmenting a once-uniform pathological entity

into multiple, overlapping conditions—breast and ovarian cancers being cases in point (Rabe-harisoa and Bourret 2009).

14. As this book goes to press, we are in the midst of the COVID-19 pandemic, which raises a different question about the generic reach of our research. Soon after COVID-19 achieved pandemic status, the CDDC mostly went "virtual" with diagnosis (excepting difficult cases, which meant a clinic visit with protective gear and other measures), adapting in a variety of ways. The ADOS could be administered virtually, according to the director of the clinic, "but the test publishers and ADOS trainers have been very strict in that we are not able to call it an ADOS in our reports." Clinicians are not able to score the ADOS because several tasks, such as the balloon-blowing exercise that we describe for Sara Brennan in chap. 7, are not adaptable to the virtual environment. As a consequence, on the basis of a review of a child's electronic medical record; behavior rating scales from parents, teachers, or other caregivers; parent interviews; and structured observations, clinicians are completing the second edition of the Childhood Autism Rating Scale (CARS-2; Schopler et al. 2010) instrument for diagnosing autism. Future research needs to document and analyze how testing is done and how the narrative structure for diagnosis that we have identified may generically adapt to the virtual environment. As Christakis (2020:267) has recently observed, "The pandemic highlighted how much of medical care could be provided at home, especially when paired with devices such as home blood pressure cuffs, glucose monitors, and oximeters to gather basic information." As part of medical care, diagnosis is now also an in-home enterprise, and what Christakis (2020:267) also says to the effect that virtual medicine is "unlikely to be abandoned as the pandemic wanes" suggests the relevance of such research.

15. For a recent study of the effectiveness of directives and what kinds of detailed markers, strategies, and relational contexts that may be more successful than others in a recreational setting, see White (2019). For an investigation of what kinds of directives may or may not work in a setting involving people with intellectual disabilities, see Antaki and Kent (2012). Other helpful studies of directives include Curl and Drew (2008), Heinemann (2006), Craven and Potter (2010), and Lindström (2005).

16. See also the ethnographic study by Tan and Eyal (2015:46) of a school for children on the autism spectrum. The school draws on the "floortime approach" of Greenspan and Wieder (2006) and teaches the instructors to "overcome their natural tendency to direct the child, and instead shape themselves into this exquisitely sensitive device that can capture, reflect, and amplify the students' faltering and idiosyncratic attempts at communication." The therapeutic approach could be said to be one in which instructors are working to make the strange more familiar. We further discuss this study below.

17. Here, *classic* refers to the experiments reported in *Studies in Ethnomethodology*. Elsewhere, Garfinkel's research focused on "natural troublemakers," including racial minorities (Black, Jewish) and people who were vision-impaired, transgender, or intellectually disabled (e.g., Garfinkel 2002; Garfinkel 2012; Turowetz and Rawls 2020). Indeed, one of the most famous chapters from *Studies* is about the sensemaking practices of a trans woman to whom he gave the pseudonym of Agnes. However, Garfinkel is perhaps best known for his breaching experiments, and these can certainly give the impression that common sense is inert and inflexible (but see our discussion of his "experiments with trust" below).

18. See the discussion in Eyal and colleagues (2010:146), which alerted us to this parable.

19. Recall John Robison's (see chap. 1) remark about his difficulties responding to other children with whom he was playing: "I was so used to living inside my own world that I answered with whatever I had been thinking."

20. This is the type of therapy implemented in the above-mentioned Tan and Eyal (2015) study of an autism-only therapy school.

21. In states like Wisconsin and others, ABA is prominent because the state will fund therapies that are "evidence-based," and ABA qualifies under that rubric. In 2008, Weiss, Fiske, and Ferraioli (2008:44) could state, "Though the amount of research on ABA as a comprehensive treatment does not provide enough support to categorize ABA as a well-established treatment, no other treatment approach comes close to ABA in empirical validation or strength of scientific evidence." More recent research concurs: while ABA, which has become a stand-in acronym for a variety of behavioral approaches or early intensive behavioral interventions (EIBIs), is the dominant approach used in clinical practice and "show[s] some evidence of effectiveness," it continues to be the case that "methodological rigor remains a pressing concern for this body of research" (Sandbank et al. 2020:21).

22. This refers to the Picture Exchange Communication Systems manual (Frost and Bondy 2002), which, to aid children in expressing themselves, depicts everyday school, home, and community activities.

23. See Wootton's (1997:chap. 2) documentation of how children are able to take sequential understandings into account by the third year of life, which matter suggests how a child's exhibits of distress may be less an expression of an internal state than a response to breaches of trajectories the child has initiated. The child's initiation and the action(s) it launches provide a moral warrant for the expression of indignation when coparticipants undermine such trajectories.

24. In more official and biological terms, Lord et al. (2020:3) observe: "More recently, phenotypic heterogeneity has been the rule in most, although not all, gene-first phenotypic studies. Thus, developmental aspects of differences in strengths, difficulties and trajectories as well as biological factors require highly personalized conceptualizations of the needs of autistic individuals and their families."

25. Although our research has concentrated on the diagnosis of children and we are discussing the design of prosthetic environments for them, that discussion has implications for longer-term autism careers. For example, programs that facilitate the transition to adulthood for teens can contribute to their social interactional skills and also help alleviate the depressive symptoms of their parents (DaWalt, Greenberg, and Mailick 2018), while independent vocational activities can improve behavioral development and functioning for adults with ASD (Taylor, Smith, and Mailick 2014), as can the structure of the family environment (e.g., Greenberg et al. 2006; Smith et al. 2008; Taylor, Smith, and Mailick 2014).

26. Some accommodations, such as curb cuts, may be costly, but as regards the workplace, one study—a survey by the University of West Virginia being conducted since 2004 (Job Accommodation Network 2020:2–3)—reports: "Most employers report no cost or low cost for accommodating employees with disabilities," and "Employers who made accommodations for employees with disabilities reported multiple benefits as a result." We are not aware of comparable studies of educational settings, where, because of disability rights mandated for schools, there already have been long-standing structural changes. Once again, we are faced with the matter of postclinical careers for autistic individuals, a topic in need of further research.

27. A quotation in note 4 from chap. 1 bears repetition here. In his book *Life Animated* about his son Owen, Ron Suskind (2014:134) observes, "What had been happening naturally and forcefully, day by day, year to year, inside our home: the judgments . . . widely accepted suppositions about those with so-called 'intellectual disabilities'—were being dislodged, often against

our will, and replaced with a much deeper understanding." See also the aforementioned Tan and Eyal (2015) research in an autism-only school and the ways in which instructors engaged in "ethical work on the self" to fully embrace a child-centered and partner-centered mode of educational interaction in which following the cues of their students was a learned, primary skill. That workplaces and other environments *are* changing to incorporate autistic individuals is documented in such studies as Silberman's (2015: chap. 12) and Grinker's (2019:256–57).

References

Abbeduto, Leonard, Andrea McDuffie, and Angela John Thurman. 2014. "The Fragile X Syndrome—Autism Comorbidity: What Do We Really Know?" *Frontiers in Genetics*. Date accessed: October 30, 2020. doi: 10.3389/fgene.2014.00355.

Abbott, Andrew. 1988. *The System of Professions: An Essay on the Division of Expert Labor.* Chicago: University of Chicago Press.

Aharoni, Eyal, Nathaniel E. Anderson, J.C. Barnes, et al. 2019. "Mind the Gap: Toward an Integrative Science of the Brain and Crime." *BioSocieties* 14:463–68.

Ainsworth-Vaughn, Nancy. 1998. *Claiming Power in Doctor-Patient Talk.* Oxford: Oxford University Press.

Alac, Morana. 2008. "Working with Brain Scans: Digital Images and Gestural Interaction in fMRI Laboratory." *Social Studies of Science* 38:483–508.

Amendah, Djesika, Scott D. Grosse, Georgina Peacock, et al. 2011. "The Economic Costs of Autism: A Review." Pp. 1347–60 in *Autism Spectrum Disorders*, edited by D. Amaral, D. Geschwind, and G. Dawson. New York: Oxford University Press.

Antaki, Charles, and Alexandra Kent. 2012. "Telling People What to Do (and, Sometimes, Why): Contingency, Entitlement, and Explanation in Staff Requests to Adults with Intellectual Impairments." *Journal of Pragmatics* 44:876–89.

Antaki, Charles, and Ray Wilkinson. 2012. "Conversation Analysis and the Study of Atypical Populations." Pp. 533–50 in *Handbook of Conversation Analysis*, edited by J. Sidnell and T. Stivers. New York: Blackwell.

APA. 1980. *Diagnostic and Statistical Manual of Mental Disorders: DSM-III.* Washington, DC: American Psychiatric Association.

———. 1987. *Diagnostic and Statistical Manual of Mental Disorders: DSM-III-R.* Washington, DC: American Psychiatric Association.

———. 2013. *Diagnostic and Statistical Manual of Mental Disorders: DSM-5.* Arlington, VA: American Psychiatric Association.

Arribas-Ayllon, Michael, Andrew Bartlett, and Jamie Lewis. 2019. *Psychiatric Genetics: From Hereditary Madness to Big Biology.* Philadelphia: Routledge.

Asperger, Hans. 1991[1944]. "'Autistic Psychopathy' in Childhood." Pp. 37–92 in *Autism and Asperger Syndrome*, edited by U. Frith. Cambridge: Cambridge University Press.

Atkinson, J. Maxwell, and John Heritage, eds. 1984. *Structures of Social Action: Studies in Conversation Analysis.* Cambridge: Cambridge University Press.

Attwood, Tony. 1998. *Asperger's Syndrome: A Guide for Parents and Professionals.* Philadelphia: Jessica Kingsley.

Auburn, Timothy, and Christianne Pollock. 2013. "Studies of Laughter in Interaction." Pp. 135–60 in *Studies of Laughter in Interaction,* edited by P. Glenn and E. Holt. London: Bloomsbury Academic.

Austin, John L. 1962. *How to Do Things with Words.* Oxford: Oxford University Press.

Bakan, Michael B. 2018. *Speaking for Ourselves: Conversations on Life, Music, and Autism.* New York: Oxford University Press.

Baker, Jeffrey P. 2013. "Autism at 70: Redrawing the Boundaries." *New England Journal of Medicine* 369:1089–91.

Bakhtin, Mikhail M. 1981. *The Dialogic Imagination.* Translated by Caryl Emerson and Michael Holquist. Austin: University of Texas Press.

Balogh, Erin P., Bryan T. Miller, and John R. Ball, eds. 2015. *Improving Diagnosis in Health Care.* Washington, DC: National Academies Press.

Bar-Hillel, Yehoshua. 1954. "Indexical Expressions." *Mind* 63:359–79.

Barker, Kristen, and Tasha R. Galardi. 2015. "Diagnostic Domain Defense: Autism Spectrum Disorder and the *DSM-5*." *Social Problems* 62:120–40.

Baron-Cohen, Simon. 2002. "The Extreme Male Brain Theory of Autism." *Trends in Cognitive Sciences* 6:248–54.

———. 2017. "Editorial Perspective: Neurodiversity—A Revolutionary Concept for Autism and Psychiatry." *Journal of Child Psychology and Psychiatry* 58(6):744–47.

Baron-Cohen, Simon, Emma Ashwin, Chris Ashwin, et al. 2009. "Talent in Autism: Hyper-Systemizing, Hyper-Attention to Detail and Sensory Hypersensitivity." *Philosophical Transactions of the Royal Society B* 364:1377–83.

Bazelon, Emily. 2007. "What Autistic Girls Are Made Of." *New York Times Magazine,* August 5.

Bearman, Peter. 2013. "Genes Can Point to Environments That Matter to Advance Public Health." *American Journal of Public Health* 103(S1):S11–S13.

Becker, Howard S., and Blance Geer. 1957. "Participant Observation and Interviewing: A Comparison." *Human Organization* 16:28–32.

Benson, Paul R., and Kristie L. Karlof. 2009. "Anger, Stress Proliferation, and Depressed Mood among Parents of Children with ASD: A Longitudinal Replication." *Journal of Autism & Developmental Disorders* 39:350–62.

Bettelheim, Bruno. 1967. *The Empty Fortress: Infantile Autism and the Birth of the Self.* New York: Free Press.

Biklen, Douglas. 2002. "Experiencing Autism: An Interview with Donna Williams." *TASH Connections* 28:15–21.

Bishop, Somer. 2015. "Seeking Precise Portraits of Girls with Autism." *Spectrum: Autism Research News.* https://www.spectrumnews.org/opinion/seeking-precise-portraits-of-girls-with-autism/.

Bishop, Somer L., Rhiannon Luyster, Jennifer Richler, et al. 2008. "Diagnostic Assessment." Pp. 23–49 in *Autism Spectrum Disorders in Infants and Toddlers: Diagnosis, Assessment, and Treatment,* edited by K. Chawarska, A. Klin, and F. R. Volkmar. New York: Guilford.

Blackman, Lucy. 1999. *Lucy's Story: Autism and Other Adventures.* Redcliffe, Queensland, Australia: Book in Hand.

———. 2005. "Reflections on Language." Pp. 144–67 in *Autism and the Myth of the Person Alone*, edited by D. Biklen. New York: New York University Press.

Bloom, Lois, Susan Merkin, and Janet Wootten. 1982. "*Wh*-Questions: Linguistic Factors That Contribute to the Sequence of Acquisition." *Child Development* 53:1084–92.

Boden, Deirdre, and Don H. Zimmerman, eds. 1991. *Talk and Social Structure*. Cambridge: Polity.

Bolden, Galina B., and Jeffrey D. Robinson. 2011. "Soliciting Accounts with Why-Interrogatives in Conversation." *Journal of Communication* 61:94–119.

Bowker, Geoffrey C., and Susan Leigh Star. 1999. *Sorting Things Out: Classification and Its Consequences*. Cambridge, MA: MIT Press.

Brigance, Albert H. 1978. *Brigance Diagnostic Inventory of Early Development*. North Billerica, MA: Curriculum Associates.

Briggs, Charles L. 1986. *Learning How to Ask: A Sociolinguistic Appraisal of the Role of the Interview in Social Science Research*. Cambridge: Cambridge University Press.

Brigham, Nicolette Bainbridge, Paul J. Yoder, Melanie A. Jarzynka, et al. 2010. "The Sequential Relationship between Parent Attentional Cues and Sustained Attention to Objects in Young Children with Autism." *Journal of Autism and Developmental Disorders* 40:200–208.

Brown, Phil. 1990. "The Name Game: Toward a Sociology of Diagnosis." *Journal of Mind and Behavior* 11:385[139]–406[160].

———. 1995. "Naming and Framing: The Social Construction of Diagnosis and Illness." *Journal of Health and Social Behavior* 28:34–52.

Bruner, Jerome. 1986. *Actual Minds, Possible Worlds*. Cambridge MA: Harvard University Press.

Buckholdt, David, and Jaber F. Gubrium. 1979. "Doing Staffings." *Human Organization* 38:255–64.

Buescher, Ariane, Cidav Zuleyha, Martin Knapp, et al. 2014. "Costs of Autism Spectrum Disorders in the United Kingdom and the United States." *JAMA Pediatrics* 168(8):721–28.

Bumiller, Kristin. 2008. "Quirky Citizens: Autism, Gender, and Reimagining Disability." *Signs* 33:967–91.

Butler, Jessica. 2019. "How Safe Is the Schoolhouse? An Analysis of State Seclusion and Restraint Laws and Policies." Retrieved March 13, 2020. http://www.autcom.org/pdf/HowSafeSchool house.pdf.

Callon, Michel. 1999. "Actor-Network Theory: The Market Test." *Sociological Review* 47S(1): 181–95.

Carlin, George. 2011. "Have a Nice Day." YouTube. Retrieved February 18, 2020. https://www .youtube.com/watch?v=on_Q16xRoxI.

Casper, Monica J., and Marc Berg. 1995. "Constructivist Perspectives on Medical Work: Medical Practices and Science and Technology Studies." *Science, Technology & Human Values* 20:395–407.

Cassirer, Ernst. 1953[1923]. *Substance and Function, and Einstein's Theory of Relativity*. Chicago: Dover.

Center for Autism Research. 2020. "Medical Diagnosis vs. Educational Eligibility for Special Services: Important Distinctions for Those Diagnosed with ASD." Children's Hospital of Philadelphia. https://www.carautismroadmap.org/medical-diagnosis-vs-educational-eligibility -for-special-services-important-distinctions-for-those-with-asd/.

Centers for Disease Control and Prevention (CDC). 2020. "Morbidity and Mortality Weekly Report." *Surveillance Summaries* 69(4):1–12.

Chamak, B., and B. Bonniau. 2013. "Changes in the Diagnosis of Autism: How Parents and Professionals Act and React in France." *Culture, Medicine, and Psychiatry* 37:405–26.

Charmaz, Kathy. 1996. "Grounded Theory." Pp. 27–49 in *Rethinking Methods in Psychology*, edited by J. A. Smith and R. Harré. London: Sage.

Charon, Rita. 2006. *Narrative Medicine: Honoring the Stories of Illness.* New York: Oxford University Press.

Chew, Kristina. 2013. "Autism and the Task of the Translator." Pp. 305–17 in *Worlds of Autism: Across the Spectrum of Neurological Difference*, edited by J. Davidson and M. Orsini. Minneapolis: University of Minnesota Press.

Christakis, Nicholas A. 2020. *Apollo's Arrow.* New York: Little, Brown.

Cicourel, Aaron V. 1974. *Cognitive Sociology.* New York: Free Press.

Clarke, Adele E., Laura Mamo, Jennifer R. Fishman, et al. 2003. "Biomedicalization: Technoscientific Transformations of Health, Illness, and U.S. Biomedicine." *American Sociological Review* 68:161–94.

Clayman, Steven E., and Virginia T. Gill. 2012. "Conversation Analysis." Pp. 120–34 in *The Routledge Handbook of Discourse Analysis*, edited by J. P. Gee and M. Handford. New York: Routledge.

Clayman, Steven E., John Heritage, and Douglas W. Maynard. Forthcoming. "The Ethnomethodological Lineage of Conversation Analysis." In *Harold Garfinkel: Praxis, Social Order, and Ethnomethodology's Legacies*, edited by D. W. Maynard and J. Heritage. New York: Oxford University Press.

Clift, Rebecca. 2001. "Meaning in Interaction: The Case of Actually." *Language* 77:245–91.

Conley, Dalton, and Jason Fletcher. 2017. *The Genome Factor: What the Social Genomics Revolution Reveals about Ourselves, Our History & the Future.* Princeton, NJ: Princeton University Press.

Corsaro, William A. 1979. "Young Children's Conception of Status and Role." *Sociology of Education* 55:160–77.

Corsaro, William A., Luisa Molinari, and Katherine Brown Rosier. 2002. "Zena and Carlotta: Transition Narratives and Early Education in the United States and Italy." *Human Development* 45:323–48.

Craven, Alexandra, and Jonathan Potter. 2010. "Directives: Entitlement and Contingency in Action." *Discourse Studies* 12:419–42.

Croen, Lisa A., Judith K. Grether, Jenny Hoogstrate, et al. 2002. "The Changing Prevalence of Autism in California." *Journal of Autism and Developmental Disorders* 32:207–15.

Curl, Traci S. 2006. "Offers of Assistance: Constraints on Syntactic Design." *Journal of Pragmatics* 38:1257–80.

Curl, Traci S., and Paul Drew. 2008. "Contingency and Action: A Comparison of Two Forms of Requesting." *Research on Language and Social Interaction* 41:129–53.

Daar, Jacob H., Stephanie Negrelli, and Mark R. Dixon. 2015. "Derived Emergence of WH Question–Answers in Children with Autism." *Research in Autism Spectrum Disorders* 19:59–71.

DaWalt, Leann S., Jan S. Greenberg, and Marsha R. Mailick. 2018. "Transitioning Together: A Multi-Family Group Psychoeducation Program for Adolescents with ASD and Their Parents." *Journal of Autism and Developmental Disorders* 48(1):251–63.

Dawson, Michelle, Isabelle Soulière, Morton Ann Gernsbacher, et al. 2007. "The Level and Nature of Autistic Intelligence." *Psychological Science* 18:657–61.

Decoteau, Claire Laurier. 2017. "The 'Western Disease': Autism and Somali Parents' Embodied Health Movements." *Social Science & Medicine* 177:169–76.

Decoteau, Claire Laurier, and Paige L. Sweet. 2016. "Psychiatry's Little Other: DSM-5 and Debates over Psychiatric Science." *Social Theory & Health* 14(4):414–35.

Dickerson, Paul, Penny Stribling, and John Rae. 2007. "Tapping into Interaction: How Children
with Autistic Spectrum Disorders Design and Place Tapping in Relation to Activities in
Progress." *Gesture* 7:271–303.

Doernberg, Ellen, and Eric Hollander. 2016. "Neurodevelopmental Disorders (ASD and ADHD):
DSM-5, ICD-10, and ICD-11." *CNS Spectrums* 21(4):295–99. doi: 10.1017/S1092852916000262.

Donaldson, Margaret. 1978. *Children's Minds*. New York: W. W. Norton.

Donvan, John, and Caren Zucker. 2010. "Autism's First Child." *Atlantic*. http://www.theatlantic
.com/magazine/archive/2010/10/autisms-first-child/308227/.

———. 2016. *In a Different Key: The Story of Autism*. New York: Crown.

Dreaver, Jessica, Craig Thompson, Sonya Girdler, et al. 2020. "Success Factors Enabling Employment for Adults on the Autism Spectrum from Employers' Perspective." *Journal of Autism &
Developmental Disorders* 50:1657–67.

Drew, Paul. 1992. "Contested Evidence in Courtroom Cross-Examination: The Case of a Trial
for Rape." Pp. 470–520 in *Talk at Work: Interaction in Institutional Settings*, edited by P. Drew
and J. Heritage. Cambridge: Cambridge University Press.

———. 2005. "Conversation Analysis." Pp. 71–102 in *Handbook of Language and Social Interaction*, edited by K. L. Fitch and R. E. Sanders. Mahwah, NJ: Lawrence Erlbaum.

Drew, Paul, and John Heritage, eds. 1992. *Talk at Work: Interaction in Institutional Settings*. Cambridge: Cambridge University Press.

Duchan, Judith F. 1998. "Describing the Unusual Behavior of Children with Autism." *Journal of
Communication Disorders* 31:93–112.

Dumont, Ron, John O. Willis, and Colin D. Elliott. 2009. *Essentials of DAS-II Assessment*. Ho-
boken, NJ: John Wiley & Sons.

Duneier, Mitchell, and Harvey Molotch. 1999. "Talking City Trouble: Interactional Vandal-
ism, Social Inequality, and the 'Urban Interaction Problem.'" *American Journal of Sociology*
104:1263–95.

Durkin, Maureen S., Matthew J. Maenner, F. John Meaney, et al. 2010. "Socioeconomic Inequality in the Prevalence of Autism Spectrum Disorder: Evidence from a U.S. Cross-Sectional
Study." *PLoS ONE* 5(7).

Durkin, Maureen S., Matthew J. Maenner, Craig J. Newschaffer, et al. 2008. "Advanced Parental Age and the Risk of Autism Spectrum Disorder." *American Journal of Epidemiology*
168(11):1268–76. doi: 10.1093/aje/kwn250.

Edwards, Derek. 2006. "Facts, Norms and Dispositions: Practical Uses of the Modal Verb *Would*
in Police Interrogations." *Discourse Studies* 8:475–501.

Elliott, Colin D. 1990. *Differential Ability Scales: Administration and Scoring Manual*. New York:
Psychological Corporation.

Engel, George. 1980. "The Clinical Application of the Biopsychosocial Model." *American Journal
of Psychiatry* 13:535–44.

Erickson, Frederick. 2007. "Some Thoughts on 'Proximal' Formative Assessment of Student
Learning." *Yearbook of the National Society for the Study of Education* 106(1):187–216.

Evans, Bonnie. 2013. "How Autism Became Autism: The Radical Transformation of a Central
Concept of Child Development in Britain." *History of the Human Sciences* 26(3):3–31.

Evers, Kris, Jarymke Maljaars, Sarah J. Carrington, et al. 2020. "How Well Are DSM-5 Diagnostic

Criteria for ASD Represented in Standardized Diagnostic Instruments?" *European Child & Adolescent Psychiatry.* doi: 10.1007/s00787-020-01481-z.

Eyal, Gil. 2013. "For a Sociology of Expertise: The Social Origins of the Autism Epidemic." *American Journal of Sociology* 118:863–907.

Eyal, Gil, and Brendan Hart. 2010. "How Parents of Autistic Children Became 'Experts on Their Own Children': Notes towards a Sociology of Expertise." In *Annual Conference of the Berkeley Journal of Sociology.*

Eyal, Gil, Brendan Hart, Emine Onculer, et al. 2010. *The Autism Matrix: The Social Origins of the Autism Epidemic.* Malden, MA: Polity.

Fein, Elizabeth. 2015. "'No One Has to Be Your Friend': Asperger's Syndrome and the Vicious Cycle of Social Disorder in Late Modern Identity Markets." *ETHOS* 43:82–107.

———. 2020. *Living on the Spectrum: Autism and Youth in Community.* New York: New York University Press.

Fein, Elizabeth, and Clarice Rios, eds. 2018. *Autism in Translation: An Intercultural Conversation on Autism Spectrum Conditions.* Cham, Switzerland: Palgrave Macmillan.

Feinstein, Adam. 2010. *A History of Autism: Conversations with the Pioneers.* Malden, MA: Wiley-Blackwell.

Feinstein, Alvan R. 1973. "An Analysis of Diagnostic Reasoning: I. The Domains and Disorders of Clinical Macrobiology." *Yale Journal of Biology and Medicine* 46:212–32.

Fitzgerald, Des. 2013. "The Affective Labour of Autism Neuroscience: Entangling Emotions, Thoughts and Feelings in a Scientific Research Practice." *Subjectivity* 6:131–52.

———. 2014. "The Trouble with Brain Imaging: Hope, Uncertainty and Ambivalence in the Neuroscience of Autism." *BioSocieties* 9:241–61.

———. 2017. *Tracing Autism: Uncertainty, Ambiguity and the Affective Labor of Neuroscience.* Seattle: University of Washington Press.

Fleck, Ludwig. 1979. *Genesis and Development of a Scientific Fact.* Chicago: University of Chicago Press.

Fombonne, Eric. 2003. "Epidemiological Surveys of Autism and Other Pervasive Developmental Disorders: An Update." *Journal of Autism and Developmental Disorders* 33:365–382.

Fortun, Mike. 2001. "Mediated Speculations in the Genomics Futures Markets." *New Genetics and Society* 20:139–256.

———. 2005. "For an Ethics of Promising, or: A Few Kind Words about James Watson." *New Genetics and Society* 24:157–73.

———. 2008. *Promising Genomics: Iceland and Decode Genetics in a World of Speculation.* Berkeley: University of California Press.

Foucault, Michel. 1973. *The Birth of the Clinic: An Archaeology of Medical Perception.* New York: Vintage.

———. 1987. *Mental Illness and Psychology.* Berkeley: University of California Press.

Frank, Arthur. 1995. *The Wounded Storyteller: Body, Illness, and Ethics.* Chicago: University of Chicago Press.

Frankel, Richard M. 1982. "Autism for All Practical Purposes: A Micro-Interactional View." *Topics in Language Disorders* 3:33–42.

Frankel, Richard M., Timothy E. Quill, and Susan H. McDaniel, eds. 2003. *The Biopsychosocial Approach.* Rochester, NY: University of Rochester Press.

Freese, Jeremy. 2008. "Genetics and the Social Science Explanation of Individual Outcomes." *American Journal of Sociology* 114:S1–S35.

Freese, Jeremy, and Douglas W. Maynard. 1998. "Prosodic Features of Bad News and Good News in Conversation." *Language in Society* 27(2):195–219.

Freese, Jeremy, and Sara Shostak. 2009. "Genetics and Social Inquiry." *Annual Review of Sociology* 35:107–28.

Freidson, Eliot. 1970. *The Profession of Medicine: A Study of the Sociology of Applied Knowledge.* New York: Dodd, Mead.

Frith, Uta. 2003. *Autism: Explaining the Enigma.* 2nd ed. Malden, MA: Blackwell.

Frost, Lori, and Andy Bondy. 2002. *The Picture Exchange Communication System Training Manual.* Newark, DE: Pyramid Educational Products.

Fujimura, Joan H. 1988. "The Molecular Biological Bandwagon in Cancer Research: Where Social Worlds Meet." *Social Problems* 35(3):261–83.

———. 1996. *Crafting Science: A Sociohistory of the Quest for the Genetics of Cancer.* Cambridge, MA: Harvard University Press.

———. 2006. "Sex Genes: A Critical Sociomaterial Approach to the Politics and Molecular Genetics of Sex Determination." *Signs: Journal of Women in Culture and Society* 32:49–82.

Fujimura, Joan H., Deborah A. Bolnick, Ramy Rajagopalan, et al. 2014. "Clines without Classes: How to Make Sense of Human Variation." *Sociological Theory* 32:208–27.

Fujimura, Joan H., and Danny Y. Chou. 1994. "Dissent in Science: Styles of Scientific Practice and the Controversy over the Cause of AIDS." *Social Science & Medicine* 38:1017–36.

Fujimura, Joan H., Troy Duster, and Ramya Rajagopalan. 2008. "Introduction: Race, Genetics, and Disease; Questions of Evidence, Matters of Consequence." *Social Studies of Science* 38:643–56.

Garb, Howard N. 1998. *Studying the Clinician: Judgment Research and Psychological Assessment.* Washington, DC: American Psychological Association.

Garcia, Angela C. 2012. "Medical Problems Where Talk Is the Problem: Current Trends in Conversation Analytic Research on Aphasia, Autism Spectrum Disorder, Intellectual Disability, and Alzheimer's." *Sociology Compass* 6:351–64.

Garfinkel, Harold. 1963. "A Conception of, and Experiments with, 'Trust' as a Condition of Stable Concerted Actions." Pp. 187–238 in *Motivation and Social Interaction*, edited by O. J. Harvey. New York: Ronald.

———. 1967. *Studies in Ethnomethodology.* Englewood Cliffs, NJ: Prentice-Hall.

———. 1996. "Ethnomethodology's Program." *Social Psychology Quarterly* 59:5–21.

———. 2002. *Ethnomethodology's Program.* Lanham, MD: Rowman & Littlefield.

———. 2012. "The 'Red' as an Ideal Object." *Etnografia: E Ricerca Qualitativa* 1:19–34.

Garfinkel, Harold, and Harvey Sacks. 1970. "On Formal Structures of Practical Actions." Pp. 337–66 in *Theoretical Sociology*, edited by J. D. McKinney and E. A. Tiryakian. New York: Appleton-Century Crofts.

Garfinkel, Harold, and D. Lawrence Wieder. 1992. "Two Incommensurable, Asymmetrically Alternate Technologies of Social Analysis." Pp. 175–206 in *Text in Context: Contributions to Ethnomethodology*, edited by G. Watson and R. M. Seiler. Newbury Park, CA: Sage.

Gernsbacher, Morton A. 2015. "Diverse Brains." *General Psychologist* 49(2):29–37.

———. 2017. "Editorial Perspective: The Use of Person-First Language in Scholarly Writing May Accentuate Stigma." *Journal of Child Psychology and Psychiatry* 58(7):859–61.

Gernsbacher, Morton A., Michelle Dawson, and H. Hill Goldsmith. 2005. "Three Reasons Not to Believe in an Autism Epidemic." *Current Directions in Psychological Science* 14:55–58.

Gernsbacher, Morton A., and Jennifer L. Frymiare. 2005. "Does the Autistic Brain Lack Core Modules?" *Journal of Developmental and Learning Disorders* 9:3–16.

Gernsbacher, Morton A., Adam R. Raimond, Jennifer L. Stevenson, et al. 2018. "Do Puzzle Pieces and Autism Puzzle Piece Logos Evoke Negative Associations?" *Autism* 22:118–25.

Gibson, David R. 2011. "Avoiding Catastrophe: The Interactional Production of Possibility during the Cuban Missile Crisis." *American Journal of Sociology* 117:361–419.

Gibson, James J. 1986. *The Ecological Approach to Visual Perception*. Hillsdale, NJ: Lawrence Erlbaum.

Gieryn, Thomas F. 2000. "A Space for Place in Sociology." *Annual Review of Sociology* 26:463–96.

Gill, Virginia Teas. 1998. "Doing Attributions in Medical Interaction: Patients' Explanations for Illness and Doctors' Responses." *Social Psychology Quarterly* 61:342–60.

Gill, Virginia Teas, and Douglas W. Maynard. 1995. "On 'Labeling' in Actual Interaction: Delivering and Receiving Diagnoses of Developmental Disabilities." *Social Problems* 42:11–37.

Gillis-Buck, Eva M., and Sarah S. Richardson. 2014. "Autism as a Biomedical Platform for Sex Differences Research." *BioSocieties* 9:262–83.

Glenn, Phillip, and Timothy Koschmann. 2005. "Learning to Diagnose: Production of Diagnostic Hypotheses in Problem-Based Learning Tutorials." Pp. 153–78 in *Diagnosis as Cultural Practice*, edited by J. F. Duchan and D. Kovarsky. New York: Mouton de Gruyter.

Goffman, Erving. 1959a. "The Moral Career of the Mental Patient." *Psychiatry* 22(2):123–42. doi: 10.1080/00332747.1959.11023166.

———. 1959b. *The Presentation of Self in Everyday Life*. Garden City, NY: Doubleday.

———. 1961. *Asylums: Essay on the Social Situation of Mental Patients and Other Inmates*. Garden City, NY: Doubleday.

———. 1963. *Behavior in Public Places: Notes on the Social Organization of Gatherings*. New York: Free Press.

———. 1964. "The Neglected Situation." *American Anthropologist* 66(pt. 2):133–36.

———. 1967. *Interaction Ritual*. New York: Doubleday.

———. 1971. *Relations in Public: Microstudies of the Public Order*. New York: Harper and Row.

———. 1978. "Response Cries." *Language* 54:787–815.

———. 1979. "Footing." *Semiotica* 25:1–29.

———. 1983. "The Interaction Order." *American Sociological Review* 48:1–17.

Goldknopf, Emily J. 2002. "Referring Indirectly to Diagnoses in a Psychiatric Clinic." *Crossroads of Language, Interaction, and Culture* 4:59–91.

Goodwin, Charles. 1984. "Notes on Story Structure and the Organization of Participation." Pp. 225–46 in *Structures of Social Action*, edited by J. M. Atkinson and J. Heritage. Cambridge: Cambridge University Press.

———. 2003a. "Introduction." Pp. 1–20 in *Conversation and Brain Damage*, edited by C. Goodwin. New York: Oxford University Press.

———. 2003b. "Pointing as Situated Practice." Pp. 217–41 in *Pointing: Where Language, Culture, and Cognition Meet*, edited by S. Kita. Hillsdale, NJ: Lawrence Erlbaum.

———. 2007. "Participation, Stance, and Affect in the Organization of Activities." *Discourse & Society* 18:53–73.

Goodwin, Marjorie H. 2006. "Participation, Affect, and Trajectory in Family Directive/Response Sequences." *Text & Talk* 26:515–43.

Goodwin, Marjorie H., and Asta Cekaite. 2013. "Calibration in Directive/Response Sequences in Family Interaction." *Journal of Pragmatics* 46(1):122–38.

Gottesman, Irving I., and Todd Gould. 2003. "The Endophenotype Concept in Psychiatry: Etymology and Strategic Intentions." *American Journal of Psychiatry* 160:636–45.

Gourdine, Ruby M., Tiffany D. Baffour, and Martell Teasley. 2011. "Autism and the African American Community." *Social Work in Public Health* 26:454–70.

Grandin, Temple. 1995. *Thinking in Pictures and Other Reports from My Life with Autism (with a Foreword by Oliver Sacks)*. New York: Vintage.

———. 2006. *Thinking in Pictures and Other Reports from My Life with Autism*. 2nd ed. New York: Vintage.

Greenberg, Jan S., Marsha M. Seltzer, Jinkuk Hong, et al. 2006. "Bidirectional Effects of Expressed Emotion and Behavior Problems and Symptoms in Adolescents and Adults with Autism." *American Journal on Mental Retardation* 111:229–49.

Greenspan, Stanley I., and Serena Wieder. 2006. *Engaging Autism: Using the Floortime Approach to Help Children Relate, Communicate, and Think*. Philadelphia: Da Capo Lifelong Books.

Grinker, Roy Richard. 2007. *Unstrange Minds: Remapping the World of Autism*. New York: Basic Books.

———. 2018. "Who Owns Autism? Economics, Fetishism, and Stakeholders." Pp. 231–50 in *Autism in Translation: Culture, Mind, and Society*, edited by E. Fein and C. Rios. Cham, Switzerland: Palgrave Macmillan.

———. 2019. "Autism, 'Stigma,' Disability: A Shifting Historical Terrain." *Current Anthropology* 61:S56–S67.

Grinker, Roy Richard, and Kyungjin Cho. 2013. "Border Children: Interpreting Autism Spectrum Disorder in South Korea." *ETHOS* 41:46–74.

Grinker, Roy Richard, and David Mandell. 2015. "Notes on a Puzzle Piece." *Autism* 19:643–45.

Grinker, Roy Richard, Marshalyn Yeargin-Allsopp, and Coleen Boyle. 2011. "Culture and Autism Spectrum Disorders: The Impact on Prevalence and Recognition." Pp. 112–36 in *Autism Spectrum Disorders*, edited by D. G. Amaral, G. Dawson, and D. H. Geschwind. New York: Oxford University Press.

Hacking, Ian. 1995. "The Looping Effects of Human Kinds." In *Causal Cognition: A Multidisciplinary Approach*, edited by D. Sperber, D. Premack, and A. J. Premack. Oxford: Clarendon.

———. 1998. *Mad Travelers: Reflections on the Reality of Transient Mental Illnesses*. Charlottesville, VA: University Press of Virginia.

———. 1999. *The Social Construction of What?* Cambridge, MA: Harvard University Press.

———. 2002. "Historical Ontology." Pp. 583–600 in *In the Scope of Logic, Methodology and Philosophy of Science*, vol. 2, edited by P. Gärdenfors, J. Woleński, and K. Kijania-Placek. Dordrecht: Springer Netherlands.

———. 2006a. "Genetics, Biosocial Groups and the Future of Identity." *Daedalus* 135(4):81–95.

———. 2006b. "Making Up People." *London Review of Books* 28:23–26.

———. 2007. "Kinds of People: Moving Targets." *Proceedings of the British Academy* 151:285–318.

———. 2009. "Autistic Autobiography." *Philosophical Transactions of the Royal Society B* 364:1467–73.

Haddon, Mark. 2003. *The Curious Incident of the Dog in the Night-Time*. New York: Vintage Books.

Haebig, Eileen, Andrea McDuffie, and Susan Ellis Weismer. 2013. "The Contribution of Two Categories of Parent Verbal Responsiveness to Later Language for Toddlers and Preschoolers on the Autism Spectrum." *American Journal of Speech-Language Pathology* 22:57–70.

Halkowski, Timothy. 2006. "Realizing the Illness: Patients' Narratives of Symptom Discovery." Pp. 86–114 in *Communication in Medical Care: Interaction between Primary Care Physicians and Patients*, edited by J. Heritage and D. W. Maynard. Cambridge: Cambridge University Press.

Halpin, Michael. 2016. "The DSM and Professional Practice: Research, Clinical, and Institutional Perspectives." *Journal of Health and Social Behavior* 57:153–67.

———. 2020. "The Brain and Causality: How the Brain Becomes an Individual-Level Cause of Illness." *Social Problems*, spaa030:1–17.

Happé, Francesca. 1999. "Autism: Cognitive Deficit or Cognitive Style?" *Trends in Cognitive Sciences* 3(6):216–22.

Haraway, Donna. 1997. "Gene: Maps and Portraits of Life Itself." Pp. 131–72 in *Modest_Witness@ Second_Millennium: Female Man©_Meets_Oncomouse*, edited by D. J. Haraway. New York: Routledge.

Harrington, Anne. 2005. "The Inner Lives of Disordered Brains." *Cerebrum: The Dana Forum on Brain Science* 7:23–36.

Hart, Brendan. 2014. "Autism Parents & Neurodiversity: Radical Translation, Joint Embodiment and the Prosthetic Environment." *BioSocieties* 9:284–303.

Hayes, Jennie, Rose McCabe, Tamsin Ford, et al. 2020. "Drawing a Line in the Sand: Affect and Testimony in Autism Assessment Teams in the UK." *Sociology of Health & Illness* 42:825–43.

Hayes, Jennie, Rose McCabe, Tamsin Ford, et al. 2021. " 'Not at the Diagnosis Point': Dealing with Contradiction in Autism Assessment Teams." *Social Science & Medicine* 268. https://doi .org/10.1016/j.socscimed.2020.113462.

Heath, Christian. 1992. "Diagnosis and Assessment in the Medical Consultation." Pp. 235–67 in *Talk at Work: Interaction in Institutional Settings*, edited by P. Drew and J. Heritage. Cambridge: Cambridge University Press.

Heath, Christian, and Paul Luff. 2012. "Embodied Action and Organizational Activity." Pp. 283– 307 in *Handbook of Conversation Analysis*, edited by J. Sidnell and T. Stivers. New York: Blackwell.

Hedgecoe, Adam. 2001. "Schizophrenia and the Narrative of Enlightened Geneticization." *Social Studies of Science* 31(6):875–911.

Heinemann, Trine. 2006. " 'Will You or Can't You?': Displaying Entitlement in Interrogative Requests." *Journal of Pragmatics* 38:1081–104.

Hepburn, Alexa, and Galina B. Bolden. 2013. "The Conversation Analytic Approach to Transcription." In *The Handbook of Conversation Analysis*, edited by J. Sidnell and T. Stivers. New York: Wiley-Blackwell.

Heritage, John. 1984a. "A Change-of-State Token and Aspects of Its Sequential Placement." Pp. 299–345 in *Structures of Social Action*, edited by J. M. Atkinson and J. Heritage. Cambridge: Cambridge University Press.

———. 1984b. *Garfinkel and Ethnomethodology*. Cambridge: Polity.

———. 1998. "Oh-Prefaced Responses to Inquiry." *Language in Society* 27:291–334.

———. 2012. "Epistemics in Action: Action Formation and Territories of Knowledge." *Research on Language and Social Interaction* 45(1):1–29.

Heritage, John, and J. Maxwell Atkinson. 1984. "Introduction." Pp. 1–16 in *Structures of Social Action*, edited by J. M. Atkinson and J. Heritage. Cambridge: Cambridge University Press.

Heritage, John, and Douglas W. Maynard. In press. "Harold Garfinkel and Ethnomethodology's Legacies: Introduction." In *Harold Garfinkel: Praxis, Social Order, and Ethnomethodology's Legacies*, edited by D. W. Maynard and J. Heritage. New York: Oxford University Press.

Heritage, John, and Amanda McArthur. 2019. "The Diagnostic Moment: A Study in US Primary Care." *Social Science & Medicine* 228:262–71.

Heritage, John, and Jeffrey D. Robinson. 2006. "Accounting for the Visit: Giving Reasons for

Seeking Medical Care." Pp. 48–85 in *Communication in Medical Care: Interaction between Primary Care Physicians and Patients*, edited by J. Heritage and D. W. Maynard. Cambridge: Cambridge University Press.

Heritage, John, and Marja-Leen Sorjonen. 1994. "Constituting and Maintaining Activities across Sequences: And-Prefacing as a Feature of Question Design." *Language in Society*:1–29.

Heritage, Margaret. 2013. *Formative Assessment in Practice: A Process of Inquiry and Action*. Cambridge, MA: Harvard Education Press.

Heritage, Margaret, and John Heritage. 2013. "Teacher Questioning: The Epicenter of Instruction and Assessment." *Applied Measurement in Education* 26:176–90.

Hester, Stephen, and Peter Eglin. 1997. *Culture in Action: Studies in Membership Categorization Analysis*. Lanham, MD: University Press of America.

Higashida, Haoki. 2013. *The Reason I Jump: The Inner Voice of a Thirteen-Year-Old Boy with Autism*. New York: Random House.

Hindmarsh, Jon, and Christian Heath. 2000. "Embodied Reference: A Study of Deixis in Workplace Interaction." *Journal of Pragmatics* 32:1855–78.

Hirstein, William, Portia Iversen, and V. S. Ramachandran. 2001. "Autonomic Responses of Autistic Children to People and Objects." *Proceedings of the Royal Society* 268:1883–88.

Hochschild, Arlie R. 1983. *The Managed Heart*. Berkeley: University of California Press.

Hollin, Gregory. 2017. "Autistic Heterogeneity: Linking Uncertainties and Indeterminacies." *Science as Culture* 26:209–31.

Hollin, Gregory, and Alison Pilnick. 2018. "The Categorisation of Resistance: Interpreting Failure to Follow a Proposed Line of Action in the Diagnosis of Autism amongst Young Adults." *Sociology of Health & Illness* 40(7):1215–32.

Holmes, David L. 1990. "Community-Based Services for Children and Adults with Autism: The Eden Family of Programs." *Journal of Autism & Developmental Disorders* 20(3):339–51.

Horwitz, Allan V. 2002. *Creating Mental Illness*. Chicago: University of Chicago Press.

Howlin, Patricia, and Anna Moore. 1997. "Diagnosis in Autism: A Survey of over 1200 Patients in the UK." *Autism* 1(2):135–62. doi: 10.1177/1362361397012003.

Hunter, Kathryn M. 1991. *Doctors' Stories: The Narrative Structure of Medical Knowledge*. Princeton, NJ: Princeton University Press.

Husserl, Edmund. 1970. *The Crisis of European Sciences and Transcendental Phenomenology*. Evanston, IL: Northwestern University Press.

Institute of Medicine. 2002. "Unequal Treatment." Washington, DC: National Academic.

Jefferson, Gail. 1974. "Error Correction as an Interactional Resource." *Language in Society* 2: 181–99.

———. 1978. "Sequential Aspects of Storytelling in Conversation." Pp. 219–48 in *Studies in the Organization of Conversational Interaction*, edited by J. Schenkein. New York: Academic.

———. 1984. "On Stepwise Transition from Talk about a Trouble to Inappropriately Next-Positioned Matters." Pp. 191–221 in *Structures of Social Action*, edited by J. M. Atkinson and J. Heritage. Cambridge: Cambridge University Press.

———. 1996. "On the Poetics of Ordinary Talk." *Text and Performance Quarterly* 16:1–16.

Job Accommodation Network. 2020. "Workplace Accommodations: Low Cost, High Impact." Morgantown, WV: Job Accommodation Network.

Jones, Lydia, Lorna Goddard, Elisabeth L. Hill, et al. 2014. "Experiences of Receiving a Diagnosis of Autism Spectrum Disorder: A Survey of Adults in the United Kingdom." *Journal of Autism & Developmental Disorders* 44:3033–44.

Jordan-Young, Rebecca M. 2011. *Brain Storm: The Flaws in the Science of Sex Differences*. Cambridge, MA: Harvard University Press.

Jutel, Annemarie Goldstein. 2009. "Sociology of Diagnosis: A Preliminary Review." *Sociology of Health and Illness* 31:278–99.

———. 2014. "When the Penny Drops: Diagnosis and the Transformative Moment." In *Social Issues in Diagnosis: An Introduction for Students and Clinicians*, edited by A. G. Jutel and K. Dew. Baltimore, MD: Johns Hopkins University Press.

Kanner, Leo. 1943. "Autistic Disturbances of Affective Contact." *Nervous Child* 2:217–50.

Kawashima, Michie, and Douglas W. Maynard. 2019. "The Social Organization of Echolalia in Clinical Encounters Involving a Child Diagnosed with Autism Spectrum Disorder." Pp. 49–67 in *Children and Mental Health Talk: Perspectives on Social Competence*, edited by J. Lamerichs, S. J. Danby, A. Bateman, and S. Ekberg. Cham, Switzerland: Palgrave Macmillan.

Kendrick, Kobin H., and Paul Drew. 2016. "Recruitment: Offers, Requests, and the Organization of Assistance in Interaction." *Research on Language and Social Interaction* 49(1):1–19. doi: 10.1080/08351813.2016.1126436.

Kent, Alexandra. 2012. "Compliance, Resistance and Incipient Compliance When Responding to Directives." *Discourse Studies* 14:711–30.

King, Marissa, and Peter Bearman. 2009. "Diagnostic Change and the Increased Prevalence of Autism." *International Journal of Epidemiology* 38:1224–34.

Kogan, Michael D., Stephen J. Blumberg, Laura A. Schieve, et al. 2009. "Prevalence of Parent-Reported Diagnosis of Autism Spectrum Disorder among Children in the US, 2007." *Pediatrics* 124:1396–403.

Köhler, Wolfgang. 1947. *Gestalt Psychology: An Introduction to New Concepts in Modern Psychology*. New York: Liveright.

Korkiagangas, Terhi. 2018. *Communication, Gaze and Autism: A Multimodal Interaction Perspective*. New York: Routledge.

Koschmann, Timothy, Phillip Glenn, and M. Conlee. 2000. "When Is a Problem-Based Tutorial Not a Tutorial? Analyzing the Tutor's Role in the Emergence of a Learning Issue." Pp. 53–74 in *Problem-Based Learning: Gaining Insights on Learning Interactions through Multiple Methods of Inquiry*, edited by C. Hmelo and D. Evensen. Mahwah, NJ: Lawrence Erlbaum.

Koshik, Irene. 2005. *Beyond Rhetorical Questions: Assertive Questions in Everyday Interaction*. Philadelphia: John Benjamins.

Kovarsky, Dana, Judith Felson Duchan, and Madeline Maxwell, eds. 1999. *Constructing (In) Competence: Disabling Evaluations in Clinical and Social Interaction*. Mahwah, NJ: Lawrence Erlbaum.

Kumagai, Arno K., and Delese Wear. 2014. "'Making Strange': A Role for the Humanities in Medical Education." *Academic Medicine* 89:1–5.

Labov, William, and Joshua Waletzky. 1967. "Narrative Analysis: Oral Versions of Personal Experience." Pp. 12–44 in *Essays on the Verbal and Visual Arts*, edited by J. Helm. Seattle, WA: University of Washington Press.

Lainhart, Janet E., and Susan E. Folstein. 1994. "Affective Disorders in People with Autism: A Review of Published Cases." *Journal of Autism and Developmental Disorders* 24:587–601.

Latour, Bruno. 1987. *Science in Action*. Cambridge, MA: Harvard University Press.

———. 1993. *The Pasteurization of France*. Boston, MA: Harvard University Press.

———. 1999. *Pandora's Hope: Essays on the Reality of Science Studies*. Cambridge, MA: Harvard University Press.

———. 2004. "Why Has Critique Run Out of Steam? From Matters of Fact to Matters of Concern." *Critical Inquiry* 30:225–48.

Law, John. 2009. "Actor Network Theory and Material Semiotics." Pp. 141–158 in *The New Blackwell Companion to Social Theory*, edited by B. S. Turner. Malden, MA: Wiley-Blackwell.

Lee, Laurie. 1959. *Cider with Rosie*. London: Hogarth.

Lerner, Gene H. 1992. "Assisted Storytelling: Deploying Shared Knowledge as a Practical Matter." *Qualitative Sociology* 15(3):247–71.

———. 1996. "Finding 'Face' in the Preference Structures of Talk-in-Interaction." *Social Psychology Quarterly* 59:303–21.

———. 2013. "On the Place of Hesitating in Delicate Formulations: A Turn-Constructional Infrastructure for Collaborative Indiscretion." Pp. 94–134 in *Conversational Repair and Human Understanding*, edited by M. Hayashi, G. Raymond, and J. Sidnell. Cambridge: Cambridge University Press.

Levinson, Stephen C. 1983. *Pragmatics*. Cambridge: Cambridge University Press.

Lindee, Susan. 2005. *Moments of Truth in Genetic Medicine*. Baltimore, MD: Johns Hopkins University Press.

Lindström, Anna. 2005. "Language as Social Action: A Study of How Senior Citizens Request Assistance with Practical Tasks in the Swedish Home Help Service." Pp. 209–30 in *Syntax and Lexis in Conversation: Studies on the Use of Linguistic Resources in Talk-in-Interaction*, edited by A. Hakulinen and M. Selting. Amsterdam: Benjamins.

Linton, Simi. 1998. "Disability Studies/Not Disability Studies." *Disability & Society* 13(4):525–40.

———. 2005. "What Is Disability Studies?" *PMLA* 120(2):518–22.

Lippman, Abby. 1991. "The Geneticization of Health and Illness: Implications for Social Practice." *Endocrinologie* 29(1–2):85–90.

Lipton, Helene L., and Bonnie L. Svarstad. 1977. "Sources of Variation in Clinicians' Communication to Parents about Mental Retardation." *American Journal of Mental Deficiency* 82:155–61.

Liu, Ka-Yuet, Marissa King, and Peter S. Bearman. 2010. "Social Influence and the Autism Epidemic." *American Journal of Sociology* 115:1387–434.

Livingston, Eric. 2008. *Ethnographies of Reason*. London: Routledge.

Loomes, Rebecca, Laura Hull, and William P. L. Mandy. 2017. "What Is the Male-to-Female Ratio in Autism Spectrum Disorder? A Systematic Review and Meta-Analysis." *Journal of the American Academy of Child & Adolescent Psychiatry* 56(6):466–74.

Lord, Catherine, Traolach S. Brugha, Tony Charman, et al. 2020. "Autism Spectrum Disorder." *Nature Reviews Disease Primers* 6(5):1–23.

Lord, Catherine, Pamela C. DiLavore, and Katherine Gotham. 2012. *ADOS-2: Autism Diagnostic Observation Schedule (Second Edition)*. Torrance, CA: Western Psychological Services.

Lord, Catherine, Susan Risi, Linda Lambrecht, et al. 2000. "The Autism Diagnostic Observation Schedule–Generic: A Standard Measure of Social and Communication Deficits Associated with the Spectrum of Autism." *Journal of Autism and Developmental Disorders* 30:205–23.

Lord, Catherine, and Michael Rutter. 2012. "ADOS-2: Module 2 (W-604c)." Torrance, CA: Western Psychological Services.

Lord, Catherine, Michael Rutter, Pamela C. DiLavore, et al. 2012. *Autism Diagnostic Observation Schedule, Second Edition (ADOS-2 Manual (Part I): Modules 1–4)*. Torrance, CA: Western Psychological Services.

Losh, Molly. 2006. "Understanding of Emotional Experience in Autism: Insights from the Personal

Accounts of High-Functioning Children with Autism." *Developmental Psychology* 42(5): 809–18.

Lovaas, O. Ivar. 1987. "Behavioral Treatment and Normal Educational and Intellectual Functioning in Young Children." *Journal of Autism and Developmental Disorders* 55:3–9.

Lutfey, Karen, and Douglas W. Maynard. 1998. "Bad News in Oncology: How Physician and Patient Talk about Death and Dying without Using Those Words." *Social Psychology Quarterly* 61:321–41.

Lynch, Michael E. 1988. "Sacrifice and the Transformation of the Animal Body into a Scientific Object: Laboratory Culture and Ritual Practice in the Neurosciences." *Social Studies of Science* 18:265–89.

Lynch, Michael E., Simon A. Cole, Ruth McNally, et al. 2008. *The Truth Machine: The Contentious History of DNA Fingerprinting.* Chicago: University of Chicago Press.

Maenner, Matthew J., Kelly A. Shaw, Jon Baio, et al. 2020. "Prevalence of Autism Spectrum Disorder among Children Aged 8 Years: Autism and Developmental Disabilities Monitoring Network, 11 Sites, United States, 2016." *Centers for Disease Control and Prevention Morbidity and Mortality Weekly Report* 69(4):1–12.

Mandelbaum, Jenny. 2003. "How to 'Do Things' with Narrative: A Communication Perspective on Narrative Skill." Pp. 595–633 in *Handbook of Communication and Social Interaction Skills,* edited by J. O. Greene and B. R. Burleson. Mahwah NJ: Lawrence Erlbaum.

———. 2013. "Storytelling in Conversation." Pp. 492–508 in *Handbook of Conversation Analysis,* edited by J. Sidnell and T. Stivers. Oxford: Blackwell.

Mandell, David S., Richard F. Ittenbach, Susan E. Levy, et al. 2007. "Disparities in Diagnoses Received prior to a Diagnosis of Autism Spectrum Disorder." *Journal of Autism and Developmental Disorders* 37:1795–802.

Mandell, David S., Lisa D. Wiggins, Laura Arnstein Carpenter, et al. 2009. "Racial/Ethnic Disparities in the Identification of Children with Autism Spectrum Disorders." *American Journal of Public Health* 99(3):493–98.

Manning, Melanie, and Louanne Hudgins. 2007. "Use of Array-Based Technology in the Practice of Medical Genetics." *ACMG Practice Guidelines* 9:650–53.

Martin, John Levi. 2011. *The Explanation of Social Action.* New York: Oxford University Press.

Mates, Andrea W., Lisa Mikesell, and Michael Sean Smith, eds. 2013. *Language, Interaction and Frontotemporal Dementia: Reverse Engineering the Social Mind.* Sheffield, UK: Equinox.

Mau, Steffen. 2019. *The Metric Society: On the Quantification of the Social.* Cambridge: Polity.

Maynard, Douglas W. 1989. "Notes on the Delivery and Reception of Diagnostic News regarding Mental Disabilities." Pp. 54–67 in *The Interactional Order: New Directions in the Study of Social Order,* edited by D. Helm, W. T. Anderson, A. J. Meehan, and A. Rawls. New York: Irvington.

———. 1992. "On Clinicians' Co-implicating Recipients in the Delivery of Diagnostic News." Pp. 331–58 in *Talk at Work: Interaction in Institutional Settings,* edited by P. Drew and J. Heritage. Cambridge: Cambridge University Press.

———. 2003. *Bad News, Good News: Conversational Order in Everyday Talk and Clinical Settings.* Chicago: University of Chicago Press.

———. 2004. "On Predicating a Diagnosis as an Attribute of a Person." *Discourse Studies* 6:53–76.

———. 2005. "Social Actions, Gestalt Coherence, and Designations of Disability: Lessons from and about Autism." *Social Problems* 52(4):499–524.

———. 2006. " 'Does It Mean I'm Gonna Die?': On Meaning Assessment in the Delivery of Diagnostic News." *Social Science & Medicine* 62:1902–16.

———. 2013. "Defensive Mechanisms: I-Mean-Prefaced Utterances in Complaint and Other Conversational Sequences." Pp. 198–233 in *Conversational Repair and Human Understanding*, edited by M. Hayashi, G. Raymond, and J. Sidnell. Cambridge: Cambridge University Press.

———. 2016. "Defending Solidarity: Self-Repair on Behalf of Other-Attentiveness." Pp. 73–107 in *Accountability in Social Interaction*, edited by J. D. Robinson. New York: Oxford University Press.

———. 2019. "Why Social Psychology Needs Autism, and Why Autism Needs Social Psychology: Forensic and Clinical Considerations." *Social Psychology Quarterly* 82(1):5–30.

Maynard, Douglas W., and Steven E. Clayman. 2018. "Mandarin Ethnomethodology or Mutual Interchange?" *Discourse Studies* 20(1):120–41.

Maynard, Douglas W., and Richard M. Frankel. 2006. "On Diagnostic Rationality: Bad News, Good News, and the Symptom Residue." Pp. 248–78 in *Communication in Medical Care: Interaction between Primary Care Physicians and Patients*, edited by J. Heritage and D. W. Maynard. Cambridge: Cambridge University Press.

Maynard, Douglas W., and Jeremy Freese. 2012. "Good News, Bad News, and Affect: Practical and Temporal 'Emotion Work' in Everyday Life." Pp. 92–112 in *Emotion in Interaction*, edited by A. Peräkylä and M.-L. Sorjonen. New York: Oxford.

Maynard, Douglas W., and Courtney L. Marlaire. 1992. "Good Reasons for Bad Testing Performance: The Interactional Substrate of Educational Exams." *Qualitative Sociology* 15:177–202.

Maynard, Douglas W., T. A. McDonald, and Trini Stickle. 2016. "Parents as a Team: Mother, Father, a Child with Autism Spectrum Disorder, and a Spinning Toy." *Journal of Autism & Developmental Disorders* 46:406–23.

Maynard, Douglas W., and Jason Turowetz. 2013. "Language Use and Social Interaction." Pp. 251–79 in *Handbook of Social Psychology*, edited by J. Delamater and A. Ward. New York: Springer Science.

———. 2017a. "Doing Diagnosis: Autism, Interaction Order, and the Use of Narrative in Clinical Talk." *Social Psychology Quarterly* 80(3):254–75.

———. 2017b. "Doing Testing: How Concrete Competence Can Facilitate or Inhibit Performances of Children with Autism Spectrum Disorder." *Qualitative Sociology* 40(4):467–91.

———. 2019. "Doing Abstraction: Autism, Diagnosis, and Social Theory." *Sociological Theory* 37(1):89–116.

———. 2020. "Sequence and Consequence: Transposing Responsive Actions to Provocations in Forensic and Clinical Encounters Involving Youths with Autism." Pp. 39–63 in *Atypical Interaction: The Impact of Communicative Impairments within Everyday Talk*, edited by R. Wilkinson, J. Rae, and G. Rasmussen. New York: Springer.

———. In press. "Ethnomethodology and Atypical Interaction: The Case of Autism." In *Harold Garfinkel: Praxis, Social Order, and Ethnomethodology's Legacies*, edited by D. W. Maynard and J. Heritage. New York: Oxford University Press.

Mazefsky, Carla A., John Herrington, Matthew Siegel, et al. 2013. "The Role of Emotion Regulation in Autism Spectrum Disorder." *Journal of the American Academy of Child & Adolescent Psychiatry* 52(7):679–88.

Merrick, Joav, Isack Kandel, and Mohammed Morad. 2004. "Trends in Autism." P. 75 in *International Journal of Adolescent Medicine and Health*, vol. 16.

Miles, Judith H. 2011. "Autism Spectrum Disorders: A Genetics Review." *Genetics in Medicine* 13:278–94.

Miles, Matthew B., and A. Michael Huberman. 1994. *Qualitative Data Analysis*. Thousand Oaks, CA: Sage.

Mirenda, Patricia L., and Anne M. Donnellan. 1986. "Effects of Adult Interaction Style on Conversational Behavior in Students with Severe Communication Problems." *Language, Speech, and Hearing Services in Schools* 17:126–41.

Mirowsky, John, and Catherine E. Ross. 1989. "Psychiatric Diagnosis as Reified Measurement." *Journal of Health and Social Behavior* 30(1):11–25.

Mishler, Elliott. 1984. *The Discourse of Medicine: Dialectics of Medical Interviews*. Norwood, NJ: Ablex.

Mitchell, David T., and Sharon L. Snyder. 2001. "Representation and Its Discontents: The Uneasy Home of Disability in Literature and Film." Pp. 47–64 in *Narrative Prosthesis and the Materiality of Metaphor*, edited by D. T. Mitchell and S. L. Snyder. Ann Arbor: University of Michigan Press.

Mol, Annemarie. 2002. *The Body Multiple: Ontology in Medical Practice*. Durham, NC: Duke University Press.

Molotch, Harvey L., and Deirdre Boden. 1985. "Talking Social Structure: Discourse, Domination and the Watergate Hearings." *American Sociological Review* 50:273–88.

Moncrieff, Joanna, and M. J. Crawford. 2001. "British Psychiatry in the 20th Century: Observations from a Psychiatric Journal." *Social Science & Medicine* 53:349–56.

Mondada, Lorenza. 2013. "The Conversation Analytic Approach to Data Collection." Pp. 32–56 in *Handbook of Conversation Analysis*, edited by J. Sidnell and T. Stivers. New York: Blackwell.

Moore, Charlotte. 2004. *George & Sam: Two Boys, One Family, and Autism*. New York: St. Martin's Griffin.

Mukherjee, Siddhartha. 2016. *The Gene: An Intimate History*. New York: Scribner.

Mukhopadhyay, Tito Rajarshi. 2003. *The Mind Tree: A Miraculous Child Breaks the Silence of Autism*. New York: Arcade.

Murray, Henry A. 1938. *Explorations in Personality: A Clinical and Experimental Study of Fifty Men of College Age*. Oxford: Oxford University Press.

Muzikar, Debra. 2019. "The Autism Puzzle Piece: A Symbol That's Going to Stay or Go?" *The Art of Autism: Connecting Through the Arts*. April 20. https://the-art-of-autism.com/the-autism-puzzle-piece-a-symbol-of-what/.

Nadesan, Majia Holmer. 2005. *Constructing Autism: Unravelling the 'Truth' and Understanding the Social*. New York: Routledge.

National Institute of Mental Health (NIMH). 2019. "NIMH Strategic Plan for Research." Retrieved November 2019. https://www.nimh.nih.gov/about/strategic-planning-reports/highlights/highlight-what-is-rdoc.shtml.

Navon, Daniel. 2011. "Genomic Designation: How Genetics Can Delineate New, Phenotypically Diffuse Medical Categories." *Social Studies of Science* 41(2):203–26.

———. 2019. *Mobilizing Mutations: Human Genetics in the Age of Patient Advocacy*. Chicago: University of Chicago Press.

Navon, Daniel, and Gil Eyal. 2016. "Looping Genomes: Diagnostic Change and the Genetic Makeup of the Autism Population." *American Journal of Sociology* 121(5):1416–71.

Nazeer, Kamran. 2006. *Send in the Idiots: Stories from the Other Side of Autism*. New York: Bloomsbury.

Nelson, Nicole C. 2018. *Model Behavior: Animal Experiments, Complexity, and the Genetics of Psychiatric Disorders*. Chicago: University of Chicago Press.

Ochs, Elinor. 1979. "Introduction: What Child Language Can Contribute to Pragmatics." Pp. 1–17 in *Developmental Pragmatics*, edited by E. Ochs and B. B. Schieffelin. New York: Academic.

Ochs, Elinor, Tamar Kremer-Sadlik, Karen G. Sirota, et al. 2004. "Autism and the Social World: An Anthropological Perspective." *Discourse Studies* 6:147–83.

Ochs, Elinor, and Olga Solomon. 2004. "Practical Logic and Autism." Pp. 140–67 in *A Companion to Psychological Anthropology*, edited by C. Casey and R. B. Edgerton. Oxford: Blackwell.

———. 2010. "Autistic Sociality." *Journal of the Society for Psychological Anthropology* 38:69–92.

O'Dell, Lindsay, Hanna Bertilsdotter Rosqvist, Francisco Ortega, et al. 2016. "Critical Autism Studies: Exploring Epistemic Dialogues and Intersections, Challenging Dominant Understandings of Autism." *Disability & Society* 31:166–79.

O'Driscoll, Aisling, Jurate Daugelaite, and Roy D. Sleator. 2013. "'Big Data,' Hadoop and Cloud Computing in Genomics." *Journal of Biomedical Informatics* 46:774–81.

O'Neill, Katherine, and Amanda LeCouteur. 2014. "Naming the Problem: A Membership Categorization Analysis Study of Family Therapy." *Journal of Family Therapy* 36:268–86.

O'Roak, Brian, and Matthew W. State. 2008. "Autism Genetics: Strategies, Challenges, and Opportunities." *Autism Research* 1:4–17.

Orsini, Michael, and Joyce Davidson. 2013. "Critical Autism Studies: Notes on an Emerging Field." Pp. 1–30 in *Worlds of Autism: Across the Spectrum of Neurological Difference*, edited by J. Davidson and M. Orsini. Minneapolis: University of Minnesota Press.

Ortega, Francisco. 2009. "The Cerebral Subject and the Challenge of Neurodiversity." *BioSocieties* 4:425–45.

Osteen, Mark. 2008. "Autism and Representation: A Comprehensive Introduction." Pp. 1–47 in *Autism and Representation*, edited by M. Osteen. New York: Taylor and Francis.

Ozand, Pinar T., Ali Al-Odaib, Hania Merza, et al. 2003. "Autism: A Review." *Journal of Pediatric Neurology* 1(2):55–67.

Paris, Joel, and James Phillips, eds. 2013. *Making the DSM-5: Concepts and Controversies*. New York: Springer.

Park, Clara Clairborne. 1967. *The Siege: The First Eight Years of an Autistic Child*. Boston: Little Brown.

———. 2001. *Exiting Nirvana*. Boston: Little, Brown.

Pellicano, Elizabeth, Ari Ne'eman, and Marc Stears. 2011. "Engaging, Not Excluding: A Response to Walsh et al." *Nature Reviews Neuroscience* 12:769.

Peräkylä, Anssi. 1998. "Authority and Accountability: The Delivery of Diagnosis in Primary Health Care." *Social Psychology Quarterly* 61:301–20.

Peräkylä, Anssi, and Sanna Vehviläinen. 2003. "Conversation Analysis and the Professional Stocks of Interactional Knowledge." *Discourse & Society* 14:727–50.

Piaget, Jean. 1952. *The Child's Conception of Number*. New York: Norton.

Pickersgill, Martyn. 2019. "Psychiatry and the Sociology of Novelty: Negotiating the US National Institute of Mental Health 'Research Domain Criteria (RDoC).'" *Science, Technology & Human Values* 44(4):567–80.

Pinch, Trevor. 1993. "'Testing—One, Two, Three . . . Testing!': Toward a Sociology of Testing." *Science, Technology & Human Values* 18:25–41.

Pinchevski, Amit. 2005. *By Way of Interruption: Levinas and the Ethics of Communication*. Pittsburgh, PA: Duquesne University Press.

Pitney, John J. 2015. *The Politics of Autism: Navigating the Contested Spectrum*. Lanham, MD: Rowman & Littlefield.

Pollner, Melvin. 1974. "Sociological and Common-Sense Models of the Labelling Process." Pp. 27–40 in *Ethnomethodology*, edited by R. Turner. Baltimore, MD: Penguin Books.

Pomerantz, Anita M. 1980. "Telling My Side: 'Limited Access' as a 'Fishing' Device." *Sociological Inquiry* 50:186–98.

Porter, Theodore M. 1995. *Trust in Numbers: The Pursuit of Objectivity in Science and Public Life.* Princeton, NJ: Princeton University Press.

Prainsack, Barbara. 2017. *Personalized Medicine: Empowered Patients in the 21st Century.* New York: New York University Press.

Prince-Hughes, Dawn. 2004. *Songs of the Gorilla Nation: My Journey through Autism.* New York: Three Rivers.

Prizant, Barry M. 1982. "Gestalt Language and Gestalt Processing in Autism." *Topics in Language Disorders* 3:16–23.

———. 2015. *Uniquely Human: A Different Way of Seeing Autism.* New York: Simon & Schuster.

Prizant, Barry M., and Judith F. Duchan. 1981. "The Functions of Immediate Echolalia in Autistic Children." *Journal of Speech and Hearing Disorders* 46:241–49.

Rabeharisoa, Vololona, and Pascale Bourret. 2009. "Staging and Weighting Evidence in Biomedicine: Comparing Clinical Practices in Cancer Genetics and Psychiatric Genetics." *Social Studies of Science* 39(5):691–715.

Rabinow, Paul. 1992. "Artificiality and Enlightenment: From Sociobiology to Biosociality." Pp. 234–52 in *Zone 6: Incorporations*, edited by J. Crary and S. Kwinter. New York: Zone.

Rajagopalan, Ramya, and Joan H. Fujimura. 2018. "Variations on a Chip: Technologies of Difference in Human Genetics Research." *Journal of the History of Biology* 51:841–73.

Ramey, Monica, and John Rae. 2015. "Parents' Resources for Facilitating the Activities of Children with Autism at Home." Pp. 459–79 in *The Palgrave Handbook of Child Mental Health*, edited by M. O'Reilly and J. N. Lester. London: Palgrave Macmillan.

Rapley, Mark. 2004. *The Social Construction of Intellectual Disability.* Cambridge: Cambridge University Press.

Rawls, Anne Warfield. 2008. "Harold Garfinkel, Ethnomethodology and Workplace Studies." *Organization Studies* 29:701–32.

Rawls, Anne Warfield, Kevin Whitehead, and Waverly Duck, eds. 2020. *Black Lives Matter: Ethnomethodological and Conversation Analytic Studies of Race and Systemic Racism in Everyday Interaction.* Philadelphia: Routledge Free Book. https://www.routledge.com/go/black-lives-matter-an-ethnomethodology-freebook.

Raymond, Chase. 2016. "Indexing a Contrast: The *Do*-Construction in English Conversation." Paper presented at the Annual Meetings of the National Communication Association, November, Philadelphia.

Reisinger, Anastasia. 2016. "Speaking Up for Students and Schools: An SLP Challenges the Use of Forced Seclusion and Restraint in Schools." *ASHA Leader* 21(12):6–7.

Rickert, Heinrich. 1986. *The Limits of Concept Formation in Natural Science: A Logical Introduction to the Historical Sciences.* Abridged ed. New York: Cambridge University Press.

Riessman, Catherine Kohler. 1991. "Beyond Reductionism: Narrative Genres in Divorce Accounts." *Journal of Narrative and Life History* 1(1):41–68.

Rimland, Bernard. 1964. *Infantile Autism: The Syndrome and Its Implications for Neural Theory of Behavior.* London: Methuen.

Rios, Clarice, and Barbara Costa Andrada. 2015. "The Changing Face of Autism in Brazil." *Culture, Medicine, and Psychiatry* 39:213–34.

Robinson, Jeffrey D. 2012. "Epistemics, Action Formation, and Other-Initiation of Repair: The Case of Partial Questioning Repeats." Pp. 261–92 in *Conversational Repair and Human Understanding*, edited by M. Hayashi, G. Raymond, and J. Sidnell. Cambridge: Cambridge University Press.

Robinson, Jeffrey D., and Galina B. Bolden. 2010. "Preference Organization of Sequence-Initiating Actions: The Case of Explicit Account Solicitations." *Discourse Studies* 12:501–33.

Robison, John Elder. 2007. *Look Me in the Eye: My Life with Asperger's*. New York: Three Rivers.

Roca-Cuberes, Carles. 2008. "Membership Categorization and Professional Insanity Ascription." *Discourse Studies* 10:543–70.

Rogge, Nicky, and Juliette Janssen. 2019. "The Economic Costs of Autism Spectrum Disorder: A Literature Review." *Journal of Autism & Developmental Disorders* 49:2873–900.

Rose, Nikolas. 2007. "Molecular Biopolitics, Somatic Ethics and the Spirit of Biocapital." *Social Theory & Health* 5:3–29.

———. 2013. "The Human Sciences in a Biological Age." *Theory, Culture & Society* 30:3–34.

Rose, Nikolas, and Joelle M. Abi-Rached. 2013. *Neuro: The New Brain Sciences and the Management of the Mind*. Princeton, NJ: Princeton University Press.

Rose, Steven P. R. 2006. "Commentary: Heritability Estimates—Long Past Their Sell-by Date." *International Journal of Epidemiology* 35:525–27.

Rossano, Federico, and Katja Liebal. 2014. " 'Requests' and 'Offers' in Orangutans and Human Infants." Pp. 335–63 in *Requesting in Social Interaction*, edited by P. Drew and E. Couper-Kuhlen. Philadelphia: John Benjamins.

Rossi, Giovanni. 2014. "When Do People Not Use Language to Make Requests?" Pp. 303–34 in *Requesting in Social Interaction*, edited by P. Drew and E. Couper-Kuhlen. Philadelphia: John Benjamins.

Rubin, Sue. 2005. "A Conversation with Leo Kanner." Pp. 82–109 in *Autism and the Myth of the Person Alone*, edited by D. Biklen. New York: New York University Press.

Rüppel, Jonas, and Torsten H. Voigt. 2019. "The Death of the Clinic? Emerging Biotechnologies and the Reconfiguration of Mental Health." *Science, Technology & Human Values* 44(4):567–80.

Rutter, Michael, and Lawrence Bartak. 1971. "Causes of Infantile Autism: Some Considerations from Recent Research." *Journal of Autism and Childhood Schizophrenia* 1:20–32.

Rutter, Michael, Ann LeCouteur, and Catherine Lord. 2003. *Autism Diagnostic Interview–Revised (ADI R)*. Torrance, CA: WPS.

Ryave, Alan. 1978. "On the Achievement of a Series of Stories." Pp. 113–32 in *Studies in the Organization of Conversational Interaction*, edited by J. Schenkein. New York: Academic.

Ryle, Gilbert. 1949. *The Concept of Mind*. New York: Barnes & Noble.

Sacks, Harvey. 1973. "On Some Puns with Some Intimations." Pp. 135–44 in *Report of the Twenty-Third Annual Round Table Meeting on Linguistics and Language Studies*, edited by R. W. Shuy. Washington, DC: Georgetown University Press.

———. 1984. "Notes on Methodology." Pp. 21–27 in *Structures of Social Action*, edited by J. M. Atkinson and J. Heritage. Cambridge: Cambridge University Press.

———. 1989[1964]. "Lecture One: Rules of Conversational Sequence." *Human Studies* 12:217–27.

———. 1992a. *Lectures on Conversation*. Vol. 1. Oxford: Blackwell.

———. 1992b. *Lectures on Conversation*. Vol. 2. Oxford: Blackwell.

Sacks, Harvey, Emanuel A. Schegloff, and Gail Jefferson. 1974. "A Simplest Systematics for the Organization of Turn-Taking for Conversation." *Language* 50:696–735.

Sacks, Oliver. 1993. "An Anthropologist on Mars." *New Yorker*, December 27, pp. 106–25.

———. 1995. *An Anthropologist on Mars*. New York: Vintage.

Saenz, Terry Irvine, Kelly Gilligan Black, and Laura Pelegrini. 1999. "The Social Competence of Children Diagnosed with Specific Language Impairment." Pp. 111–24 in *Constructing (In) Competence: Disabling Evaluations in Clinical and Social Interaction*, edited by D. Kovarsky, J. F. Duchan, and M. Maxwell. Mahwah, NJ: Lawrence Erlbaum.

Sandbank, Micheal, Susanne A. Albarran, Kristen Bottema-Beautel, et al. 2020. "Project AIM: Autism Intervention Meta-analysis for Studies of Young Children." *Psychological Bulletin* 146:1–29.

Schegloff, Emanuel A. 1986. "The Routine as Achievement." *Human Studies* 9:111–51.

———. 1987a. "Analyzing Single Episodes of Interaction: An Exercise in Conversation Analysis." *Social Psychology Quarterly* 50(2):101–14.

———. 1987b. "Between Macro and Micro: Contexts and Other Connections." Pp. 207–34 in *The Micro-Macro Link*, edited by J. Alexander, R. M. B. Giesen, and N. Smelser. Berkeley: University of California Press.

———. 1995. "Discourse as an Interactional Achievement III: The Omnirelevance of Action." *Research on Language and Social Interaction* 28(3):185–211.

———. 2003a. "Conversation Analysis and Communication Disorders." Pp. 21–55 in *Conversation and Brain Damage*, edited by C. Goodwin. New York: Oxford University Press.

———. 2003b. "On ESP Puns." Pp. 531–40 in *Studies in Language and Social Interaction: In Honor of Robert Hopper*, edited by P. Glenn, C. LeBaron, and J. Mandelbaum. Mahwah, NJ: Lawrence Erlbaum.

———. 2003c. "The Surfacing of the Suppressed." Pp. 241–62 in *Studies in Language and Social Interaction: In Honor of Robert Hopper*, edited by P. Glenn, C. LeBaron, and J. Mandelbaum. Mahwah, NJ: Lawrence Erlbaum.

———. 2007a. "Categories in Action: Person-Reference and Membership Categorization." Pp. 70–96 in *Roots of Human Sociality*, edited by S. C. Levinson and N. J. Enfield. New York: Berg.

———. 2007b. *Sequence Organization in Interaction*. Cambridge: Cambridge University Press.

———. 2007c. "A Tutorial on Membership Categorization." *Journal of Pragmatics* 39(3):462–82.

Schegloff, Emanuel A., Gail Jefferson, and Harvey Sacks. 1977. "The Preference for Self-Correction in the Organization of Repair in Conversation." *Language* 53:361–82.

Schegloff, Emanuel A., and Harvey Sacks. 1973. "Opening Up Closings." *Semiotica* 8:289–327.

Schnittker, Jason. 2017. *The Diagnostic System: Why the Classification of Psychiatric Disorders Is Necessary, Difficult, and Never Settled*. New York: Columbia University Press.

Schopler, Eric, and Robert Jay Reichler. 1979. *Individualized Assessment and Treatment for Autistic and Developmentally Disabled Children*. Vol. 1, *Psychoeducational Profile*. Baltimore, MD: University Park.

Schopler, Eric, Mary E. Van Bourgondien, Glenna Janette Wellman, et al. 2010. *Childhood Autism Rating Scale*. 2nd ed. Los Angeles: Western Psychological Services.

Schelly, David, Patricia Jiménez, and Pedro J. Solis. 2015. "The Diffusion of Autism Spectrum Disorder in Costa Rica: Evidence of Information Spread or Environmental Effects?" *Health and Place* 35:119–27.

Schuetz, Alfred. 1944. "The Stranger: An Essay in Social Psychology." *American Journal of Sociology* 49(6):499–507.

Schutz, Alfred. 1962. *Collected Papers*. Vol. 1, *The Problem of Social Reality*. The Hague: Martinus Nijhoff.

Schwarze, Katharina, James Buchanan, Jenny C. Taylor, et al. 2018. "Are Whole-Exome and Whole-Genome Sequencing Approaches Cost-Effective? A Systematic Review of the Literature." *Genetics in Medicine* 20:1122–30.

Searle, John R. 1969. *Speech Acts: An Essay in the Philosophy of Language*. Cambridge: Cambridge University Press.

Seedhouse, Paul, Penny Stribling, and John Rae. 2007. "Tapping into Interaction: How Children with Autistic Spectrum Disorders Design and Place Tapping in Relation to Activities in Progress." *Gesture* 7:271–303.

Sharon, Gil, Nikki Jamie Cruz, Dae-Wook Kang, et al. 2019. "Human Gut Microbiota from Autism Spectrum Disorder Promote Behavioral Symptoms in Mice." *Cell* 177(May 30):1600–1618.

Sheffer, Edith. 2018. *Asperger's Children: The Origins of Autism in Nazi Vienna*. New York: W. W. Norton.

Shields, Kenneth, and David Beversdorf. 2020. "A Dilemma for Neurodiversity." *Neuroethics*. https://doi.org/10.1007/s12152-020-09431-x.

Shklovsky, Viktor. 1990[1929]. *Theory of Prose*. Elmwood Park, IL: Daily Archive Press.

Shore, Stephen. 2003. *Beyond the Wall: Personal Experiences with Autism and Asperger Syndrome*. 2nd ed. Shawnee Mission, KS: AAPC.

Shumer, Daniel E. 2016. "Evaluation of Asperger Syndrome in Youth Presenting to a Gender Dysphoria Clinic." *LGBT Health* 3:387–90.

Sidnell, Jack. 2007. " 'Look'-Prefaced Turns in First and Second Position: Launching, Interceding and Redirecting Action." *Discourse Studies* 9:387–408.

Sidnell, Jack, and N. J. Enfield. 2014. "The Ontology of Action, in Interaction." Pp. 423–46 in *The Cambridge Handbook of Linguistic Anthropology*, edited by N. J. Enfield, P. Kockelman, and J. Sidnell. Cambridge: Cambridge University Press.

Siegel, Bryna. 2018. *The Politics of Autism*. New York: Oxford University Press.

Silberman, Steve. 2015. *Neurotribes: The Legacy of Autism and the Future of Neurodiversity*. New York: Avery.

Siller, Michael, and Marian Sigman. 2002. "The Behaviors of Parents of Children with Autism Predict the Subsequent Development of Their Children's Communication." *Journal of Autism and Developmental Disorders* 32(2):77–89. doi: 10.1023/A:1014884404276.

Silverman, Chloe. 2012. *Understanding Autism: Patients, Doctors, and the History of a Disorder*. Princeton, NJ: Princeton University Press.

Silverman, Chloe, and Martha Herbert. 2003. "Autism and Genetics." *GeneWatch* 16(1).

Simmel, Georg. 1950. "The Stranger." Pp. 402–8 in *The Sociology of Georg Simmel*, edited by K. Wolff. New York: Free Press.

Singh, Jennifer S. 2011. "The Vanishing Diagnosis of Asperger's Disorder." Pp. 235–57 in *Sociology of Diagnosis*, vol. 12, *Advances in Medical Sociology*, edited by P. J. McGann and J. H. David. Bingley, UK: Emerald Group.

———. 2016. *Multiple Autisms: Spectrums of Advocacy and Genomic Science*. Minneapolis: University of Minnesota Press.

Singh, Jennifer S., Judy Illes, Laura Lazzeroni, et al. 2009. "Trends in US Autism Research Funding." *Journal of Autism & Developmental Disorders* 39:788–95.

Siromaa, Maarit. 2012. "Resonance in Conversational Second Stories: A Dialogic Resource for Stance Taking." *Text & Talk* 32(4):525–45.

Smith, Leann E., Jan S. Greenberg, Marsha M. Seltzer, et al. 2008. "Symptoms and Behavior

Problems of Adolescents and Adults with Autism: Effects of Mother-Child Relationship Quality, Warmth, and Praise." *American Journal on Mental Retardation* 113:387–402.

Solomon, Andrew. 2012. *Far from the Tree: Parents, Children, and the Search for Identity*. New York: Scribner.

Solomon, Olga. 2010. "Sense and the Senses: Anthropology and the Study of Autism." *Annual Review of Anthropology* 39:241–59.

Solomon, Olga, and Nancy Bagatell. 2010. "Introduction: Autism; Rethinking the Possibilities." *ETHOS* 38:1–7.

Speer, Susan A., and Elizabeth Stokoe. 2011. "An Introduction to Conversation and Gender." Pp. 1–27 in *Conversation and Gender*, edited by S. A. Speer and E. Stokoe. Cambridge: Cambridge University Press.

State, Matthew W., and Nenad Šestan. 2012. "The Emerging Biology of Autism Spectrum Disorders." *Science* 337:1301–3.

Sterponi, Laura, Kenton de Kirby, and Jennifer Shankey. 2015. "Rethinking Language in Autism." *Autism* 19:517–26.

Sterponi, Laura and Jennifer Shankey. 2014. "Rethinking Echolalia: Repetition as Interactional Resource in the Communication of a Child with Autism." *Journal of Child Language* 41:275–304.

Stickle, Trini, Waverly Duck, and Douglas W. Maynard. 2017. "Children's Use of 'I Don't Know' during Clinical Evaluations for Autism Spectrum Disorder: Responses to Emotion Questions." Pp. 247–74 in *A Practical Guide to Social Interaction Research in Autism Spectrum Disorders*, edited by M. O'Reilly, J. N. Lester, and T. Muskett. London: Palgrave Macmillan.

Stigler, Kimberly A., Brenna C. McDonald, Amit Anand, et al. 2011. "Structural and Functional Magnetic Resonance Imaging of Autism Spectrum Disorders." *Brain Research* 1380:146–61.

Stivers, Tanya. 2002. "Presenting the Problem in Pediatric Encounters: 'Symptoms Only' versus 'Candidate Diagnosis' Presentations." *Health Communication* 14:299–338.

———. 2008. "Stance, Alignment, and Affiliation during Storytelling: When Nodding Is a Token of Affiliation." *Research on Language and Social Interaction* 41(1):31–57.

Stivers, Tanya, and Stefan Timmermans. 2016. "Negotiating the Diagnostic Uncertainty of Genomic Test Results." *Social Psychology Quarterly* 79(3):199–221.

———. 2017. "Always Look on the Bright Side of Life: Making Bad News Bivalent." *Research on Language and Social Interaction* 50(4):404–18.

Stribling, Penny, and John Rae. 2010. "Interactional Analysis of Scaffolding in a Mathematical Task in ASD." Pp. 185–208 in *Analysing Interactions in Childhood: Insights from Conversation Analysis*, edited by H. Gardner and M. Forrester. London: Palgrave Macmillan.

Stribling, Penny, John Rae, and Paul Dickerson. 2007. "Two Forms of Spoken Repetition in a Girl with Autism." *International Journal of Language & Communication Disorders* 42:427–44.

Sturrock, Alexandra, Natalie Yau, Jenny Freed, et al. 2020. "Speaking the Same Language? A Preliminary Investigation, Comparing the Language and Communication Skills of Females and Males with High-Functioning Autism." *Journal of Autism & Developmental Disorders* 50:1639–56.

Suskind, Ron. 2014. *Life Animated: A Story of Sidekicks, Heroes, and Autism*. New York: Kingswell.

Svarstad, Bonnie L., and Helene L. Lipton. 1977. "Informing Parents about Mental Retardation: A Study of Professional Communication and Parent Acceptance." *Social Science and Medicine* 11:645–51.

Sweet, Paige L., and Claire Laurier Decoteau. 2017. "Contesting Normal: The DSM-5 and Psychiatric Subjectivation." *BioSocieties* 13(1):103–22.

Tan, Catherine D., and Gil Eyal. 2015. "'Two Opposite Ends of the World': The Management of Uncertainty in an Autism-Only School." *Journal of Contemporary Ethnography* 44:34–62.

Talkington, Adam, and Douglas W. Maynard. 2021. "Transitions as a Series of Sequences: Implications in Testing for and Diagnosing Autism." *Research on Language and Social Interaction* 54(4):in press. doi: 10.1080/08351813.2021.1974741.

Tarplee, Clare, and Elizabeth Barrow. 1999. "Delayed Echoing as an Interaction Resource: A Case Study of a 3-Year-Old Child on the Autistic Spectrum." *Clinical Linguistics and Phonetics* 13:449–82.

Tartter, Vivien C. 1980. "Happy Talk: Perceptual and Acoustic Effects of Smiling on Speech." *Perception and Psychophysics* 27:24–27.

Tattersall, Robert B. 2010. "The History of Diabetes Mellitus." Pp. 3–33 in *Textbook of Diabetes*, edited by R. Holt, C. Cockram, A. Flyvbjerg, and B. Goldstein. New York: Blackwell.

Taylor, Julie Lounds, Leann E. Smith, and Marsha R. Mailick. 2014. "Engagement in Vocational Activities Promotes Behavioral Development for Adults with Autism Spectrum Disorders." *Journal of Autism & Developmental Disorders* 44:1447–60.

Thapar, Anita, and Michael Rutter. 2020. "Genetic Advances in Autism." *Journal of Autism and Developmental Disorders.* https://doi.org/10.1007/s10803-020-04685-z.

Thunberg, Greta, Svante Thunberg, Malena Ernman, et al. 2020. *Our House Is on Fire: Scenes of a Family and a Planet in Crisis.* London: Penguin Books.

Timmermans, Stefan. 2015. "Trust in Standards: Transitioning Clinical Exome Sequencing from Bench to Bedside." *Social Studies of Science* 45:77–99.

Timmermans, Stefan, and Mara Buchbinder. 2013. *Saving Babies: The Consequences of Newborn Genetic Screening.* Chicago: University of Chicago Press.

Timmermans, Stefan, and Steven Epstein. 2010. "A World of Standards but Not a Standard World: Toward a Sociology of Standards and Standardization." *Annual Review of Sociology*, 69–89.

Timmermans, Stefan, and Steven Haas. 2008. "Towards a Sociology of Disease." *Sociology of Health & Illness* 30:659–76.

Torres, Elizabeth B., Richa Rai, Sejal Mistry, et al. 2020. "Hidden Aspects of the Research ADOS Are Bound to Affect Autism Science." *Neural Computation* 32:515–61.

Turowetz, Jason J. 2015a. "Citing Conduct, Individualizing Symptoms: Accomplishing Autism Diagnosis in Clinical Case Conferences." *Social Science and Medicine* 142:214–22.

———. 2015b. "The Interactional Production of a Clinical Fact in a Case of Autism." *Qualitative Sociology* 38:57–78.

Turowetz, Jason, and Douglas W. Maynard. 2016. "Category Attribution as a Device for Diagnosis: Fitting Children to the Autism Spectrum." *Sociology of Health and Illness* 38:610–26.

———. 2017. "Narrative Methods for Differential Diagnosis in a Case of Autism." *Symbolic Interaction* 41(3):357–83.

———. 2019. "Documenting Diagnosis: Testing, Labelling, and the Production of Medical Records in an Autism Clinic." *Sociology of Health & Illness* 41(6):1023–39.

Turowetz, Jason, and Anne W. Rawls. 2020. "The Development of Garfinkel's 'Trust' Argument from 1947 to 1967: Demonstrating How Inequality Disrupts Sense and Self-Making." *Journal of Classical Sociology.* doi: 10.1177/1468795X19894423.

Ungar, Wendy J. 2015. "Next Generation Sequencing and Health Technology Assessment in Autism Spectrum Disorder." *Journal of Canadian Academy of Child & Adolescent Psychiatry* 24(2):123–27.

Vermeulen, Peter. 2001. *Autistic Thinking: This Is the Title*. London: Jessica Kingsley.

Vivanti, Giacomo. 2020. "Ask the Editor: What Is the Most Appropriate Way to Talk about Individuals with a Diagnosis of Autism?" *Journal of Autism & Developmental Disorders* 50:691–93.

Waye, Mary M. Y., and Ho Yu Cheng. 2018. "Genetics and Epigenetics of Autism: A Review." *Psychiatry and Clinical Neuroscience* 72:228–44.

Weiss, Lauren A., and Dan E. Arking. 2009. "A Genome-Wide Linkage and Association Scan Reveals Novel Loci for Autism." *Nature* 461(October):802–8.

Weiss, Mary Jane, Kate Fiske, and Suzannah Ferraioli. 2008. "Evidence-Based Practice for Autism Spectrum Disorders." Pp. 33–63 in *Clinical Assessment for Intervention for Autism Spectrum Disorders*, edited by J. Matson. Boston: Elsevier/Academic.

Werling, Donna M., and Daniel H. Geschwind. 2013. "Sex Differences in Autism Spectrum Disorders." *Current Opinion in Neurology* 26(2):146–53.

White, Anne. 2019. "Authority and Camaraderie: The Delivery of Directives Amongst the Ice Floes." *Language in Society* 49:207–30.

Whitehead, Kevin A. 2009. "'Categorizing the Categorizer': The Management of Racial Common Sense in Interaction." *Social Psychology Quarterly* 72:325–42.

WHO. 2018. *International Classification of Diseases for Mortality and Morbidity Statistics*. 11th Ed.

Whooley, Owen, and Allan V. Horwitz. 2013. "The Paradox of Professional Success: Grand Ambition, Furious Resistance, and the Derailment of the DSM-5 Revision Process." Pp. 75–94 in *Making the DSM-5: Concepts and Controversies*, edited by J. Paris and J. Phillips. New York: Springer.

Wieder, D. Lawrence. 1974. *Language and Social Reality: The Case of Telling the Convict Code*. The Hague: Mouton.

Wilkinson, Ray, John Rae, and Gitte Rasmussen, eds. 2020. *Atypical Interaction: Impacts of Communicative Impairments within Everyday Talk*. New York: Palgrave Macmillan.

Williams, Donna. 1992. *Nobody Nowhere*. New York: Avon Books.

Wing, Lorna. 1973. "The Handicaps of Autistic Children: A Review of Some Aspects of Work in the UK." Pp. 106–22 in *Research and Education: Top Priorities for Mentally Ill Children*, edited by C. C. Park. Rockville, MD: National Institute of Mental Health.

———. 1991. "The Relationship between Asperger's Syndrome and Kanner's Autism." Pp. 93–121 in *Autism and Asperger Syndrome*, edited by U. Frith. Cambridge: Cambridge University Press.

Wiscons, Lucas. 2020. "Particularizing the Picture: Clinicians' Use of Instantiation Stories in Autism Diagnosis." Unpublished master's thesis, University of Wisconsin, Madison, WI.

Wittgenstein, Ludwig. 1958. *Philosophical Investigations*. Translated by G. E. M. Anscombe. New York: Macmillan.

Wolff, Sula. 2004. "The History of Autism." *European Child & Adolescent Psychiatry* 13:201–8.

Woodcock, Richard W., and M. Bonner Johnson. 1977. *Woodcock-Johnson Psycho-Educational Battery: Examiner's Manual*. Allen, TX: DLM Teaching Resources.

Wootton, Anthony J. 1997. *Interaction and the Development of Mind*. Cambridge: Cambridge University Press.

———. 1999. "An Investigation of Delayed Echoing in a Child with Autism." *First Language* 19:359–81.

———. 2002. "Interactional Contrasts between Typically Developing Children and Those with Autism, Asperger's Syndrome, and Pragmatic Impairment." *Issues in Applied Linguistics* 13:133–59.

Yeargin-Allsopp, Marshalyn, Catherine Rice, Tanya Karapurkar, et al. 2003. "Prevalence of Autism in a US Metropolitan Area." *Journal of the American Medical Association* 289:49–55.

Yuen, Tracy, Melissa T. Carter, Peter Szatmari, et al. 2018. "Cost-Effectiveness of Genome and Exome Sequencing in Children Diagnosed with Autism Spectrum Disorder." *Applied Health Economics Health Policy* 16:481–93.

Zimmerman, Don H. 1970. "The Practicalities of Rule Use." Pp. 221–38 in *Understanding Everyday Life*, edited by J. Douglas. Chicago: Aldine.

———. 1988. "On Conversation: The Conversation Analytic Perspective." Pp. 406–32 in *Communication Yearbook II*. Newbury Park, CA: Sage.

Name Index

Page numbers set in italics refer to tables or figures.

Subject Index

Milton Keynes UK
Ingram Content Group UK Ltd.
UKHW010120280923
429506UK00003B/24

9 780226 815985